Antibodies

STRUCTURE, SYNTHESIS,
FUNCTION, AND IMMUNOLOGIC
INTERVENTION IN DISEASE

University of South Florida International Biomedical Symposia Series

ANTIBODIES: Structure, Synthesis, Function, and
Immunologic Intervention in Disease
Edited by Andor Szentivanyi, Paul H. Maurer, and Bernard W. Janicki

IMMUNOBIOLOGY AND IMMUNOPHARMACOLOGY OF
BACTERIAL ENDOTOXINS
Edited by Andor Szentivanyi, Herman Friedman, and Alois Nowotny

VIRUSES, IMMUNITY, AND IMMUNODEFICIENCY
Edited by Andor Szentivanyi and Herman Friedman

A Continuation Order Plan is available for this series. A continuation order will bring delivery of each new volume immediately upon publication. Volumes are billed only upon actual shipment. For further information please contact the publisher.

Antibodies

STRUCTURE, SYNTHESIS, FUNCTION, AND IMMUNOLOGIC INTERVENTION IN DISEASE

Edited by
Andor Szentivanyi
University of South Florida College of Medicine
Tampa, Florida

Paul H. Maurer
Jefferson Medical College
Thomas Jefferson University
Philadelphia, Pennsylvania

and
Bernard W. Janicki
National Institute of Allergy and Infectious Disease
National Institutes of Health
Bethesda, Maryland

PLENUM PRESS • NEW YORK AND LONDON

Library of Congress Cataloging in Publication Data

University of South Florida College of Medicine International Symposium on Antibodies: Structure, Synthesis, Function, and Immunologic Intervention in Disease (1986: Clearwater, Fla.)
   Antibodies: structure, synthesis, function, and immunologic intervention in disease.

   (University of South Florida international biomedical symposia series)
   "Proceedings of the University of South Florida College of Medicine International Symposium on Antibodies: Structure, Synthesis, Function, and Immunologic Intervention in Disease, held February 19–21, 1986, in Clearwater, Florida"—T.p. verso.
   Includes bibliographies and index.
   1. Immunoglobulins—Congresses. 2. Immunoglobulins—Therapeutic use—Congresses. I. Szentivanyi, Andor. II. Maurer, Paul H. III. Janicki, Bernard W. IV. Title. V. Series. [DNLM: 1. Antibodies—congresses. QW 575 U58a 1986]
   QR186.7.U55   1986   616.07'93   87-2457
   ISBN-13: 978-1-4612-9044-5   e-ISBN-13: 978-1-4613-1873-6
   DOI: 10.1007/978-1-4613-1873-6

Proceedings of the University of South Florida College of Medicine
International Symposium on Antibodies: Structure, Synthesis, Function,
and Immunologic Intervention in Disease, held February 19–21, 1986,
in Clearwater, Florida

© 1987 Plenum Press, New York
Softcover reprint of the hardcover 1st edition 1987
A Division of Plenum Publishing Corporation
233 Spring Street, New York, N.Y. 10013
Softcover reprint of the hardcover 1st edition 1987

PREFACE

This publication is based on a Symposium that has been held in Clearwater, Florida on February 19-21, 1986, on antibodies, their structure, synthesis, function, and clinical applicability in disease.

Organization of this symposium by the University of South Florida College of Medicine was prompted by the unparalleled current expansion of information on these topics in general, and in the field of antibody diversity, in particular. The issues that surround the last named dimension of this field, began to surface in the late 1950's with the first conclusive genetic studies having been answered, and a new set of concepts has been defined. As we see it from the material presented in this volume, now new and different questions are being raised and answered by studies in progress, and it may be expected that there will be other questions that will be with us for a considerably longer time.

We believe that the symposium brought together many prominent investigators with different backgrounds and training experiences such as immunologists, microbiologists, biochemists, molecular biologists, and clinical scientists, thus providing an excellent example of the interdisciplinary value of modern immunology and modern biomedical science in general. We believe, therefore, that bringing these complex topics to a wide audience of biomedical scientists through this symposium as well as this volume is of value to the scientific and to the medical community.

We also take this opportunity to express our gratitude to Mrs. Christine Abarca for her outstanding editorial assistance and contributions, as well as to Dr. Pierre Bouis, Associate Dean for Continuing Medical Education, and his office for their support and organization of this symposium.

Paul H. Maurer, Ph.D.
Chairman and Professor
Department of Biochemistry
Jefferson Medical College of
Thomas Jefferson University
Philadelphia, Pennsylvania

Andor Szentivanyi, M.D.
Dean of the College of Medicine
Deputy Vice President for Medical Affairs
Chairman and Professor, Department of
   Pharmacology and Therapeutics
University of South Florida
Tampa, Florida

Bernard W. Janicki, Ph.D.
Deputy Director
Immunology, Allergic and Immunologic
   Diseases Program
National Institute of Allergy and
   Infectious Disease
National Institutes of Health
Bethesda, Maryland

September 30, 1986

CONTENTS

SECTION I
STRUCTURES OF ANTIBODIES AND THE COMBINING SITE

The Three Dimensional Structure of Immunoglobulin G and Its Relationship
to the Expression of Biological Functions
Keith J. Dorrington and Michel H. Klein

New Concepts in Antibody Structure
Heinz Kohler and Thomas Kieber-Emmons

Nature of the Antibody Combining Site
Elvin A. Kabat

THE THREE-DIMENSIONAL STRUCTURE OF IMMUNOGLOBULIN G AND ITS

RELATIONSHIP TO THE EXPRESSION OF BIOLOGICAL FUNCTIONS

Keith J. Dorrington and Michel H. Klein

Departments of Immunology and Biochemistry
University of Toronto
Toronto, Canada

INTRODUCTION

The immunoglobulin G (IgG) molecule has evolved to participate in two distinct types of interaction. Approximately two-thirds of the molecule is dedicated to antigen binding, the primary or adaptive function of antibodies, with one combining site being located in each Fab region. More precisely, the combining site is formed from complementarity-determining regions (CDR's) contained within the variable regions of the paired heavy and light chains (see chapter by Kabat in this volume). The remaining one-third of the molecule, termed the Fc region, contains the sites by which IgG is recognized by non-antigen-specific, biological effector mechanisms which play a central role in homeostasis. The complex organizational features of immunoglobulin genes reflect the need to link a large number of antigen-binding specificities to a limited number of biological effector mechanisms.

This brief review will summarize our current knowledge regarding the three-dimensional structure of immunoglobulin domains, the basic building block of all antibodies, and how these domains interact. This will be followed by a discussion of where the sites responsible for the expression of effector functions are located within Fc and how these are related to the conformation of the IgG molecule.

CONFORMATION AND INTERACTIONS OF DOMAINS

A "domain" may be defined as the compact, folded structure formed from approximately 110 amino acid residues and possessing one intrachain disulfide band. The amino acid sequence forming each domain corresponds to one of the homology regions which are clearly apparent when immunoglobulin sequences are analyzed. Thus, the light chain contains two domains (corresponding to V_L and C_L) and the heavy (γ) chain contains four domains (V_H, $C\gamma 1$, $C\gamma 2$, and $C\gamma 3$). The $C\gamma 1$ and $C\gamma 2$ domains of each γ chain are linked by a specialized stretch of polypeptide termed the "hinge" region containing the disulfide bonds which link the γ chains (see below).

Figure 1 shows diagrammatically the folding of the polypeptide backbone corresponding to the variable and constant domains of an L chain as determined by x-ray crystallography of an L-chain dimer (5). Each domain is an approximately cylindrical structure formed from two sheets of anti-parallel β structure; a four-chain layer on one side and three-chain layer on the other. The interior of each domain contains tightly-packed hydrophobic side-chains and the two β sheets are linked by a disulfide bridge. The polypeptides linking the β sheets are relatively unstructured. It is noteworthy that although the V and C regions are not homologous in sequence, their three-dimensional structures are clearly similar, although the β sheets in the V domain are more irregular. A comparison of the relative dispositions of the β sheets in V and C domains shows that the V domain is rotated 160-170° relative to the C domain. Consequently, interactions between V domains involve the three-chain β sheets, whereas C-C interactions are mediated by four-chain structures. The unique mode of interaction between V domains allows for the formation of antigen-binding sites having widely differing shapes and dimensions, with binding specificities dictated by the CDR's located on the polypeptide loops linking the elements of the three-chain layer.

X-ray diffraction data have been solved to high resolution for a number of Fab fragments as well as the Bence Jones L chain dimer. In contrast, it has not been possible to determine the structure of an entire IgG molecule. This appears to be due to the fact that, within crystals of intact IgG, the Fc region can take up a number of different orientations relative to the Fab regions. Consequently, only diffraction corresponding to the latter is observed. Moderate resolution data have been obtained for IgG(Dob), a human myeloma protein in which the hinge region is deleted (12). This suggests that the failure to detect Fc during x-ray analysis of intact IgG is due to

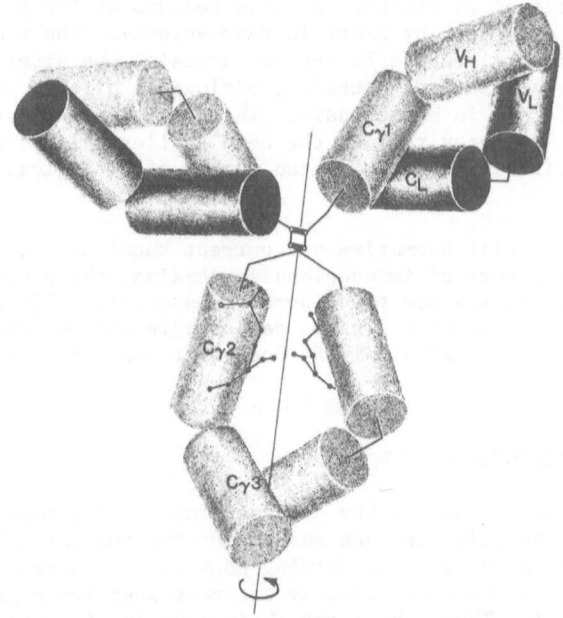

Figure 1. Diagrammatic representation of the polypeptide conformation of one of the monomers in a light chain dimer as determined by x-ray crystallographic analysis. Regions of the polypeptide in β conformation are represented by arrows; four-chain layers by white and three-chain by cross-hatched arrows. In each domain the two layers are connected by a disulfide bond (black bar). Note that the homologous β sheets face in different directions in the V and C domains. [From (5) with permission.]

flexibility mediated by the hinge region. We shall return to this phenomenon below.

Information on the conformation of the Fc region of IgG has been obtained from x-ray diffraction analyses of Fc fragments and of the complex formed between Fc and Fragment B derived from Protein A of <u>Staphylococcus aureus</u> (3). Figure 2 shows that the Fc region has some unique structural features. The paired Cγ3 regions show the same mode of interaction as seen between C_L domains and C_L–Cγ1 domains, i.e., mediated through the four-chain-β- sheets. In marked contrast, the Cγ2 domains do not associate and are separated by a solvent-filled channel. Although the four-chain β sheets of the Cγ2 regions do face each other across the two-fold axis of Fc, the oligosaccharide chain linked to ASN 297 of each Cγ2 interacts for much of its length with side chains of residues forming part of the four-chain layer. However, in addition to the role played by the carbohydrate in blocking domain association, the residues forming the outer surface of the four-chain layer in Cγ2 are less hydrophobic than seen in a typical C-domain. It is also worthy of note that the Cγ2 and Cγ3 regions within each chain interact more extensively than V and C domains in the Fab region. Each Cγ2-Cγ3 contact involves a surface area of 778Å^2 or about one third of the size of the Cγ3-Cγ3 contact. The x-ray data also show the Cγ2 regions to have a more motile conformation than other C domains.

In summary, x-ray crystallographic analyses show that all immunoglobulin domains so far studied have the same basic conformation (the immunoglobulin fold) but exhibit significant differences in the ways they associate with each other both within the same polypeptide chain (<u>cis</u> interactions) and across local two-fold axes (<u>trans</u> interactions).

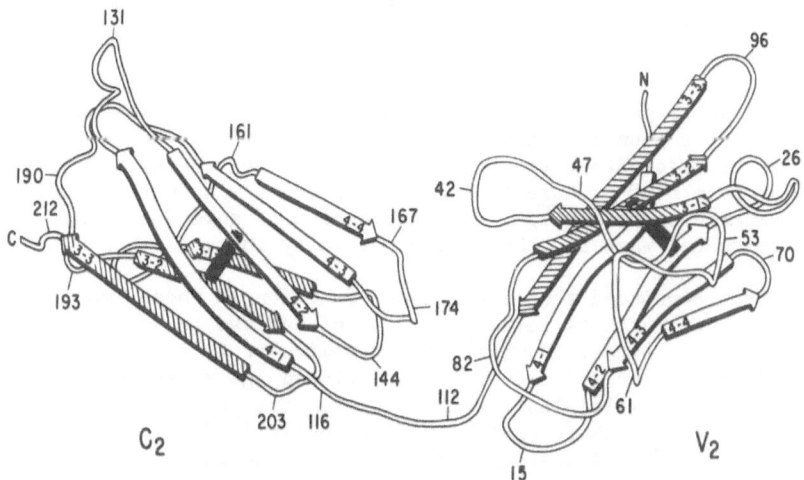

Figure 2.   Model of human IgG1 illustrating the arrangement of the compact of domains. Note that, with the exception of the Cγ2 domains, pairs of domains interact across local two-fold rotation axes. The carbohydrate prosthetic groups linked to Asn 297 of each Cγ2 domain are shown as linked-filled circles. The two heavy bars at the center of the molecule represent the inter-γ chain disulfide bonds contained within hinge region. Segmental motion of the Fab regions is mediated by the polypeptide immediately amino-terminal to these disulfides. [From (4) with permission.]

As noted above, the hinge region links the $C\gamma 1$ and $C\gamma 2$ domains within each of the paired chains (Figure 1). This region is encoded by a separate DNA exon (10), contains the half-cystine residues which form the inter-γ-chain disulfide bonds, is rich in proline and shows no sequence homology with other regions of the molecule. It is also the source of extreme polymorphism between immunoglobulin classes and subclasses. For example, the four human IgG subclasses show differences in the number of disulfide bonds contained in this region (two bonds in IgG1 and IgG4, four in IgG2 and eleven in IgG3) as well as its length (fifteen residues in IgG1 and sixty in IgG3). Based on currently available data, some of which will be discussed below, it is possible to identify three functions for the hinge region (4).

1. Mediates segmental motion which allows the Fab regions to assume a variety of spacial orientations relative to each other and to Fc. Since the effect of such motion is to modulate the distance between the two combining sites, it allows for bivalent attachment of antibodies to epitopes immobilized on a surface (e.g., bacterial membrane).

2. The disulfide bonds serve to maintain the quaternary relationship between the paired $C\gamma 2$ domains which do not associate noncovalently.

3. Serves as a "spacer" thus minimizing the population of conformational states in which close association between Fab and Fc regions is achieved.

The role played by the hinge region in the expression of effector functions has been explored following reduction of hinge-region disulfides and using variant, human IgG1 monoclonal proteins which lack the hinge region (7). The structural defect in the latter molecules involves the deletion of residues 216-230 of the normal $\gamma 1$ sequence, corresponding to the entire hinge region (13). X-ray crystallographic studies (12) suggested that the folding of the Fab and Fc regions in one of these hinge-deleted proteins (IgGDob) was normal but that unusually close association between the Fab regions and the $C\gamma 2$ domains existed.

Table 1 summarizes the effects of reduction and alkylation and of deletion of the hinge region on a number of effector functions known to be mediated by sites located within the Fc region. With the single exception of binding to protein A of S. aureus, the modified molecules were functionally deficient compared to normal IgG. The expression of some functions was completely abrogated whereas others were partially lost.

It has been concluded that the loss of function in these two types of molecules is due to contacts between regions of Fab and Fc leading to steric blockade of effector sites. However, the dynamics of this putative blockade seem to be different for reduced and hinge-deleted IgG molecules. The latter are essentially rigid molecules, otherwise x-ray analysis would not have been possible, and the Fab-Fc contacts are essentially "static." In contrast, reduction of the hinge-region disulfides is known to increase segmental motion as determined by fluorescence depolarization (2) and change in the quaternary relationship between the $C\gamma 2$ domains as determined by electron microscopy (11). Reduction, therefore, seems to lead to a dynamic relationship between portions of the Fab and Fc regions. This dynamic relationship, however, does not appear to allow for exposure of Fc binding sites to effector systems to any greater extent than in the static hinge-deleted proteins.

Reduction of the hinge-region disulfides in Fc fragment can also lead to significant loss of biological activity (Table 1). These effects are

Table 1. Effects of Reduction and Hinge Deletion on a Variety of
Biological Effector Functions Exhibited by IgG

Effector Function	Effects of Reduction on Activity of:		Activity of Hinge-Deleted IgG Proteins
	IgG	Fc	
C1q binding	lost	none	absent
Interaction with Fc receptors on:			
a) human B-cells	lost	?	absent
b) human neutrophils	lost	lost	absent
c) human monocytes, alveolar macrophages & U-937 cells	partially lost	partially lost	diminished
d) placental syncitiotrophoblast	partially lost	partially lost	diminished
e) murine P388D$_1$ macrophages	partially lost	partially lost	diminished
Binding to Protein A of S. aureus	none	none	normal

obviously not due to steric interference per se but probably result from
either changes in the relative orientation of the Cγ2 domains or conformational changes in these regions due to the loss of the stabilizing influence
of the intact hinge region.

LOCATION OF EFFECTOR SITES WITHIN Fc

    Compared with our detailed understanding of the chemistry of the anti-
body-combining site, information regarding structure-function relationships
with Fc is sparse. A number of strategies have and are being used to explore
these relationships.

    1. Fragmentation of Fc to yield-isolated domains or sub-domains and
determining whether these species are active in assays for specific
effector functions (6).

    2. The use of variant immunoglobulin molecules of known structure.
These may be deletion mutants, such as those lacking the hinge region as
described above or lacking entire domains, or recombinant molecules carrying
domains derived from different immunoglobulin classes or subclasses produced
by rare natural mutational events or deliberately by "exon shuffling" (see
chapter by Morrison in this volume).

    3. The synthesis of peptides corresponding to exposed regions of the
Cγ2 and Cγ3 regions (1).

    4. The use of chemical modifications using either site-specific re-
agents or site-specific mutagenesis at the genetic level.

    5. Topographical mapping in which the effects of binding molecules of
known binding specificity (e.g., protein A or monoclonal antibodies) on the
expression of effector functions are assessed.

The most notable success in using fragments corresponding to Fc domains has been the demonstration that the site responsible for binding the C1q subcomponent of the classical complement system is located on the Cγ2 domain (14). A variety of studies suggest that the C1q binding site involves residues 279 to 295 in the Cγ2 region (8).

With a few exceptions, all attempts to allocate other effector sites (principally those involved in binding to Fc receptors) to either Cγ2 or Cγ3 have failed (4). This failure may be explained in a number of ways: 1) binding sites involve residues from both domains; 2) the conformations of Cγ2 or Cγ3, or both, are significantly different when isolated; or 3) the sites depend upon the native quaternary relationship between the paired Cγ2 domains.

The only effector site which has been completely delineated is that responsible for binding protein A of Staphylococcus aureus. As noted above, the structure of the complex formed between Fc and the monovalent fragment B of protein A has been determined by x-ray crystallography. The interaction involves residues derived from both the Cγ2 and Cγ3 regions at the interface between the two domains. This information has been useful for the interpretation of data obtained in studies on the location of other effector sites.

It was noted above (Table 1) that for all effector functions studied, their expression was compromised at least to some extent upon reduction of IgG or deletion of the hinge region. The single exception was protein A binding which was fully expressed in both types of modified IgG. One can conclude that the putative steric blockade does not extend to the Cγ2-Cγ3 interface. Furthermore, the protein A binding data suggest that the Cγ3 regions play little or no direct binding roles for those functions partially or completely abrogated by reduction or hinge-region deletion. The failure of isolated Cγ2 domains to participate in effector mechanisms (except C1 binding) suggests that they do not exist in a native conformation. The latter may depend upon a crucial supporting function provided by the contacts with the Cγ3 regions further stabilized by the disulfides in the hinge region. The conformational motility of Cγ2 has been noted in x-ray crystallographic studies and contrasts with the rigid conformation of the Cγ3 regions both in Fc and as isolated fragments (9).

The studies with hinge-deleted proteins and reduced IgG showed that their ability to interact with Fc receptors was bimodal. These molecules showed no measurable affinity for receptors on human B-lymphocytes or neutrophils. In contrast, the binding affinity to receptors on human monocytes, alveolar macrophages and V-937 cells, and murine P388D$_1$ macrophages was reduced by about one order of magnitude compared to normal IgG (Everett, MacFadden, Dorrington and Klein, to be published). These data strongly suggest that there are at least two topographically distinct sites on Cγ2 which recognize Fc receptors. Some direct evidence for two sites has been obtained using the hinge-deleted proteins as inhibitors of murine IgG2a and IgG2b binding to P388D$_1$ cells (7). The two murine IgG subclasses bind to different receptors on P388D$_1$ cells. Only IgG2b binding was inhibitable by the hinge-deleted proteins.

A further interesting correlation may exist between the existence of two Fc receptor recognition sites on Cγ2 and the affinity of the receptors on human cell types with which they interact. Low affinity receptors ($K_A \sim 10^5 M^{-1}$) present on neutrophils and B lymphocytes do not interact with reduced or hinge-deleted IgG whereas the high-affinity receptors ($K_A \sim 10^8 M^{-1}$) on mononuclear phagocytes are recognized by the modified proteins albeit with a lower affinity. This possible correlation deserves further study.

CONCLUSION

Although immunoglobulin domains have highly homologous three-dimensional structures, they have evolved to participate in a variety of different intra- and intermolecular associations. Thus V domains interact via their three-chain β sheets whereas C domains utilize their four-chain layers. However, the Cγ2 domains do not associate, their four-chain layers showing affinity for oligosaccharide residues. The predominant sites for intermolecular interactions are the V regions, which jointly form the antibody-combining site, and the Cγ2 domains. The latter may mediate these interactions alone (i.e., Cl binding), although more commonly they require the Cγ2 region to be stabilized by _cis_ interactions with the Cγ3 domains and disulfide bonds within the hinge region. This dependence of many effector functions on the precise three-dimensional structure of the Fc region will complicate the chemical definition of the binding sites. Answers will probably require the concentrated application of the techniques of molecular genetics, such as site-specific mutagenesis and exon shuffling.

ACKNOWLEDGEMENTS

Work from the author's laboratory was supported by the Medical Research Council of Canada (grant MT4259).

REFERENCES

1. D. R. Burton, Immunoglobulin G: Functional sites. Molec. Immunol. 22:161 (1985).
2. L. Chan and R. Cathou, The role of inter-heavy chain disulfide bond in modulating the flexibility of immunoglobulin G antibody, J. Molec. Biol. 112:653 (1977).
3. J. Deisenhofer, Crystallographic refinement and atomic models of a human Fc fragment and its complex with fragment B of protein A from Staphylococcus aureus at 2.9 and 2.8A resolution, Biochemistry 20:2361 (1981).
4. K. J. Dorrington and M. J. Klein, Binding sites for Fc receptors on immunoglobulin G and factors influencing their expression, Molec. Immunol. 19:1215 (1982).
5. A. B. Edmundson, K. R. Ely, E. E. Abola, M. Schiffer, and N. Panagiotopoulos, Rotational allomerism and divergent evolution of domains in immunoglobulin light chains, Biochemistry 18:3953 (1975).
6. J. R. Ellerson, D. Yasmeen, R. H. Painter, and K. J. Dorrington, Structure and function of immunoglobulin domains. III. Isolation and characterization of a fragment corresponding to the Cγ2 homology region of human immunoglobulin G, J. Immunol. 116:510 (1976).
7. M. Klein, N. Haeffner-Cavaillon, D. E. Isenman, C. Rivat, M. A. Navia, D. R. Davies, and K. J. Dorrington, Expression of biological effector functions by IgG molecules lacking the hinge region, Proc. Natl. Acad. Sci. U.S.A. 78:524 (1981).
8. R. H. Painter, The Clq receptor site on human immunoglobulin G, Can. J. Biochem. Cell Biol. 62:418 (1984).
9. R. P. Phizackerley, B. C. Wishner, S. H. Bryant, L. M. Amzel, J. A. Lopez de Castro, and R. J. Poljak, The three-dimensional structure of the pFc' fragments of guinea pig IgG1, Molec. Immunol. 16:841 (1979).
10. H. Sakano, J. H. Rogers, K. Hoppi, C. Brack, A. Trannecker, R. Maki, R. Wall, and S. Tonegawa, Domains and the hinge region of an immunoglobulin heavy chain are encoded in separate DNA segments, Nature (London) 277:627 (1979).

11. G. W. Seegan, C. A. Smith, and V. N. Schumaker, Changes in quaternary structure of IgG upon reduction of the inter-heavy chain disulfide bond, Proc. Natl. Acad. Sci. U.S.A. 76:907 (1979).
12. E. W. Silverton, M. A. Navia, and D. R. Davies, Three-dimensional structure of an intact human immunoglobulin, Proc. Natl. Acad. Sci. U.S.A. 74:5140 (1977).
13. L. A. Steiner and A. D. Lopes, The crystallizable human myeloma protein Dob has a hinge-region deletion, Biochemistry 18:4054 (1979).
14. D. Yasmeen, J. R. Ellerson, K. J. Dorrington, and R. H. Painter, The structure and function of immunoglobulin domains. IV. The distribution of some effector functions among the $C\gamma2$ and $C\gamma3$ homology regions of human immunoglobulin G, J. Immunol. 116:518 (1976).

NEW CONCEPTS IN ANTIBODY STRUCTURE

Heinz Kohler and Thomas Kieber-Emmons

Department of Molecular Immunology
Roswell Park Memorial Institute
Buffalo, New York

INTRODUCTION

The accepted view of the three-dimensional structure of the antibody molecule is derived from our understanding of how enzymes work and from the known structure of enzyme-substrate complexes. X-ray crystallographic analysis of enzymes and their substrates have given us ample evidence for the existence of pockets or tunnels in which substrates enter and undergo enzymatically mediated chemical changes. This view has greatly influenced the models for how antibodies bind their antigens, although antibodies do not change anything of the chemistry of antigens. The pocket or groove concept was reinforced by several X-ray crystallographic studies (2,26,29) of Fab fragments of myeloma proteins which had defined hapten specificities. In these structures the relevant hapten are indeed embraced by a pocket in the immunoglobulin structure. These pockets or grooves fit quite well into the concept of antibody binding sites which represent concave areas of the antibody molecule present on the tip of the Fab arms. However, this classical concept of antibody structure based on concave impressions for holding antigen, runs into difficulties in the structural interpretation of the immune network hypothesis of Niels Jerne (14).

PARADOX OF POCKET MODEL

According to the network theory, idiotypes and anti-idiotypes have complementary structures and engage in functional interactions. In the view which has been influenced by the pocket concept of the antibody binding site, the anti-idiotypic antibody attaches via its binding site to an idiotypic determinant or idiotope of another antibody. Experimental data in many idiotypic systems, however, indicate that the target idiotope is very near or actually must be in the binding site of the second antibody. This clearly creates the paradox of two binding sites interacting, having both pocket or concave structures.

Although it is possible to draw models of two interacting binding sites, none of these models are very satisfactory in terms of the original structural three-dimensional concept of antibody binding sites. More serious than the finding of anti-idiotypes directed against other antibody binding sites is

the demonstration that anti-idiotypes and idiotypes are functionally completely interchangeable and only defined by the experimental protocol of the
investigator. Depending on the situation, the idiotype may behave like an
anti-idiotype or vice versa (22,28). The functional interchangeability of
the terms idiotype and anti-idiotype is inherent in the network concept.

Facing the dilemma in the incompatibility of the network hypothesis
with the current structural models of antibodies, one has either the choice
to abandon the network concept or change the models for antibody structures.
It appears that experimental evidence for the network hypothesis is overwhelm-
ing and does not allow us to give up the network concept. On the other hand,
the [3]pocket' model of antibody binding sites is supported only by a handful
of data on structures of Fab fragments and their haptens. Recently two new
immunoglobulin structures have been obtained (1,7) which do not conform to
the [3]pocket' binding site models. Thus, it may be time to change our view
as to how antibodies bind their antigens and to develop new ideas for understanding the function and structure of antibody molecules. In the following
we present a novel approach to analyze the structure and function of antibodies. A model is developed for the antibody structure which creates no
conflict with the network hypothesis and allows a general interpretation of
the biological activities of antibodies in the immune system.

Analysis of the Immunoglobulin Surface

We approach the relationship between network and antibody structure by
asking which parts of the antibody molecule are most likely to be recognized
by network interactions; this is the same as asking, where are idiotopic
structures located? By definition of the network hypothesis, idiotopes are
self-antigens recognized by the immune system. This implies that anti-idiotypes are autoantibodies and idiotypes are autoantigens. The question can
therefore be reduced to the issue of which sequence regions on the antibody
molecule are autoreactive or autoantigenic. Recently, (19) we have analyzed
autoantigenic sequence regions on cytochrome c and lysozyme using a statistical approach which is based on the relation of self-recognition and evolutionary structural variability. This evolutionary link of autoantigenicity
was first noted by Jemmerson and Margoliash (12) who predicted autoantigenic
sequence regions on rabbit cytochrome c by describing the sequence variability
of evolutionary different cytochrome c species. It became clear from their
analysis that sequence regions which are highly variable in mammalian cytochrome c are also best recognized by the rabbit on its own cytochrome c. We
have refined the statistical approach of evolutionary instable sequence
regions and derived an almost perfect correlation to experimentally observed
autoantigenic regions (19). Since idiotopes are autoantigens we can apply
the same approach for determining idiotopic sequence regions on the antibody
molecule.

For the idiotopes on antibodies an important difference exists. While
for proteins like cytochrome c or lysozyme, the structural variability is
confined to the evolutionary established variation, the antibody molecule
has the potential to undergo numerous changes due to extensive somatic variations. Thus, the relationship between the evolutionary (germline encoded)
variability of antibodies and the potential of the immune system to be recognized is augmented by the added-on variability generated by somatic mutational
events.

Description of the Immunoglobulin Surface

The first step in our statistical approach toward identifying idiotopic
regions is to describe the surface of the antibody molecule using established
physico-chemical methods. The importance of surface accessible structures
for antigenicity should be obvious from what is known about antibodies and

antigen targets (3,25). A general approach to such a description is the calculation of hydropathy profiles (11,12). The "goodness" of such plots depends largely on the choice of hydrophilicity/hydrophobic indices for amino acids (10,27,33), and we have used the parameters of Wolfenden and associates (33). Such hydropathy plots describe the surface of individual antibodies, but do not necessarily indicate autoantigenic regions of the antibody surface.

The second step in the analysis of the autoantigenicity of immunoglobulin structures is simply the determination of the degree of variability in the surface features of light and heavy chains within the antibody molecule as described by the hydropathy profiles. The alogrithm of Wu and Kabat (34) was followed. Wu and Kabat determined the primary sequence variability of heavy and light chains and observed regions of high and low variability which they interpreted in terms of structural and functional properties of the antibody molecule. They identified for each chain three so-called hypervariable regions which should be involved in determining the complementary structures for antigens. Less variable regions, called framework regions, were thought to provide stabilizing and common structures for the antibody. This approach is in contrast to our analysis of the variability of the Ig surface which produces different plots than the variability plots of Wu and Kabat (18).

Relation Between Surface Variability and Idiotypy

Generating such surface variability plots for randomly selected light and heavy chain sequences (15) reveals some new regions of high variability which are not detected by the Wu-Kabat plots. These peaks of variability include regions which are previously defined as framework regions and believed not to be involved in determining antigen complementarity. We will return to this finding later and its meaning for the network. When the surface variable regions are compared to regions which are experimentally identified as idiotypic, very good agreement is seen (18). This agreement is often also seen in quantitative terms relating peak height of variability to strength in idiotypic expression (30). Thus, we have defined these variable surface regions as "Idiotope Determining Regions " or IDR (18,20).

Overlap Between IDR and CDR

Inspection of the IDR plots of heavy and light chains shows that IDR's and CDR's overlap (18). However, there are more IDR's than CDR's. The interpretation of the overlap for the structure and function of antibodies is that CDR's are indeed idiotopes recognized by auto-antiidiotypic antibodies. This finding is not easily reconciled with the classical [3]pocket-view' of the antibody molecule, but it does conform with the network hypothesis and with several experimental idiotype data. Since our approach of identifying IDR's is statistical in nature, it follows that not every region classified as IDR in every antibody must be an idiotope. That means, in terms of structure, that there are [3]pocket-type' and [3]non-pocket-type' antibody molecules. Recently, such non-pocket type Ig structures have been observed (1,7) and these support our conclusions.

Where, in the three-dimensional models of known antibody structures are these IDR's located and what is their relationship to the position of CDR's? We have labeled the IDR's in the three dimensional representation of the alpha-carbon tracing of MCPC603, NEWM and KOL Fab structures. The IDR's in these three structures are all of similar spatial relationships. This might have been predicted since all three structures are of the [3]pocket-type'. It would be interesting to look at the IDR's in LOC which does not have a pocket (7). Another lambda chain dimer, MCG (8) which is homologous to LOC possess a typical pocket binding site. This indicates that changes of only a few key residues in the antibody structure have a dramatic influence on the overall shape of the molecule. It is also interesting to note that our simple statistical analysis of the antibody surface has predicted the existence of other than [3]pocket-type' structures.

Structural Interpretation of the Surface Variability Concept

What is the meaning of defining idiotypic regions which overlap to a great extent with regions which obviously can bind to antigens. It appears that a new concept of the antibody structure emerges, in which the surface of the antibody molecule has several biologically important sites. The function of these sites are twofold; to provide the target sites (idiotopes) in the immune network and to bind to external and internal antigens (internal images). The new model also predicts that each IDR site may participate in either of these functions depending on the difference of its basic structure. We should also keep in mind, that other antibody structures may exist which are still different from the pocket-type and the LOC-type forms. This potential repertoire of different basic folds of the antibody molecule, however, would still conform with the concept of variable and structurally conserved biologically active sites.

Consequences for the Immune Network

The picture which now emerges from these considerations shows an antibody structure which has the potential to express several biologically important sites on its surface. These sites are the glue which holds the immune network together and which also allows the immune network to respond to stimulation. The multiple active sites may have different shapes, pockets, flat areas or protrusions, and they may either interact with an antigen or another antibody molecule. It is understood that these considerations also include T cell receptors because of their structural and serological similarities with immunoglobulins. The key question to be asked here is whether or not all active sites are equal in their functional importance.

In the original network concept of Niels Jerne (13) a hierarchy of idiotypes was postulated. Idiotypes and anti-idiotypes formed primary interactive loops and so-called parallel sets. Recently Jerne (14) elaborated on the hierarchic structure of the network and distinguished anti-idiotypic antibodies as Ab2alpha and Ab2beta. Ab2alpha is the classical anti-idiotype while Ab2beta represents an internal antigen image. The binding of Ab2alpha and beta are thought to be reciprocal. This concept of the network clearly establishes two kinds of idiotopic interactions, thereby implying qualitative differences between idiotopes and paratopes. The division of structures or domains on the antibody molecule into two classes, paratopes and idiotopes, is incompatible with our view of multiple active sites on antibodies which essentially can do both, bind antigen and being idiotopes, i.e., being bound to by another antibody. As mentioned earlier, the distinction of paratope and idiotope creates great difficulties for a structural interpretation of the immune network. Thus, to avoid this dilemma, we propose the abandonment of any functional hierarchic distinction of antibodies being either Ab2alpha, beta, gamma or epsilon (6,14,21). While these terms may be helpful in describing certain unusual antibodies such as epibodies (4,5) or autobodies (16), they confuse the understanding of the antibody structure and of the molecular basis of its biology.

Multiple Active Site Hypothesis

From the foregoing discussion, a new concept of the structures of the antibody molecule which are important for its function in the network and in the defense against disease emerges. The concept can briefly be described as the multiple variable surface model. This model places no restrictions as to the conformation or shapes of binding sites or idiotopes; it removes a

hitherto existing dilemma to understand the molecular basis of network interactions and may facilitate and stimulate new research into the structure-
function relationship of antibodies.

Molecular Mimicry of Antigens

One of the new developments in the field of exploiting the antibody
molecule is their use as substitutes for antigens (24,26). These surrogate
antigens, which are operationally anti-idiotypic antibodies, can stimulate
specific immune responses and have already been used as material to produce
experimental vaccines against model infections (17). The next step in this
line of work on so-called idiotype vaccines will be the synthesis of active
idiotypic peptides which work like the original anti-idiotypic antibody as
vaccine. It will be important here to have predictive methods available
which indicate which sequence regions of the entire variable antibody structure needs to be synthesized in order to obtain an active peptide vaccine.
The demonstration of potential idiotope expressing regions certainly will be
helpful here leading to the rational design of idiotope derived vaccines
(20).

Variable Surfaces and Regulatory Idiotopes

The other interesting new insight into the biology of antibodies and
the network, derived from the multiple variable surface model, concerns the
so-called regulatory idiotopes, as defined by Bona (32) for B cells and found
on T cells (9). The relatively ubiquitous nature of these special idiotopes
in antibodies of different specificities and variable subgroups, postulates
an involvement of other than the classical CDR or hypervariable structures.
Our demonstration of IDR's involving the so-called framework regions provides
a molecular basis for the existence of regulatory idiotopes. Possibly, regulatory idiotopes represent antibody structures which belong to different
structural subclasses which are not yet defined at present but their existence
is predicted by our model. An understanding of these important idiotopes
which can cross-stimulate entire sets of different antibodies will be another
step forward into therapeutic applications of the antibody molecule to regulate or modify an immune response.

SUMMARY

In this chapter we have outlined a new statistical analysis of the antibody structure as it relates to its antigen binding and interaction in the
immune network. With this approach we recognize certain surface accessible
areas of the Ig molecule which express idiotypic determinants. These Idiotope Determining Regions (IDR) overlap to a large extent with previously defined CDR's implicated in providing contact residues for the antigen. Experimental data on idiotypic sequence regions are in excellent agreement with
the predicted location of IDR's. The establishment of IDR's leads to the
development of a new concept of the antibody structure-function relationship
and provides a better rationale for immuno-modulatory approaches based on
the use of antibodies.

Another advantage of the proposed multiple variable surface model relates
to a reconciliation of previous views on the antibody structure with models
of an immune network. According to these views the interaction of two concave
or "female" binding sites would have to take place during network interactions. Removing the restriction for a binding site to be concave and for an
idiotope to be protrusive allows to build a better molecular model for the
immune network. As a consequence of this, we propose to abandon the idiotype
terminology of Ab2 alpha, beta, gamma and epsilon.

ACKNOWLEDGMENTS

This work was supported in part by Grant No. IM-405 from the American
Cancer Society, by Grant No CTR1565R2 from The Council for Tobacco Research-
U.S.A., Inc., by Institutional Research Grant IN-54X of the American Cancer
Society and by the Center for Applied Molecular Biology and Immunology,
State University of New York at Buffalo. We thank Dr. Robert Rein of the
Theoretical Biology Unit at RPMI for providing the Units Evans and
Sutherland graphic system and the molecular display program MOSES at our
disposal. We thank Mr. Joseph McDonald of the Theoretical Biology Unit for
the photography.

REFERENCES

1. A. G. Amit, R. A. Mariuzza, S.E.V. Phillips, and R. J. Poljak, Three-
   dimensional structure of an antigen-antibody complex at 6 Angstrom
   resolution, Nature 313:156 (1985).
2. L. M. Amzel and R. J. Poljak, Three dimensional structure of immunoglobulins, Ann. Rev. Biochem. 48:961 (1979).
3. J. A. Berzofsky, Intrinsic and extrinsic factors in protein antigenic-
   structure, Science 22:932 (1985).
4. C. A. Bona, Epibodies: A particular set of anti-idiotypes specific for
   autoantibodies. Clin. Immunol. Newletter 6:87 (1985).
5. C. A. Bona, S. Finley, S. Waters, and H. G. Kunkel, Anti-immunoglobulin
   to heterologous anti-gamma globulins. Detection of reactivity of anti-
   idiotype antibodies with epitopes of Fc fragments (homobodies) and with
   epibodies and idiotopes (epibodies), J. Exp. Med. 156:986 (1982).
6. C. A. Bona and H. Kohler, Anti-idiotypic antibodies and internal images,
   in: "Receptor Biochemistry and Methodology, Vol. 4," Venter, Fraser,
   and Lindstrom, eds., A. R. Liss, New York (1984).
7. C.-H. Chang, M. T. Short, F. A. Westholm, F. J. Stevens, B.-C. Wang,
   Jr., W. Furey, A. Solomon, and M. Schiffer, Novel arrangement of immunoglobulin variable domains: X-ray crystallographic analysis of the
   lambda chain dimer Bence-Jones Protein Loc, Biochemistry 24:4890 (1985).
8. A. B. Edmundson, M. Schiffer, K. R. Ely, and M. K. Wood, Structure of a
   lambda-type Bence-Jones protein at 6-A resolution, Biochemistry 11:1822
   (1972).
9. K. Gleason and H. Kohler, Regulatory idiotypes. T helper cells recognize
   a shared VH idiotope on phosphorylcholine-specific antibodies, J. Exp.
   Med. 156:539 (1982).
10. R. H. Guy, Amino acid side-chain partition energies and distribution of
    residues in soluble proteins, Biophys. J. 47:61 (1985).
11. T. P. Hopp and K. R. Woods, Prediction of protein antigenic determinants
    from amino acid sequences, Proc. Natl. Acad. Sci. 78:3824 (1981).
12. R. Jemmerson and E. Margoliash, Germ-line deletion of genes coding for
    self-determinants, Nature 288:303 (1980).
13. N. K. Jerne, Towards a network theory of the immune system, Ann.
    Immunol. (Institute Pasteur) 125C:373 (1974).
14. N. K. Jerne, J. Roland, P.-A. Cazenave, Recurrent idiotopes and internal
    images, EMBO J. 1:243 (1982).
15. E. A. Kabat, T. T. Wu, H. Bilofsky, M. Reid-Miller, and H. Perry,
    Sequence of proteins of biological interest, U.S. Department of Health
    and Human Services, National Institutes of Health, Bethesda, Maryland
    (1983).
16. C.-Y. Kang and H. Kohler, A novel chimeric antibody with circular
    network characteristics: autobody, Ann. N.Y. Acad. Sci., in press
    (1986).
17. R. C. Kennedy, G. R. Dreesman, and H. Kohler, Vaccines utilizing
    internal image anti-idiotypic antibodies that mimic antigens of infec-
    tious organisms, Biotechniques 3:4040 (1985).

18. T. Kieber-Emmons and H. Kohler, Towards a unified theory of immunoglobulin structure-function relations, _Immunological Reviews_ 90:29 (1986).
19. T. Kieber-Emmons and H. Kohler, Evolutionary origin of autoreactive determinants (autogens), _Proc. Natl. Acad. Sci. U.S.A._, in press (1986).
20. T. Kieber-Emmons, R. E. Ward, S. Raychaudhuri, R. Rein, and H. Kohler, Rational design and application of idiotope vaccines, _Inter. Rev. Immunol._ 1:1 (1985).
21. H. Kohler, S. Muller, and C. Bona, Internal antigen and the immune network, _Proc. Soc. Exp. Biol. Med._ 178:189 (1985).
22. H. Kohler, D. A. Rowley, T. Duclos, and B. Richardson, Complementary idiotypy in the regulation of the immune response, _Fed. Proc._ 36:221 (1977).
23. J. Kyte and R. F. Doolittle, A simple method for displaying the hydropathic character of proteins, _J. Mol. Biol._ 157:105 (1982).
24. M. K. McNamara, R. E. Ward, and H. Kohler, Monoclonal idiotope vaccine against Streptococcus pneumoniae infection, _Science_ 226:1325 (1984).
25. J. Novotny, H. Handschumacher, E. Haber, R. E. Bruccoleri, W. Carlson, D. W. Fanning, J. A. Smith, and G. Rose, Antigenic determinants in proteins coincide with surface regions accessible to large probes (antibody domains) _Proc. Natl. Acad. Sci. U.S.A._ 83:226 (1986).
26. R. J. Poljak, L. M. Amzel, H. P. Avey, B. L. Chen, R. P. Phizackerly, and F. Saul, Three-dimensional structure of the Fab' fragment of a human immunoglobulin at 2.8-A resolution, _Proc. Natl. Acad. Sci. U.S.A._ 70:3305 (1973).
27. G. D. Rose, A. R. Geselowitz, G. J. Lesser, R. H. Lee, and M. H. Zehfus, Hydrophobicity of amino acid residues in globular proteins, _S ience_ 229:834 (1985).
28. D. A. Rowley, H. Kohler, H. Schreiber, S. T. Kaye, and I. Lorbach, Suppression by autogenous complementary idiotypes: the priority of the first response, _J. Exp. Med._ 144:946 (1976).
29. S. Rudikoff, M. Potter, D. M. Segal, E. A. Padlan, and D. R. Davies, Crystals of phosphorylcholine-binding Fab fragments from mouse myeloma proteins: preparation and X-ray analysis, _Proc. Natl. Acad. Sci._ 69:3689 (1972).
30. M. V. Seiden, R. Heuckeroth, B. Clevinger, S. McMillan, R. Lerner, and J. M. Davie, Hypervariable region peptides variably induce specific anti-idiotypic antibodies: an approach to determining antigenic dominance, _J. Immunol._ 136:582 (1986).
31. S. Srinivasan, D. McGroder, N. Shibata, and R. Rein, Biomolecular stereodynamics. III. Proceedings of the Fourth Conversation in Biomolecular Stereodynamics MOSES: A Computer Graphics Simulation Program in Real Time, R. H. Sarma, M. H. Sarma, eds., Adenine Press, Albany (1985).
32. C. Victor-Korbin, F. A. Bonilla, B. Bellon, and C. A. Bona, Immunochemical and molecular characterization of regulatory idiotopes expressed by monoclonal antibodies exhibiting or lacking beta2,6 fructosan binding activity, _J. Exp. Med._ 162:647 (1985).
33. R. V. Wolfenden, P. M. Cullis, and C.C.F. Southgate, Water, protein folding and the genetic code, _Science_ 206:575 (1979).
34. T. T. Wu and E. A. Kabat, An analysis of the sequences of the variable regions of Bence-Jones proteins and myeloma light chains and their implications for antibody complementarity, _J. Exp. Med._ 132:211 (1970).

NATURE OF THE ANTIBODY COMBINING SITE

Elvin A. Kabat

Departments of Microbiology, Genetics and Development,
and Neurology, College of Physicians and Surgeons
Columbia University and National Institute of Allergy and
Infectious Diseases, National Institutes of Health
Bethesda, Maryland

Despite the enormous progress of molecular biology in bringing under-standing of the generation of antibody complementarity and diversity to the gene level, we do not yet have a comprehensive picture of which individual amino acid side chains are functionally important, e.g., involved in deter-mining antibody complementarity either by contacting the antigenic deter-minant directly, or by playing a conformational role, or are neutral non-contacting residues, or are involved in idiotypic specificity, or may reduce ability of the determinant to enter the site.

So many mechanisms have been suggested or implicated in the generation of diversity that it is possible to explain almost anything and so in effect explain nothing about the detailed basis for the binding of an antigenic determinant with a given antibody combining site. Diversity is not equatable with complementarity--differences in amino acid or nucleotide composition may not lead to significant differences in antibody complementarity, e.g., defined as the existence of a set of interactions between small areas of the antigenic determinant and a corresponding small region of the antibody combining site. Since it is agreed that there are an extraordinarily large number of antibodies of distinguishable specificity, somewhere between 10^8 and 10^{10}, one has employed numerology to create such a number based on the two chain structure of antibody combining sites, e.g., 10^4 assembled V_K x 10^4 assembled V_H = 10^8 distinct antibody combining sites; there is no way to estimate how many of such combinations would generate functional sites. A second multiplication involves the product of germline V_K (23,40) genes by the number of J_K minigenes. Thus, if there are 100 mouse V_K genes and four functional mouse J_K minigenes, there could be 400 light chain variable regions; however, it has clearly been shown by Nishi and associates (76) that there is preferential utilization; J_K1 and J_K2 minigenes were used two to five times more frequently than J_K4 and J_K5 [see also (35)]. The same approach is used to estimate the number of V_H chains as the product of the estimated numbers of V_H and the D_H and J_H minigene segments. It would seem that such calculations must be taken with a grain of salt in terms not only of numbers of different combining sites generated but there are no data pro-vided as to the functionality of such combinations. A considerable number of pseudogenes have also been found in immunoglobulin chains.

If we discount the effectiveness of numerology in accounting for the repertoire, we may look at the other mechanisms involved in the generation of diversity and examine available data as to how much complementarity may be ascribed to such other mechanisms. Evidently in a structure involving domains as V_L and V_H, it is important to locate the regions of the sequence involved in binding the antigenic determinant. This was accomplished by the variability plot (54,106) which defined the three hypervariable regions of the V_L and V_H chains from amino acid sequences aligned for homology and it was predicted that they would fold to form the walls of the antibody combining site and contain the complementarity determining segments (CDR) with the rest of the residues in the V-domains forming the framework (FR). The verification by high resolution x-ray crystallography that the hypervariable regions as defined formed the walls and surface of the antibody combining site, now established for four Fab and four V_L dimers (25,52), confirmed the validity of the approach of relating specificity in binding

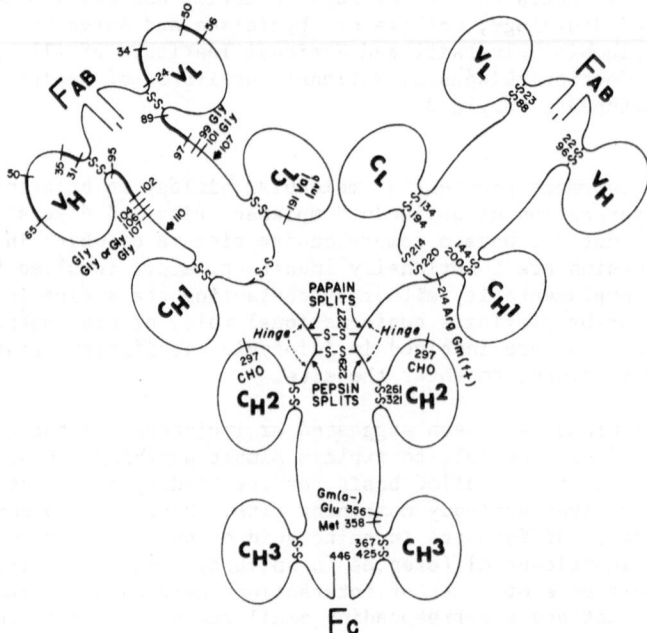

Figure 1.   Schematic view of 4-chain structure of human IgGκ molecule.
Number on right side: actual residue number in protein Eu
(28,29); numbers of Fab fragment on left side aligned for maximum homology; light chains numbers as in (54) and (106). Heavy
chains of Eu have residue 52A, 3 residues 82A,B,C and lack
residues termed 100 A,B,C,D,E,F,G,H and 35A,B. Thus residue
110 (end of variable region is 114 in actual sequence. Hypervariable regions, e.g., complementarity-determining segments
of regions (CDR): heavier lines. V_L and V_H: light- and
heavy-chain variable region; C_H1, C_H2 and C_H3: domains of
constant region of heavy chain; C_L: constant region of light
chain. Hinge region in which two heavy chains are linked by
disulfide bonds is indicated approximately. Attachment of carbohydrate is at residue 297. Arrows at residues 107 and 110
denote transition from variable to constant regions. Sites of
action of papain and pepsin and location of a number of genetic
factors are given. [From Kabat (46). Reproduced with permission of Academic Press. Modified from E. A. Kabat, Proc. 3rd
Int. Convocation Immunology, S. Karger, Basel (1972).]

of antigenic determinants to side chain differences in the amino acids of the CDR. Figure 1 is a schematic representation of an IgG molecule showing the location of the three CDRs in the variable regions of each chain.

This formulation opened the way to attempt immunochemically to correlate established differences in specificity with differences in the amino acids making up the CDRs. If a sufficient number of different antibodies whose combining sites differed in sequence in the CDRs could be associated with differences in binding properties, association constants, idiotypic specificities, etc., it should be possible to make a topographic map of the amino acid differences and attempt to evaluate the contributions to specificity and binding of the individual amino acid side chains.

Such studies are now being attempted in many laboratories. The development of the hybridoma technique by Köhler and Milstein (59) has provided access to monoclonal antibodies with an ease which would never have been thought possible. The antigens used involve: 1) Various determinants coupled to protein such as nitrophenyl (NP), diazotized arsenilic acid, 2-phenyloxazolone, etc. These, however, suffer from the added complexity resulting from the addition of the determinant to different sites on the carrier protein to create not one, but a set of antigenic determinants all containing the introduced haptenic group but attached to regions of the protein of different amino acid sequence. Thus, identifying the exact structure of the combining site of any determinant to which a hybridoma antibody is obtained is an almost impossible task. This might be overcome by attaching groups of a size sufficient to provide a site filling determinant. This does not seem to have been done and such studies are sorely needed. 2) Antibodies to protein antigens. Several series of monoclonal antibodies to crystalline lysozyme have been obtained (24,98) and two laboratories have obtained crystals of lysozyme interacting with an anti-lysozyme Fab fragment (1,24). The very important lesson learned from mapping the location of the antigenic determinants on lysozyme and other protein antigens is that almost any area of the surface of a protein molecule may be a portion of an antigenic determinant [reviewed in (3)]. Indeed the immunodominant groups may differ even when the same amino acids make up the determinant itself. This may seriously complicate efforts to characterize the sites of such antiprotein antibodies by methods other than high resolution x-ray crystallography since only by seeing the nature of the contacts could one determine which amino acids were immunodominant in the determinants. 3) Antibodies to homopolymeric carbohydrates and to other homopolymers. I believe these offer the greatest promise for evaluating the repertoire of antibodies to a simple antigenic determinant, their range of sizes and shapes, and the relative contributions of each amino acid in the CDRs to binding.

Several such antigen-antibody systems have been described including the $\alpha(1\rightarrow6)$dextrans (20,45,46,49,50), the $\beta(1\rightarrow6)$galactans (88), the $\beta(2\rightarrow1)$-fructosans and the $\beta(2\rightarrow6)$fructosans (21,80,107). In the earliest studies, the anti-$\alpha(1\rightarrow6)$dextrans were obtained from individuals immunized with dextrans and although the antisera were pauciclonal, important information as to the size and heterogeneity of the combining sites was obtained (44). Studies in the other systems as well as with the anti-$\alpha(1\rightarrow6)$dextrans were with monoclonal mouse myeloma and Waldenstrom macroglobulin antibodies (80). Use of the hybridoma technique (59) made possible attempts to define the repertoire of distinct antibody combining sites in systems involving a single antigenic determinant and to determine functional parameters such as the size, shape, binding constants and the relative contribution of each sugar of the determinant to the total binding energy (64,73,94,95). When such data on the repertoire are combined with the amino acid sequences, a topographic map of the determinant becomes possible and hopefully one or more of these monoclonal antibodies would yield a crystalline Fab or an Fc fragment suitable for high resolution x-ray studies. From the nucleotide sequences of cDNA clones (97) one can learn which germ-line V genes as well as D and J minigenes are used, their relation to the germ-line V-region families (10,27), and gain some insights into the contributions of various genetic mechanisms, somatic mutation, gene conversion, etc. in generating functionally distinct sites. One may also estimate mutational noise not affecting site complementarity.

I shall endeavor to describe the $\alpha(1\to6)$dextran system in detail, the extent of our progress to date, where we intend to go and what we expect to accomplish.

THE AVAILABLE REPERTOIRE OF ANTI-$\alpha(1\to6)$DEXTRANS

$\alpha(1\to6)$dextran is considered to be a T-independent antigen in the mouse (33). Two IgA myeloma anti-$\alpha(1\to6)$dextrans, W3129 and QUPC52, were available (20). The former has been shown to have a combining site complementary to five $\alpha(1\to6)$-linked glucoses with most of the binding energy directed toward the one or two sugars at the terminal non-reducing end; such sites have been loosely termed cavity-type sites since the binding data imply that these two terminal sugars are more likely held by the side chains of the site in three rather than in two dimensions. QUPC52 on the other hand has a combining site complementary to a chain of six $\alpha(1\to6)$-linked glucoses but the two sugars at the non-reducing end contribute only about five percent of the total binding energy. Moreover, a synthetic linear $\alpha(1\to6)$dextran containing 200 glucoses (86) actually precipitates QUPC52 antidextran indicating that the linear $\alpha(1\to6)$dextran is multivalent toward QUPC52 and that QUPC52 has a groove-type site (20). The anti-$\beta(1\to6)$galactan also has a groove-type site (7). In contrast since it has but one non-reducing end, the synthetic linear dextran inhibits precipitation of W3129 by native dextran.

In addition to the two myeloma anti-$\alpha(1\to6)$dextrans, a considerable number of hybridomas have been obtained; 11 of these were in BALB/c, seven IgM and four IgA and a twelfth IgA in a C57BL/6 mouse, all immunized with B512 dextran 96); an additional eight, four IgM and four IgA in C57BL/6 mice immunized with B512 dextran (73); and 12, four IgM and eight IgA in C57BL/6 mice immunized with synthetic glycolipids prepared by coupling stearylamine to the various isomaltose oligosaccharides, nine to stearylisomaltotetraose, two to stearylisomaltopentaose and one to stearylisomaltohexaose (64). Several additional hybridomas to stearylisomaltotetraose have been obtained in C58 mice, one of which is an IgG3 (Chen, Makover, and Kabat, in preparation). The stearylisomaltosyl oligosaccharides also are T-independent antigens giving a good response in nude mice (64).

These findings give some insight into the difficulties and limitations of defining the repertoire even to this simple homopolymeric $\alpha(1\to6)$-linked linear polysaccharide--dextran and to synthetic glycolipids containing precisely defined short oligosaccharide chains of $\alpha(1\to6)$-linked glucoses. The existence of one, W3129, or possibly two IgA myeloma anti-dextrans with cavity-type sites (W3434; 21) suggests that there might be a large number of clones expressing these types of sites as do fractionation studies on human pauciclonal anti-dextrans (20). It is not clear why hybridomas with such sites have not yet been obtained. Numerous reasons might be advanced such as the sensitivity of the assay for cavity--relative to groove-type combining sites, different rates of cell growth or of antibody synthesis, different optimal conditions for synthesizing cavity-type combining sites, etc. Since the partial amino acid sequence data on W3129 (55) indicate that different germ-line genes are used for its V_K and V_H genes than those for groove-type sites (97), we are subject to very serious limitations of interpretation about the repertoire.

A second question as to the repertoire arises from the extremely skewed nature of the classes of hybridoma antibodies obtained, e.g., almost all are IgM or IgA (64,73,96) although earlier studies of murine antisera to polysaccharide antigens gave predominantly IgM and IgG3 (79). Why are there not more of the various IgG classes which tend to occur overwhelmingly with other antigens and to some extent with anti-polysaccharide antibodies [see (38)]? Numerous factors might be involved--mode of immunization and screening for hybridomas, effects of adjuvants, etc. It is of interest that when IM6 was coupled to KLH to produce a thymus-dependent antigen, an antibody response paralleled the development of the Lyb-5$^+$ subset of lymphocytes (101); male mice with the xid defect produced very low levels of anti-α (1→6)dextran to this antigen (100). Soluble factors from T-cell clones selectively stimulated IgG1 antibodies (6).

An important finding as to the repertoire emerged from mapping the combining sites of the hybridomas produced in C57BL/6 mice immunized with stearylisomaltotetraose (64). Surprisingly, although the structure of the immunizing determinant is unequivocally defined as made up of three intact glucose rings linked α(1→6) plus an α(1→6)-linkage to an open chain joined by the coupling reaction to stearylamine, two of the hybridomas had combining sites complementary to six glucoses and seven had sites complementary to seven glucoses. Similarly the hybridoma antibodies from one mouse immunized with stearylisomaltopentaose and one immunized with sterylisomaltohexaose each had sites complementary to seven glucoses. Only one of the twelve hybridomas from a mouse immunized with stearylisomaltopentaose had a site size compatible with that of the original antigen. This is a striking instance of the phenomenon described by Davenport and associates (26) and later by Fazekas de St. Groth and co-workers (32) in influenza viruses and termed Original Antigenic Sin; namely, that a cross-reacting virus could trigger a preexisting clone and thus stimulate an antibody response. Earlier studies in rabbits with isomaltotriosyl-BSA (2) and the stearylisomaltose oligosaccharides (104,105) had indicated that occasionally animals made anti-α(1→6) dextrans with site sizes larger than the immunizing determinant. The present findings with hybridomas obtained after immunizing with antigenic determinants of known size and structure extend this concept and clearly show that a determinant with fewer sugar residues can trigger proliferation of preexisting clones of site size complementary to a determinant substantially larger than it contains.

The implications of this finding for the problem of elucidating the repertoire are very serious. The previous immunological history of the animal may determine to a very large extent the kinds of antibody obtained. One can no longer infer automatically that the specificity of the antibody following immunization with an antigen represents the response to the determinant structures of the antigen itself. This, plus the uncertainties in selection in obtaining hybridomas that represent a random sample of the antibodies produced, may mean that we may have substantial difficulties in knowning all of the germ-line genes which may be used and the range of V-J, V-D-J choices in assembling complete V_L and V_H chains and hence the extent of the repertoire.

THE α(1→6)DEXTRAN - ANTI-α(1→6)DEXTRAN SYSTEM

To broaden our insights based on the mapping of the fine structure of anti-α(1→6)dextran combining sites, we have been making cDNA from mRNA using C-region primers of our various hybridoma antibodies and sequencing the cDNA to obtain nucleotide and derived amino acid sequences (97).

A number of very informative and significant findings have emerged. Figure 2 gives the sequences of two BALB/c and one C57BL/6 κ chains. All three are identical throughout the V-region and correspond nucleotide for nucleotide with the V_K-Ox1 germ-line gene found in antibodies obtained on primary immunization of BALB/c mice with 2-phenyloxazolone chicken serum albumin (5). Moreover, although our BALB/c anti-α(1→6)dextrans use J1, the BALB/c anti-2-phenyloxazolone and our C57BL/6 anti-α(1→6)dextran both use J3 and the nucleotide sequences are identical throughout the entire V-region including the nucleotide at the site of V-J recombination.

In gel diffusion by the Ouchterlony method none of the 32 anti-α(1→6) dextrans cross-reacted with 2-phenyloxazolone BSA nor did four ascitic fluids containing hybridoma antibodies to 2-phenyloxazolone precipitate with native α (1→6)dextran. However, by ELISA assays, ascitic fluid diluted 10^{-2} to 10^{-4} from a number of anti-α(1→6)dextrans bound to Ox-BSA as measured on microtiter plates coated with 1 μg/ml solutions of Ox-BSA; the four anti-2-phenyloxazolone ascitic fluids showed no binding to microtiter plates coated with 1 μg/ml of α(1→6)dextran. The four anti-2-phenyloxazolones also showed no cross reactions with dextran B1355S with alternating α(1→3)α(1→6) linkages.

The findings with the heavy α chains have also been very informative (97). Since the two BALB/c antidextrans 14.6b.1 and 26.4.1 have identical V_K chains, any differences in specificity must be due to amino acid differences between them. The data show that there are only three differences in CDR2 and two in CDR3 (Figure 3 and Table 1). These are for 14.6b.1 and 26.4.1 a Ser → Asn, Thr → Ser, Lys → Asn, His → Tyr and Ser → His at posi-

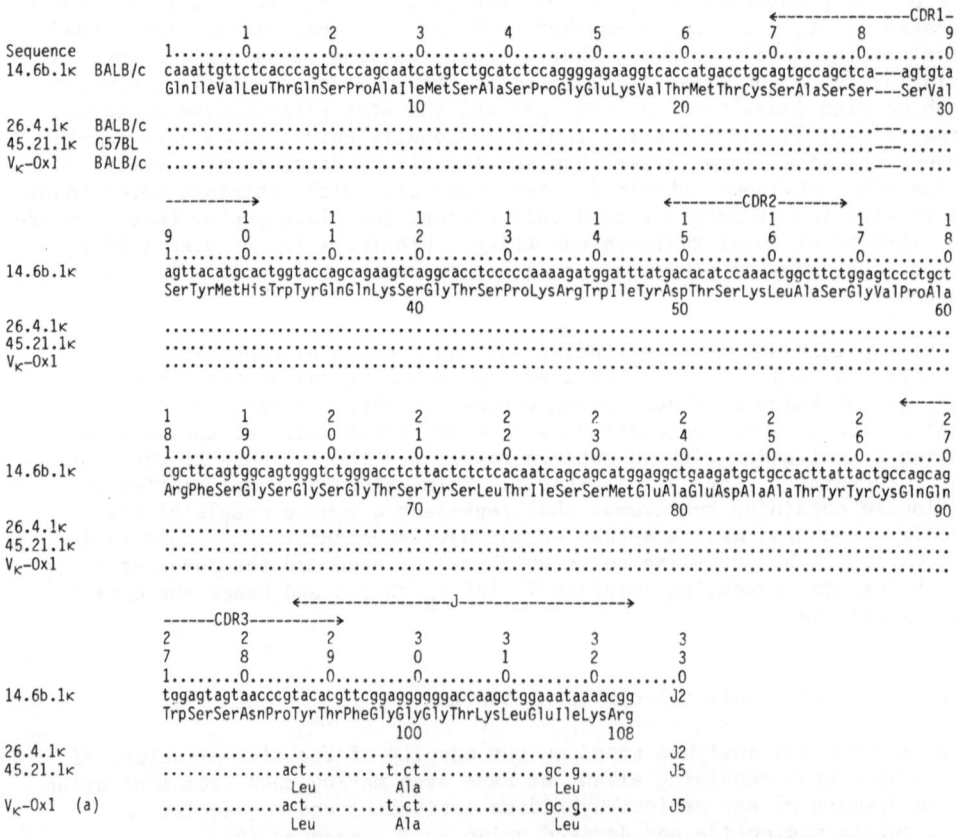

Figure 2. Nucleotide sequences of V_K cDNA from anti-α-(1→6)dextrans and amino acids deduced from them. [From (97). Reproduced with permission of the Journal of Immunology.]

tions 56, 60, 62, 95, and 100A [numbering as in (55)]; both use J_H3. There are no significant differences in site size, and K^a for dextran or for IM7. However, there are two functional differences, in the ratio of IM4 to IM3 as inhibitors, 7.5 for 14.6b.1 and 14.9 for 26.4.1 and a difference in idiotypic specificity with a rabbit antiserum to QUPC52. Since many idiotypes have been associated with CDR3, the differences probably may be ascribed to

```
                    1         2         3         4         5         6         7         8         9
Sequence   1........0.........0.........0.........0.........0.........0.........0.........0.........0
14.6b.1α   caggttcagctgcagcagtctggagctgagctgatgaagcctgggggcctcagtgaagatatcctgcaaggctactggctacacattcagt
           GlnValGlnLeuGlnGlnSerGlyAlaGluLeuMetLysProGlyAlaSerValLysIleSerCysLysAlaThrGlyTyrThrPheSer
                    10                            20                            30
26.4.1α    ..........................................................................................

45.21.1α   g....c.........a.........c.........g..........................t....t....a.....g....c.
           Glu                 Pro       Val                                 Ser          Thr
pCH 105 (a) .....c.........c.........g.........t....................t....t.c....ca
                               Pro       Val                                 Ser          Thr
B1-8    (b) .....c..a.........c....g........tg.......t.........c.g..........t........c....cc
                               Pro       Val       Leu                       Ser          Thr
VH-Ox1 (c) .....g......a..g...a...c...gc...g..gc...ctcacagagcc..tcc..ca.t....ct.tct...g.ttt:...a.cc
           LysGlu      ProGly      ValAla  SerGlnSerLeuSer   Thr   ThrValSer   PheSerLeuThr

           ←---CDR-1-----→
                    1         1         1         1         1         1         1         1         1
           9        0         1         2         3         4         5         6         7         8
           1........0.........0.........0.........0.........0.........0.........0.........0.........0
14.6b.1α   agctactggatagagtgggttaagcagaggcctggacatggccttgagtggattggagagattttacctggaagtggtagtactaactac
           SerTyrTrpIleGluTrpValLysGlnArgProGlyHisGlyLeuGluTrpIleGlyGluIleLeuProGlySerGlySerThrAsnTyr
                                    40                        50      52A
26.4.1α    .................................a................................................a....
                                                                                              Asn
45.21.1α   ga.....ac..ga.c.....g........c.a....a.ga..............t...aat...aac.ac...g..........g....
           Asp    TyrMetAsn           SerHis   LysSer          Asp   Asn   AsnAsn  Gly   Ser
pCH 105    ......at...c.c.....g................g.............t.t...at...a..ga............t...
           Tyr    His                         Gln                   Tyr   Tyr   ArgAsp
B1-8       ........gc..c.....g...............ga.............ag....gat...aat.....g....g...
               MetHis                        Arg                    Arg   Asp   Asn   Gly
VH-Ox1     .....tggtg.ac.c......cgc...cct..a.g..t..g.......c.g...ta..a.gg---.ctg....a..c..a..t..t
           GlyValHis        Arg   Pro       Lys         Leu   Val   Trp   AlaGly

           ------------------→
           1        1         2         2         2         2         2         2         2         2
           8        9         0         1         2         3         4         5         6         7
           1........0.........0.........0.........0.........0.........0.........0.........0.........0
14.6b.1α   accgagaagttcaagggcaaggccacattcactgcagatacatcctccaacacagcctacatgcaactcagcagcctgacatctgaggac
           ThrGluLysPheLysGlyLysAlaThrPheThrAlaAspThrSerSerAsnThrAlaTyrMetGlnLeuSerSerLeuThrSerGluAsp
                    60                    70                        80      82A82B82C
26.4.1α    .gt.....t...................................................................
           Ser   Asn
45.21.1α   .a.c...........t.......g....t....c.ag......g.........gg....c.........
           AsnGln              Leu   Val   Lys    Ser          Gly   Arg
pCH 105    .at.....................c.g.......c........g............g.........
           Asn                 Leu               Ser
B1-8       .at.....a...........c.g...t....c.a.c.....g...........g.........
           Asn       Ser       Leu   Val   LysPro   Ser
VH-Ox1     .attc.gctc...t.tc..gactg.gca...gcaa..c.ac....aag.g.ca..tt.t.t.aa..a.g.a...t..ca.a....t...
           AsnSerAlaLeuMetSerArgLeuSerIleSerLys   Asn   LysSerThrValPheLeuLysMetAsn   GlnThrAsp

                                    ←-----------------J------------------→
                          ←---------CDR-3---------------→
           2        2         2         3         3         3         3         3         3         3
           7        8         9         0         1         2         3         4         5         6
           1........0.........0.........0.........0.........0.........0.........0.........0.........0
14.6b.1α   tctgccgtctattactgtgcaagacattactacggtagtagctccttt------gcttactgggccaaggggactctggtcactgtctctgca J3
           SerAlaValTyrTyrCysAlaArgHisTyrTyrGlySerSerSerPhe------AlaTyrTrpGlyGlnGlyThrLeuValThrValSerAla
                    90                        100 A B                                 110
26.4.1α    ..................................ca.......------.............................. J3
                                            Tyr       His
45.21.1α   .....a............tc.ct..............-----------ctagt.......ac......cac..........ct.. J1
                             Tyr                       LeuVal    Thr      Thr           Ser
pCH 105    .....a.......t..........
                    Phe
B1-8       .....g.......t........t.cg.t...tacg....tag..acttt---.ac..............c...cactc.c..a.....ct.. J2
                                            TyrAsp    TyrGly  SerTyrPhe---Asp                 ThrLeu    Ser
VH-Ox1     a.a...a.g..c........c...g..cggggg---------------------..............................-. J3
           Thr   Met          AspArgGly
```

Figure 3. Nucleotide sequences of V_K cDNA from anti-α-(1→6)dextrans and amino acids deduced from them. [From (97). Reproduced with permission of the Journal of Immunology.]

Table 1. Amino Acids in CDRs of the V_H Chains. Physico-chemical and Immunological Properties of the Hybridoma Antibodies to α(1→6)Dextran

Residue		BALB/c 14.6b.1	BALB/c 26.4.1	C57BL 45.21.1
CDR1	31	Ser	Ser	Asp
	32	Tyr	Tyr	Tyr
	33	Trp	Trp	Tyr
	34	Ile	Ile	Met
	35	Glu	Glu	Asn
CDR2	50	Glu	Glu	Asp
	51	Ile	Ile	Ile
	52	Leu	Leu	Asn
	52A	Pro	Pro	Pro
	53	Gly	Gly	Asn
	54	Ser	Ser	Asn
	55	Gly	Gly	Gly
	56	Ser	Asn	Gly
	57	Thr	Thr	Thr
	58	Asn	Asn	Ser
	59	Tyr	Tyr	Tyr
	60	Thr	Ser	Asn
	61	Glu	Glu	Gln
	62	Lys	Asn	Lys
	63	Phe	Phe	Phe
	64	Lys	Lys	Lys
	65	Gly	Gly	Gly
CDR3	95	His	Tyr	Tyr
	96	Tyr	Tyr	Tyr
	97	Tyr	Tyr	Tyr
	98	Gly	Gly	Gly
	99	Ser	Ser	Ser
	100	Ser	Ser	Ser
	100A	Ser	His	---[a]
	100B	Phe	Phe	---
	101	Ala	Ala	Leu
	102	Tyr	Tyr	Val
		J3	J3	J1
Reaction with Ox-Bsa		-	-	-
Site Size[b]		6	6	7
Ratio IM4/IM3[b]		7.5	14.9	6.7
Ka Dextran x 10^{-5b}		4.43	4.14	2.09
Ka IM7 x 10^{-4b}		5.76	7.01	1.78
Idiotypic Specificity[c]				
QUPC52 anti-QUPC52		0.06	0.26	0
14.6b.1 anti-QUPC52		0.72	0.54	0

[a]deletion; [b] from (94,95); [c] from (94,97)

the amino acid differences at positions 95 and 100A. Positions 96 and 97 have been shown to be associated with individual idiotypic differences among myelomas and hybridomas to the α(1→3)α(1→6)dextrans as determined with anti-idiotype to IgA myeloma proteins J558 and MOPC 104E (22,74,75) and both 95 and 100A are in the D_H region.

The findings with the heavy chain 45.21.1 from the C57BL/6 mouse are of great significance. It is clear that the C57BL/6 mouse uses a different V_H germ-line gene than the BALB/c although both come from the same V_HJ558 family. Thus, 45.21.1 is 85 percent identical in nucleotide sequence and 82 percent identical in amino acid sequence to B1-8, a member of the V_hJ558 family (10) with anti-NP activity (8) whereas it is only 83 and 82 percent identical with 14.6b.1 and 26.4.1 in nucleotide and 73 and 72 percent identical in amino acid sequence. There are only five amino acid differences in the V_H germ-line gene from J558, positions 20, 25, 35, 81, 82A (Figure 3). All three anti-α(1→6)dextrans are only about 56 and 40 percent identical in nucleotide and amino acid sequence to the germ-line V_H-Ox1 sequence or to MOPC 141, a member of the V_HQ52 family used for the heavy chains of anti-2-phenyloxazolone hybridomas (5,37). Table 1 compares the amino acids in the three CDRs for the C57BL/6, 45.21.1 anti-α(1→6)dextran with those of the two BALB/c mice. There are striking differences. Only one of the five residues in CDR1; eight of 15 in CDR2; and six of ten residues in CDR3 are identical between 45.21.1 and one or both of the two BALB/c anti-α(1→6)dextrans. Moreover, 45.21.1 does not have two amino acids, 101A and 101B, present in the two BALB/c anti-α(1→6)dextrans and it uses J3 rather than J1. 45.21.1 binds α(1→6)dextran and IM7 about two and three times less strongly than do the two BALB/c anti-α(1→6)dextrans; these differences are probably not significant. It does show complete absence of the QUPC52 idiotype. This is not surprising since the deletion of two residues 100A and 100B would be expected to result in major conformational differences in CDR3 in addition to the other differences in amino acid sequence in CDR3.

An important and exciting conclusion from these findings is that two very different amino acid sequences can generate combining sites which are essentially very similar in functional properties, e.g., size, shape, binding constant and ratio of IM4/IM3, etc. Since antibody combining sites represent surface areas which are complementary to the antigenic determinant there is no a priori reason why different amino acid side chains might not create similar binding surfaces. Using another T-independent antigen NP-Ficoll and a T-dependent antigen NP-CGG, Maizels and Bothwell (67) have also found large repertoires of V_H and V_L genes. Somatic mutation did not occur with antibodies to DNP-Ficoll.

In studies on ligands interacting with Bence Jones dimers in the crystal, Edmundson and associates (30) have found that a heterodimer of 5- and 6-carboxytetramethylrhodamine and a homodimer of 6-carboxytetramethylrhodamine both bound in the site but in different conformations. The second and third CDRs were seen to be very flexible and moved in ways to expand or change the binding site. Although the Bence Jones V_L dimers may have more flexibility in their combining sites than do the Fab or Fv molecules, the possibility must be considered that groove-type combining sites could show directional specificity, e.g., the antigen might enter one combining site in one direction and another in the opposite direction. Functionally the two might be equivalent and yet the amino acids in the CDR could be quite different. Whether this will prove to be so is for the future. It seems clear, however, that there are many possibilities to be considered in accounting for the generation of very similar combining sites by very different germ-line genes. Additional data permitting more complete evaluation of the repertoire of antibody combining sites to a site-filling ligand will come as sequences of the remaining hybridomas become available.

The α-(1→6)-linked oligosaccharides may exist in different conformations due to the relatively free rotation around each --OCH_2--; it is perfectly possible that antibodies could be formed to a variety of such conformations and that the hexasaccharide molecules would be free to adapt into these various sites (43). No new information has been obtained about this. Conceivably x-ray crystallography could reveal such differences in conformation; one would require a number of crystalline monoclonal anti-α(1→6)dextrans with ligand in the site to establish this.

An additional potential difference in the nature of antibody combining sites derives from the recent study by Chang et al. (15) of a Bence Jones dimer in which the CDRs exist as a convex male type of combining site; this possibility had earlier been suggested (47). This raises the question of whether such a site might be reacting with a pocket or depression on an antigen. Alternatively it was noted that the two sides of the convex site might constitute the functional sites (15). Of course, the data on Bence Jones dimers do not necessarily indicate that such a convex site might exist on intact Fab or Fv fragments.

UNUSUAL CROSS REACTIONS DUE TO CHARGED GROUPS

Extensive studies over many decades with various antisera to a wide variety of antigens have generally shown a high degree of specificity of antibody molecules and as protein chemistry and carbohydrate chemistry advanced, cross reactions have been ascribable to similarities in sequence and structure which were readily apparent. However, in an effort to reduce the vastly increasing number of different antibody specificities, the concept of multispecificity was introduced (84) which hypothesized that one antibody combining site or its subsites might be capable of binding a number of structurally unrelated antigenic determinants. This hypothesis remained highly controversial, most suggested instances of multispecificity being subject to alternative interpretations based on unappreciated structural similarities [see Kabat (46)]. However, Lafer et al. (63) have ascribed the cross reactions of anti-lupus hybridoma autoantibodies with DNA, polynucleotide and phospholipids to structural similarities involving the ionized phosphates.

In the last few years a variety of lines of evidence have tended to indicate that part of what has been termed multispecificity may be a real phenomenon but restricted to antibodies to charged groups with carboxyl, phosphate and sulfate groups being responsible in a number of instances for the cross reactivity rather than the existence of distinct non-contiguous sites proposed (84). Thus, the contribution to the repertoire of multi-specific antibody combining sites may be limited to a small but important group of specificities since these cross reactions frequently involve poly-nucleotides, DNA, etc. This would account for the earlier results (11)* using rabbit antibody fractions to AMP oxidized with periodate and coupled to gramicidin S and with poly-A coupled to BSA (57).

Manjula and associates (69) reported an IgG2a with λ3 chains, SAPC15, which precipitated a variety of negatively charged polysaccharides in 0.05M Tris buffer, or in a buffer made isotonic with sucrose, including dextran sulfate, heparin, chondroitin sulfates A, B and C, denatured calf thymus DNA, Klebsiella K63, poly-L-glutamic acid and H. influenza type b polysaccharide; the pepsin Fab' did not precipitate but heparin quenched the tryptophanyl fluorescence.

---

*Their inhibition data suggest that their antibody fractions were still mixtures, some involving the phosphate of the AMP and others specific for the purine ring or portions of it analogous to findings of Winkel-hake and Voss (103).

In studies of cross reaction among various pneumococcal types, Heidelberger pointed out that the reciprocal extensive cross reactions of type 8 polysaccharide with anti-type 19 horse serum and the type 19 polysaccharide with type 8 antiserum were ascribable to interactions involving the COO⁻ groups on the cellobiuronic acid residues of S8 and the phosphorylated β(1→4)-N-acetyl-D-mannosamine of S19 (39).

One unusual instance of such cross reactivity emerged from our studies on a group of five human monoclonal IgM antibodies specific for certain Klebsiella polysaccharides containing 3,4-pyruvylated-β-D-galactose or 4,6-pyruvylated-D-glucose (82). Their specificities were established by quantitative precipitin and precipitin inhibition assays in 0.15M NaCl. All were different in specificity as determined by the varying extents of precipitation with a collection of Klebsiella and other polysaccharides of different structures, by differences in the pH at which certain Klebsiella polysaccharides (81) precipitated, and by the differing abilities of various oligosaccharides to inhibit precipitation (51).

The surprising finding was that of the four antibodies specific for 3,4-pyruvylated galactose, one precipitated with poly-G and another with poly-G, poly-I and with single stranded DNA and not with a variety of other polynucleotides (71). The reaction with the polynucleotides was specifically inhibited by the Klebsiella polysaccharide. Moreover, all four showed strong cross reactivity with antiserum to an idiotype 16/6 present in monoclonal lupus autoantibodies to DNA. If one looks at the structures of both the Klebsiella polysaccharides and the polynucleotides which react, one sees only a set of negatively charged carboxylate ions in the former and of ionized phosphate in the latter which if similarly distributed in the two molecules might account for the cross specificity.

A second pair of monoclonal IgMs from Dr. Elliott Osserman's collection showed specificity for chondroitin sulfates (53). One of these IgM^{MAC} precipitated with chondroitin sulfate C (6-sulfated) and not with A and B (4-sulfated). The second IgM^{FIS} precipitated equally well with chondroitin sulfates A, B and C. Inhibition studies with three disaccharides from chondroitin sulfates, one (2-acetamido-2-deoxy-3-0-(4-deoxy-β-L-threo-hex-4-enopyranosyluronic acid)-D-galactose) without sulfate, one with 6-linked and another with 4-linked sulfate confirmed these specificities. That these were not merely charge effects was evident since the sulfate-free disaccharide itself was a good inhibitor of precipitation by chondroitin sulfate C in both IgM^{MAC} and IgM^{FIS}. Both antisera precipitation by chondroitin sulfate could be inhibited by glucose-6-sulfate, galactose-1- or 6-phosphates and by sodium sulfate, sodium pyruvate, etc. IgM^{FIS} did not show any cross reaction with polynucleotides or denatured DNA nor did it have the 16/6 idiotype. Most likely the distribution of charges in the polynucleotides and the chondroitin sulfates was not equivalent to that of the carboxyls in the Klebsiella polysaccharides or of the phosphates in the polynucleotides or denatured DNA. It is of special significance that Padlan et al. (78) observed in a phosphorylcholine binding myeloma protein McPC603 crystallized from 42 percent ammonium sulfate, that a sulfate ion occupied the phosphate binding region in the crystal and had displaced the phosphate residue of the phosphorylcholine. Some of the monoclonal IgMs of patients with polyneuropathy reacted with acidic glycolipids of nerve and with a myelin-associated glycoprotein (41); two IgM's that did not react with myelin-associated glycoprotein did not react with chondroitin sulfate C.

Yet another unusual cross reaction involving charged groups is the finding with IgM^{NOV}, a human myeloma protein specific for α(2→8)-linked poly-N-acetylneuraminic acid (NeuNAc), the specific capsular polysaccharide of the group B meningococcus and of E. coli K1 (52). This monoclonal antibody gives precipitin curves with poly-A and poly-I superimposable on those to poly-α(2→8)NeuNAc; with denatured DNA and poly-G, larger amounts are needed to precipitate equivalent amounts of antibody. Native DNA or other polynucleotides did not precipitate. Again it would seem that the only reasonable basis for this cross reactivity would be the charged phosphates of denatured DNA and the various polynucleotides and the carboxyls of the N-acetylneuraminic acids. Thus multispecificity would contribute selectively to the total population of antibody combining sites. If this analysis is correct, the conformations of those combining sites in which such multispecificity occurs should show similarities of charge distribution, whereas those in which it is absent would be expected not to have such conformations. The basis for shared idiotypes will have to await sequence data in several of those systems.

IDIOTYPIC DETERMINANTS

An idiotypic determinant may be defined as an antigenic determinant located on the Fv fragment of an antibody molecule (48). They appear to be important in the regulation of the immune network (13,42,89,102) and a substantial body of evidence has shown that anti-idiotypic antibodies to antibodies to various hormones, agonists and antagonists show specificity structurally resembling a portion of the hormone (31,85,92 and this volume). Moreover a substantial number of instances have been accumulating to show that anti-idiotypic antibody (antibody 2) may induce the formation of immunoglobulins bearing the idiotype (antibody 3), a proportion of which may have combining sites for the antigen which induced the original idiotypic antibody (antibody 1) used to obtain the anti-idiotype (antibody 2). This is an area requiring much insight especially as to how a sequence of amino acids can exhibit a structural contour which would be accommodated in an anticarbohydrate combining site; this now seems to have been found with an anti-idiotypic antibody to the carbohydrate of a parasite system but the polysaccharide involved has not yet been characterized (90).

In relating idiotypic determinants to antibody combining sites, there are certain basic observations which have determined current ideas about idiotypic determinants. A most crucial one was the finding (14,77) that, on immunization with crystalline ovalbumin, similar idiotypic determinants appeared on antibodies to different antigenic determinants of the ovalbumin as well as on immunoglobulin molecules with no detectable anti-ovalbumin specificity; these idiotypic determinants were not detected in preimmunization serum from the animal. Those findings established that there were two distinct but overlapping universes of determinants on Fv fragments, a universe of antibody combining sites and a universe of idiotypic specificities (48) and added significance to the old observation that immunization often induced a rise in immunoglobulin which did not react with the antigen (9).

With respect to the basic problem of understanding the three-dimensional structure of antibody combining sites, the existence of two universes offers advantages and disadvantages. Those idiotypic determinants associated with CDR1 and CDR2 could prove helpful in identifying germ-line genes used for various antibody specificities and for the detection of gene conversions; those associated with CDR3 or the D-minigenes could provide insight into the basis of D-minigene usage and of the role of the N-region nucleotides. A major difficulty would appear to be the dependence of many idiotypes on both V_L and V_H rather than on a single chain; determining the amino acids making up these complex idiotypes is far more complicated than for those associated with a single chain. The relationship between the idiotype and individual idiotopes requires extensive study. In two instances, the same idiotypic determinant has been found on both V_H and V_L of a single immunoglobulin molecule, a monoclonal cold agglutinin with blood group i specificity (58) and a monoclonal autoantibody to thyroglobulin (108) and was expressed on both the separated chains. The location and sequence of such idiotypic determinants on each chain might lead to important genetic insights.

Idiotypic determinants have been divided into two groups, cross reacting (IdX) and individual (IdI). Human antibodies to blood group A substance from four different individuals were used to produce anti-idiotypic sera in rabbits (61). Each anti-idiotypic serum was entirely different in specificity reacting only with the immunizing anti-A and not with 28 other isolated human anti-A's. Mouse monoclonal proteins with specificities for $\beta(2\rightarrow6)$ and $\beta(2\rightarrow1)$ fructosans yielded ten distinct anti-IdI and 11 IdX patterns (66).

The earliest definitive localization of idiotypic determinants was made in mouse hybridoma antibodies to $\alpha(1\rightarrow3)\alpha(1\rightarrow6)$dextrans (22,91) of which dextran B1355S is the prototype (70) and for which a number of V_H nucleotide sequences had been done. Quantitative precipitin studies with $\alpha(1\rightarrow3)\alpha(1\rightarrow6)$-dextrans and with a large number of dextrans not having the alternating structure (74,75) showed the antibodies to fall into five groups depending on the number of dextrans not having $\alpha(1\rightarrow3)\alpha(1\rightarrow6)$ structure which cross reacted and the extent of their cross reactivities--group 1 showing no cross reactivity and group 5 showing the most extensive cross reactivity. Two types of rabbit anti-IdI to myeloma antibodies J558 and MOPC104E as well as an anti-IdX serum were available.

Table 2 shows that IdX specificity was present in all monoclonals with Asn-Asn at positions 53 and 54 [numbering as in (55)]; the sole protein, Hdex14, which did not express IdX, had Lys-Lys at these positions.

The findings with the two IdI specific sera were quite striking; IdI J558 specificity was present in all five precipitin groups and was associated with Arg-Tyr or Asn-Tyr at positions 96 and 97 of V_H. Anti-IdI MOPC104E, however was associated exclusively with precipitin group 5 and with residues Tyr-Asp at these positions. Probably the hybridomas with other amino acid residues at positions 96 and 97 would show additional distinct idiotypic specificities. It would also be of great importance to obtain monoclonal anti-idiotypic antibodies to these other hybridomas. A number of other studies on myeloma and hybridoma proteins specific for $\beta(1\rightarrow6)$ galactans (87,88) associated IdI and IdX with CDR3(D) in all but one instance. In a variety of other cases inferences as to the role of residues in CDR1 and CDR2 has been more indirect. For a more detailed discussion see (48).

Another important association indicating the predominant role of D was established in the Ars system for the cross reacting idiotype Id^{CR+} in a selected population of hybridomas one of which 45-49, although Id^{CR-}, was derived from the same germ-line V_H and V_K genes (36). A suitably absorbed rabbit antiserum to the 45-49 antibody reacted with seven Ars Id^{CR+} hybridoma proteins; all 11 bound Ars protein conjugates to about the same extent. Sequences of the D-region showed that the Id^{CR+} proteins reacting with the 45-49 antiserum used a selected set of D-segments similar to the D of 36-65 having the consensus amino acid sequence from 95 through 100B of Ser-X-Tyr-Tyr-Gly-Gly-Ser-Tyr; Tyr-Tyr-Gly-Ser-Ser-Tyr is coded for by the DFL16.1 minigene (62,99). However, those reacting with the 45-49 antiserum but which were Id^{CR-} used D segments which differed from the consensus by an insertion of a single amino acid between position 95 and 96 in two D segments and between residue 100A and 100B in three D segments plus additional substitutions; one D segment had a deletion at position 96. Thus the D minigene again appears to be determining Id^{CR+} in the Ars system. Berek (5) has also found the D minigene in mice immunized with pneumococci to be associated with the T15 idiotype.

Table 2. Association of Group Specificity, Sequence, Idiotype and Affinity in Anti-α(1→3)α(1→6)dextrans

Specificity	V_H a	V_H 1-99 (1-95) 16	34	39	40	50	54	55	63	73	77	78	80	D_H 100,101 (96,97)	J_H 102-117 (98-113)		IdX	IdI (J558)	IdI (MOPC104E)	Affinity Ka B1355S (ml/g)
Group 1																				
CAL20TEPC1035				N										GN	YR-AY--Q-----		++	-	-	4.18×10^3
Hdex 12	1'*													SY	-------------	J_3	++	-	-	N.D.*
Hdex 25	1														-------------	J_1	++	++	-	6.03×10^3
Hdex 31	1													RY	YAM-Y-Q--S---	J_4	++			1.97×10^3
Group 2																				
Hdex 36	?													?	Y----?-------		++	++	-	2.1×10^5
Hdex 37	1													RY	Y---Y-Q--L---	J_2	?	++?	-	5.3×10^5
Group 3																				
J558	1													RY	Y---Y-Q--L---	J_1	++	++	-	1.4×10^5
Hdex 4	1													KD	Y---Y-Q--L---	J_2	++	-	-	3.47×10^3
Hdex 5	1													SN	-------------	J_2	++	-	-	8.54×10^3*
Hdex 6	1													SH	-------------	J_1	++	-	-	
Hdex 9	3						K							RY	-------------	J_1	++	++	-	2.0×10^4
Hdex 10	4						K		R	H	N		F	VN	-------------	J_1	?			3.0×10^3
Hdex 13	1*										N?			GN	-------------	J_1	?	?	?	1.63×10^3
Group 4																				
Hdex 1	1													NY	H---V--------	J_1*	++	+	-	1.74×10^3
Hdex 3	1													RD	-------------	J_1	++	-	-	5.39×10^3
Hdex 24	1													SS	Y---Y-Q--L---	J_2	++	-	-	1.18×10^3
Group 5																				
MOPC104E	1	A	M		Q	S	D	N		D	S	T	Y	YD	WYFDVWGAGTTVTVSS	J_1	++	-	++	1.31×10^3
Hdex 2	1													NY	-------------	J_1	++	+	+	6.79×10^3
Hdex 7	1													AD	-------------	J_1	+?	-	++	6.86×10^3
Hdex 8	2	T	V	H	P	T	S						G	YD	-------------	J_1	++	-	++	6.78×10^3
Hdex 11	1					K	K							YD	F---Y-Q--L---	J_2	++	-	++	4.71×10^3
Hdex 14	4					K	K							YD	-------------	J_1	-	-	++	2.08×10^3

A very powerful approach to identifying idiotypic determinants is the use of antisera to peptides of CDR1, CDR2, and CDR3 of V_H and V_L (16-19). These have proven especially useful in identifying IdI on human rheumatoid factors. Peptides coding for all six CDRs and frequently containing one N-terminal FR residue and a Gly-Gly-Cys at the C-terminus for coupling to KLH (keyhole limpet hemocyanin) were used to immunize rabbits. All produced antibody to the peptides and half reacted with either the L or H chains of the parent protein. Using these antisera two major CRI were found on L chains of human rheumatoid factors (RF). Thirteen of 17 monoclonal IgM RF (75%) had a determinant detected by an antiserum (PSL2) to the peptide in CDR2 of V_L of IgM^{SIE}, the proportion 76 percent corresponding closely to the 65 percent of light chains with the Wa-CRI$^+$ detected with a rabbit anti-idiotypic serum (60) suggesting the association of the Wa-CRI$^+$ idiotype with CDR2. Although 69 percent of the RFs reacted with an antiserum PSL3 to the peptide from CDR3 of V_L, blotting studies showed the specificity of this antiserum not to correlate with the Wa-CRI$^+$.

Two antisera PPH2 and PPH3 made to V_H peptides of CDR2 and CDR3 of a human RF POM, which has a cross reacting idiotype designated PO-CRI$^+$, reacted only with POM and not with other rheumatoid factors; similar results were obtained with antisera to CDR2 and CDR3 of another RF Wol with its unique CRI$^+$. Thus the two anti-CDR2 and three anti-CDR3 sera recognize individual antigenic determinants in V_H in the RFs studied suggesting, unlike the findings with V_L, a large number of human V_H genes encoding IgM-RF autoantibodies. It is not clear, however, why RF LAY with the identical sequence as POM in CDR2 and CDR3 did not react with PPH2 and PPH3; indeed the LAY and POM V_H chains differ only at amino acid 31 in CDR1, all other FRs and CDR2 being identical; blotting with LAY was not reported (12).

Using antisera to synthetic peptides CDR3 of V_H of RF autoantibodies was also established as defining an immunodominant idiotype in the intact protein (34). Anti-peptide sera with the sequence of CDR3 of three V_H chains, POM, SIE, and WOL reacted strongly in blotting assays with the corresponding intact proteins and heavy chains whereas anti-peptide sera to CDR1 and CDR2 reacted weakly; all antisera reacted very strongly with the synthetic peptide used for immunization. A somewhat different approach utilized two synthetic peptides for J1 and J2 of mouse V_H spanning residues 101 through 113, the three N-terminal amino acids plus a C-terminal Lys for coupling to KLH were synthesized (93). Rabbit and rat antisera reacted with the peptide and with myeloma proteins MOPC-104E, J558, both anti-$\alpha(1{\to}3)$ $\alpha(1{\to}6)$dextrans; with TEPC15, anti-phosphorylcholine; and with hybridoma protein GAC34, anti-group A streptococcal carbohydrate. Specificity of binding by RIA of a rabbit anti-J1 was determined for a variety of mouse myeloma and hybridoma proteins with anti-$\alpha(1{\to}3)\alpha(1{\to}6)$dextran, anti-phosphorylcholine, anti-group A carbohydrate, anti-DNP and anti-$\beta(2{\to}1)$ fructosan and anti-DNP. Only the anti-$\alpha(1{\to}3)\alpha(1{\to}6)$dextran specifically blocked binding of anti-J1 to MOPC104E; only three or four of six anti-phosphorylcholines blocked binding of anti-J1 to TEPC15 and six of six antibodies to the group A carbohydrate blocked binding of anti-J1 to GAC34. Of interest, however, were the findings that one anti-levan, M47A, inhibited binding of anti-J1 to TEPC15 and one anti-$\beta(2{\to}1)$fructosan inhibited binding of anti-J1 to GAC34 to the same extent as did the homologous TEPC15 and GAC34, respectively.

It will be of great importance to obtain monoclonal antibodies to the synthetic peptides specific for the CDR and J segments. The inhibition data with anti-J1 and the various anti-$\alpha(1{\to}3)\alpha(1{\to}6)$dextrans whose IdI specificity has been associated with amino acid residues in the D segment, residues 96 and 97 (Table 2), raises the question as to whether the J1 peptide was not triggering clones of anti-$\alpha(1{\to}3)\alpha(1{\to}6)$dextran to respond (see Original Antigenic Sin above). This could be resolved using monoclonal antibodies to the synthetic J peptides and determining their sequence to see whether they contained the appropriate amino acids at positions 96 and 97. Padlan (78) has developed a procedure, when the three dimensional structure of a protein is known, of using structural parameters to estimate the immunogenic potential of a protein antigen which should prove useful in designing synthetic peptides.

Inhibition by antigen of the idiotype anti-idiotype reaction is the usual way of attempting to locate idiotypic determinants in relation to the binding site. However, with three RF, two IgG and one IgM (72), only partial inhibition was obtained by very large amounts of the antigen, normal IgG. With these three RFs, the association constants for monomeric IgG were about 10^5 whereas those for the idiotype-anti-idiotype reactions using monomeric Fab' fragments were 7.0 and 0.4 X $10^7 M^{-1}$. With so great a difference, it is not surprising that complete inhibition was not obtainable. This could mean that some non-inhibitable idiotype-anti-idiotype reactions could still be site-associated.

The success in obtaining antibodies to peptides from CDR3 and J which react with the intact immunoglobulin makes it of special interest to study the properties of the D-J-C miniproteins described by Reth and Alt (83). These investigators found transcriptional promoter elements in several cell lines 5' to the D minigene segments and showed mRNAs coding for Dμ J-C miniproteins with short V-regions. These miniproteins were expressed. Their function is unknown. Antisera to CDR3 might prove very valuable for detecting these miniproteins and a study of antisera to the mini-V-D-J epitopes might shed light on their possible role and functions. It is conceivable that they may function by inducing antibodies regulating expression of idiotypic determinants.

ACKNOWLEDGMENTS

Aided in part by grants PCM81-02321 from the National Science Foundation, and 1R01 AI-19042 from the National Institute of Allergy and Infectious Diseases to E. A. Kabat; by Cancer Support Grant CA 13696 to Columbia University and Program Project Grant CA 21112 to Elliott F. Osserman. Work with the PROPHET computer system is supported by the National Cancer Institute, National Institute of Allergy and Infectious Diseases, National Institute of Arthritis, Diabetes and Digestive and Kidney Diseases, the National Institute of General Medical Sciences, and the Division of Research Resources (Contract N01-RR-8-2118) of the National Institutes of Health.

The author thanks Drs. Rose G. Mage and Sherie Morrison for comments upon reading the manuscript and Mr. Darryl J. Guinyard for his excellent typing.

REFERENCES

1. A. G. Amit, R. A. Mariuzza, S.E.V. Phillips, and R. J. Poljak, Three-dimensional structure of an antigen-antibody complex at 6 A resolution, Nature 313:156 (1984).
2. Y. Arakatsu, G. Ashwell, and E. A. Kabat, Immunochemical studies on dextrans. V. Specificity and cross-reactivity with dextrans of the antibodies formed in rabbits to isomaltonic and isomaltotrionic acids coupled to bovine serum albumin, J. Immunol. 97:858 (1966).
3. D. C. Benjamin, J. A. Berzofsky, I. J. East, F.R.N. Gurd, C. Hannum, S. J. Leach, E. Margoliash, J. G. Michael, A. Miller, E. M. Prager, M. Reichlin, E. E. Sercarz, S. J. Smith-Gill, P. E. Todd, and A. C. Wilson, The antigenic structure of proteins. A reappraisal, Ann. Rev. Immunol. 2:67 (1984).

4. C. Berek, The D-segment defines the T15 idiotype. The immune response of A/J mice to Pneumococcus pneumoniae, Eur. J. Immunol. 14:1043 (1984).

5. C. Berek, G. M. Griffiths, and C. Milstein, Molecular events during maturation of the immune response to oxazolone, Nature 316:412 (1985).

6. S. Bergstedt-Lindquist, P. Sideras, and H. R. MacDonald, Regulation of Ig class secretion by soluble products of certain T cell lines, Immunol. Rev. 78:25 (1984).

7. A. K. Bhattacharjee, M. K. Das, A. Roy, C.P.J. Glaudemans, The binding sites of the two monoclonal immunoglobulins as J539 and W3129. Thermodynamic mapping of a groove- and cavity-type immunoglobulin, both having antipolysaccharide specificity, Mol. Immunol. 18:277 (1981).

8. A.L.M. Bothwell, M. Paskind, M. Reth, T. Imanishi-Kari, K. Rajewsky, and D. Baltimore, Heavy chain variable region contribution to the NP^b family of antibodies: somatic mutations evident in a γ2a variable region, Cell 24:625 (1981).

9. W. C. Boyd and H. Bernard, Quantitative changes in antibodies and globulin fraction in sera of rabbits injected with several antigens, J. Immunol. 33:111 (1937).

10. P. H. Brodeur and R. Riblet, The immunoglobulin heavy chain variable region (Igh-V) locus in the mouse. I. One hundred Igh-V genes comprise seven families of homologous genes, Eur. J. Immunol. 14:922 (1984).

11. D. J. Cameron and B. F. Erlanger, Nucleic acid-reactive antibodies of restricted heterogeneity, Immunochemistry 13:263 (1976).

12. J. D. Capra and J. M. Kehoe, Structure of antibodies with shared idiotype: the complete sequence of the heavy chain variable regions of two immunoglobulin M anti-gamma globulins, Proc. Natl. Acad. Sci. 71:4032 (1974).

13. P.-A. Cazenave, Idiotypic anti-idiotypic regulation of antibody synthesis in rabbits, Proc. Natl. Acad. Sci. 74:5122 (1977).

14. P.-A. Cazenave, T. Ternynck, and S. Avrameas, Similar idiotypes in antibody-forming cells and in cells synthesizing immunoglobulins without detectable antibody function, Proc. Natl. Acad. Sci. 71:4500 (1974).

15. C. Chang, M. T. Short, F. A. Westholm, F. J. Stevens, B. Wang, W. Furey, A. Solomon, and M. Schiffer, A novel arrangement of immunoglobulin variable domains: x-ray crystallographic analysis of the λ chain dimer, Bence Jones protein Loc., Biochemistry 24:4890 (1985).

16. P. P. Chen, S. Fong, R. A. Houghten, and D. A. Carson, Characterization of an epibody, J. Exp. Med. 161:323 (1985).

17. P. P. Chen, S. Fong, D. Normansell, R. A. Houghten, J. G. Karras, J. H. Vaughan, and D. A. Carson, Delineation of a cross-reactive idiotype on human autoantibodies with antibody against a synthetic peptide, J. Exp. Med. 159:1502 (1984).

18. P. P. Chen, F. Goni, R. A. Houghten, S. Fong, R. Goldfien, J. H. Vaughan, B. Frangione, and D. A. Carson, Characterization of human rheumatoid factors with seven anti-idiotypes induced by synthetic hypervariable region peptides, J. Exp. Med. 162:487 (1985).

19. P. P. Chen, R. A. Houghten, S. Fong, G. H. Rhodes, T. A. Gilbertson, J. H. Vaughan, R. A. Lerner, and D. A. Carson, Anti-hypervariable region antibody induced by a defined peptide. A new approach for studying the structural correlates of idiotypes, Proc. Natl. Acad. Sci. 81:1784 (1984).

20. J. Cisar, E. A. Kabat, M. Dorner, and J. Liao, Binding properties of immunoglobulin combining sites specific for terminal or non-terminal antigenic determinants in dextran, J. Exp. Med. 142:435 (1975).

21. J. O. Cisar, E. A. Kabat, J. Liao, and M. Potter, Immunochemical studies on mouse myeloma proteins reactive with dextrans or with

fructosans and on human antilevans, J. Exp. Med. 139:159 (1974).

22. B. Clevinger, J. Schilling, L. Hood, and J. M. Davie, Structural correlates of cross-reactive and individual idiotypic determinants on murine antibodies to α(1→3)dextran, J. Exp. Med. 151:1059 (1980).

23. S. Cory, Immunoglobulin variable region genes, Surv. Synth. Path. Res. 3:149 (1984).

24. M. J. Darsley and A. R. Rees, Nucleotide sequences of five anti-lysozyme monoclonal antibodies, EMBO J. 4:393 (1985).

25. D. R. Davies and H. Metzger, Structural basis of antibody function, Ann. Rev. Immunol. 1:87 (1983).

26. F. M. Davenport, A. V. Hennessy, and T. Francis, Jr., Epidemiological and immunologic significance of age distribution of antibody to antigenic variant of influenza virus, J. Exp. Med. 98:641 (1953).

27. R. Dildrop, A new classification of mouse V_H sequences, Immunology Today 5:85 (1984).

28. G. M. Edelman, The covalent structure of a human γG-immunoglobulin XI. Functional implications, Biochemistry 9:3197 (1970).

29. G. M. Edelman, B. A. Cunningham, W. E. Gall, P. D. Gottlieb, V. Rutishauser, M. J. Waxdal, The covalent structure of an entire γG immunoglobulin molecule, Proc. Natl. Acad. Sci. 63:78 (1968).

30. A. B. Edmundson, K. R. Ely, and J. N. Herron, A search for site-filling ligands in the Mcg Bence Jones dimer: crystal binding studies of fluorescent compounds, Mol. Immunol. 21:561 (1984).

31. B. F. Erlanger, Anti-idiotypic antibodies: what do they recognize? Immunology Today 6:10 (1985).

32. S. Fazekas de St. Groth and R. G. Webster, Disquisitions on original antigenic sin. I. Evidence in Man; II. Proof in lower vertebrates, J. Exp. Med. 124:331 (1966).

33. C. Fernandez and G. Moller, The immune response against two epitopes on the same thymus-independent polysaccharide carrier, Immunology 33:59 (1977).

34. R. D. Goldfien, P. P. Chen, S. Fong, and D. A. Carson, Synthetic peptides corresponding to third hypervariable region of human monoclonal IgM rheumatoid factor heavy chains define an immunodominant idiotype, J. Exp. Med. 162:756 (1985).

35. F. Goni, P. P. Chen, B. Pons-Estel, D. A. Carson, and B. Frangione, Sequence similarities and cross-idiotypic specificity of L chains among human monoclonal IgM_K with anti-γ-globulin activity, J. Immunol. 135:4073 (1985).

36. T. Gridley, M. N. Margolies, and M. L. Gefter, The association of various D elements with a single immunoglobulin V_H gene segment: influence on the expression of a major cross-reactive idiotype, J. Immunol. 134:1236 (1985).

37. G. M. Griffiths, C. Berek, M. Kaartinen, and C. Milstein, Somatic mutation and the maturation of immune response to 2-phenyl oxazolone, Nature 312:271 (1984).

38. L. Hadjipetrou-Kourounakis and E. Moller, Adjuvants influence the immunoglobulin subclass distribution of immune responses in vivo, Scand. J. Immunol. 19:219 (1984).

39. M. Heidelberger, Precipitating cross-reactions among pneumococcal types, Infection and Immunity 41:1234 (1983).

40. T. Honjo, Immunoglobulin genes, Ann. Rev. Immunol. 1:499 (1983).

41. A. A. Ilyas, R. H. Quarles, M. C. Dalakas, and R. O. Brady, Polyneuropathy with monoclonal gammopathy: glycolipids are frequently antigens for IgM paraproteins, Proc. Natl. Acad. Sci. 82:6697 (1985).

42. N. K. Jerne, Towards a network theory of the immune system, Ann. Immunol. (Inst. Pasteur) 125C:373 (1974).

43. E. A. Kabat, Size and heterogeneity of the combining sites on an antibody molecule, J. Cell Comp. Physiol. Suppl. 50:79 (1957).

44. E. A. Kabat, The nature of an antigenic determinant, J. Immunol. 97:1 (1966).

45. E. A. Kabat, "Structural Concepts in Immunology and Immunochemistry," Second Edition, Holt, Rinehart and Winston, New York (1976).

46. E. A. Kabat, The structural basis of antibody complementarity, _Adv. Protein Chemistry_ 32:1 (1978).

47. E. A. Kabat, The antibody combining site, _in_: "Fifth International Congress of Immunology," Academic Press, New York (1983).

48. E. A. Kabat, Idiotypic determinants, minigenes and the antibody combining site, _in_: "The Biology of Idiotypes," M. I. Greene and A. Nisonoff, eds., Plenum Publishing Corporation, New York (1984).

49. E. A. Kabat, Antibody combining sites--past, present and future, _in_: "Ninth International Subcellular Methodology Forum," Plenum Publishing Corporation, New York (1986).

50. E. A. Kabat, Antibody combining sites: how much of the antibody repertoire are we seeing? How does it influence our understanding of the structural and genetic basis of antibody complementarity, _in_: "Symposium on Molecular Immunology of Complex Carbohydrates," A. M. Wu, ed., Plenum Publishing Corporation, New York, in press (1986).

51. E. A. Kabat, J. Liao, H. Bretting, E. C. Franklin, D. Geltner, B. Frangione, M. E. Koshland, J. Shyong, and E. F. Osserman, Human monoclonal macroglobulins with specificity for _Klebsiella_ K polysaccharides that contain 3,4-pyruvylated-_D_-galactose and 4,6-pyruvylated-_D_-galactose, _J. Exp. Med._ 152:979 (1980).

52. E. A. Kabat, J. Liao, L. Grossbard, E. F. Osserman, K. Nickerson, E. Glickman, L. Chess, J. B. Robbins, R. Schneerson, and Y. Yang, A human macroglobulin with specificity for α(2→8)-linked poly-N-acetylneuraminic acid, the capsular polysaccharide of group B meningococci and _E. coli_ K1, which cross reacts with polynucleotides and with denatured DNA (in preparation, 1986).

53. E. A. Kabat, J. Liao, W. H. Sherman, and E. F. Osserman, Immunochemical characterization of the specificities of two human monoclonal IgM's reacting with chondroitin sulfates, _Carbohydrate Res._ 130:289 (1984).

54. E. A. Kabat and T. T. Wu, Attempts to locate complementarity-determining residues in the variable positions of light and heavy chains of immunoglobulins, _in_: "Immunoglobulins," S. Kochwa and H. G. Kunkel, eds., _Ann. N.Y. Acad. Sci._ 190:382 (1971).

55. E. A. Kabat, T. T. Wu, H. Bilofsky, M. Reid-Miller, and H. Perry, "Sequences of Proteins of Immunological Interest. Tabulation and Analysis of Amino Acid and Nucleic Acid Sequences of Precursors, V-regions, C-regions, J-chain, β_2-microglobulins, Major Histocompatibility Antigens, Thy-2, Complement, C-reactive Protein, Thymopoietin, Post-gamma Globulin, and α_2-macroglobulin," U. S. Department of Health and Human Services, Public Health Service, National Institutes of Health, Bethesda, Maryland (1983).

56. E. A. Kabat, T. T. Wu, M. Reid-Miller, H. Perry, and K. Gottesman, "Sequences of Proteins of Immunological Interest," Second Edition, National Institutes of Health, Bethesda, Maryland (1986).

57. Z. E. Kahana and B. F. Erlanger, Immunochemical study of the structure of poly(adenylic acid), _Biochemistry_ 2:320 (1980).

58. L. Kobzik, M. C. Brown, and A. G. Cooper, Demonstration of a idiotypic antigen on a monoclonal cold agglutinin and on its isolated heavy and light chains, _Proc. Natl. Acad. Sci._ 73:1702 (1976).

59. G. Kohler and C. Milstein, Continuous cultures of fused cells secreting antibody of predefined specificity, _Nature_ 256:495 (1975).

60. H. G. Kunkel, V. Agnello, F. G. Joslin, R. J. Winchester, and J. D. Cooper, Cross-idiotypic specificity among monoclonal IgM proteins with anti-gamma globulin activity, _J. Exp. Med._ 137:331 (1973).

61. H. G. Kunkel, J. Killander, and M. Mannik, Current trends in immune globulin research, _Acta. Med. Scand._ Suppl. 445:63 (1966).

62. Y. Kurosawa and S. Tonegawa, Organization, structure, and assembly of immunoglobulin heavy chain diversity DNA segments, _J. Exp. Med_. 155:201 (1982).

63. E. M. Lafer, J. Rauch, C. Andrzejewski, D. Mudd, B. Furie, B. Furie, R. S. Schwartz, and B. D. Stollar, Polyspecific monoclonal lupus autoantibodies reactive with both polynucleotides and phospholipids, _J. Exp. Med_. 153:897 (1981).

64. E. Lai and E. A. Kabat, Immunochemical studies of conjugates of isomaltosyl oligosaccharides to lipid: production and characterization of mouse hybridoma antibodies specific for stearyl-isomaltosyl oligosaccharides, _Mol. Immunol_. 22:1021 (1985).

65. E. Lai, E. A. Kabat, and L. Mobraaten, Genetic and nongenetic control of the immune response of mice to a synthetic glycolipid, stearyl-isomaltotetraose, _Cellular Immunol_. 92:172 (1985).

66. R. Lieberman, M. Potter, W. Humphrey, Jr., E. B. Mushinski, and M. Vrana, Multiple individual and cross-specific idiotypes on 13 levan-binding myeloma proteins of BALB/c mice, _J. Exp. Med_. 142:106 (1975).

67. N. Maizels and A. Bothwell, The T cell independent immune response to the hapten NP uses a large repertoire of heavy chain genes, _Cell_ 43:715 (1985).

68. S. D. Makover, H. C. Chen, and E. A. Kabat (in preparation, 1986).

69. B. N. Manjula, M. Potter, C.P.J. Glaudemans, The interaction of mouse myeloma immunoglobulin S15 with negatively charged polysaccharide antigens, _Molecular Immunol_. 19:913 (1982).

70. A. Misaki, M. Torii, T. Sawai, and I. J. Goldstein, Structure of the dextran of Leuconostoc mesenteroides B-1355, _Carbohydrate Res_. 84:273 (1980).

71. Y. Naparstek, D. Duggan, A. Schattner, M. P. Madaio, F. Goni, B. Frangione, B. D. Stollar, E. A. Kabat, and R. S. Schwartz, Immuno-chemical similarities between monoclonal antibacterial Waldenstrom's macroglobulins and monoclonal anti-DNA lupus autoantibodies, _J. Exp. Med_. 161:1525 (1985).

72. J. L. Nelson, F. A. Nardella, and M. Mannik, Competition between antigen and anti-idiotypes for rheumatoid factors, _J. Immunol_. 135:2357 (1985).

73. B. A. Newman and E. A. Kabat, An immunochemical study of the combining site specificities of C57BL/6J monoclonal antibodies to an $\alpha(1\rightarrow6)$-linked dextran B512, _J. Immunol_. 135:1220 (1985).

74. B. A. Newman, J. Liao, F. Gruezo, S. Sugii, E. A. Kabat, M. Torii, B. L. Clevinger, J. M. Davie, J. Schilling, M. Bond, and L. Hood, Immunochemical studies of mouse monoclonal antibodies to dextran B1355S. II. Combining site specificity sequence, idiotype and affinity, _Mol. Immunol_., in press (1986).

75. B. Newman, S. Sugii, E. A. Kabat, M. Torii, J. Clevinger, J. Schilling, J. M. Davie, and L. Hood, Combining site specificites of mouse hybridoma antibodies to dextran B1355, _J. Exp. Med_. 157:130 (1983).

76. M. Nishi, T. Kataoka, and T. Honjo, Preferential rearrangment of the immunoglobulin κ chain joining region $J_\kappa 1$ and $J_\kappa 2$ segments in mouse spleen DNA, _Proc. Natl. Acad. Sci_. 82:6399 (1985).

77. J. Oudin and P.-A. Cazenave, Similar idiotypic specificities in immuno-globulin fractions with different antibody functions or even without detectable antibody function, _Proc. Natl. Acad. Sci_. 68:2616 (1971).

78. E. A. Padlan, D. M. Segal, T. F. Spande, D. R. Davies, S. Rudikoff, and M. Potter, Structure at 4.5 resolution of a phosphorylcholine-binding Fab, _Nature_ (London) _New Biol_. 145:165 (1973).

79. R. M. Pearlmutter, D. Hansburg, D. E. Briles, R. A. Nicolotti, and J. M. Davie, Subclass restriction of murine anti-carbohydrate anti-bodies, _J. Immunol_. 121:566 (1978).

80. M. Potter, Antigen-binding myeloma proteins of mice, _Adv. Immunol_. 25:141 (1977).

81. A. S. Rao, E. A. Kabat, W. Nimmich, and E. F. Osserman, Effect of pH
     on the precipitin reaction of human monoclonal macroglobulins with
     specificity for klebsiella K polysaccharides containing 3,4-
     pyruvylated D-galactose and 4,6-pyruvylated D-galactose, Molecular
     Immunol. 19:609 (1982).
82. A. S. Rao, J. Liao, E. A. Kabat, E. F. Osserman, M. Harboe, and W.
     Nimmich, Immunochemical studies on human monoclonal macroglobulins
     with specificities for 3,4-pyruvylated D-galactose and 4,6-
     pyruvylated D-glucose, J. Biol. Chem. 259:1018 (1984).
83. M. G. Reth and F. W. Alt, Novel immunoglobulin heavy chains are pro-
     duced from DJ$_H$ gene segment rearrangements in lymphoid cells,
     Nature 312:418 (1984).
84. F. F. Richards and W. H. Konigsberg, Speculations how specific are
     antibodies? Immunochemistry 10:545 (1973).
85. I. M. Roitt, D. K. Thanavala, and F. C. Hay, Anti-idiotypes as surro-
     gate antigens: structural considerations, Immunology Today 6:265
     (1985).
86. E. R. Ruckel and C. Schuerch, Chemical synthesis of a dextran model,
     poly-α-(1→6)-anhydro-D-glucopyranose, Biopolymers 5:515 (1967).
87. S. Rudikoff, Immunoglobulin structure-function correlates: antigen
     binding and idiotypes, Contemp. Topics Molecular Immunol. 9:169
     (1983).
88. S. Rudikoff, M. Pawlita, J. Pumphrey, E. Mushinski, and M. Potter,
     Galactan-binding antibodies. Diversity and structure of idiotypes,
     J. Exp. Med. 158:1385 (1983).
89. D. H. Sachs, Genetic control of idiotype expression, in: "Immunology
     80," Academic Press, New York (1980).
90. D. L Sacks, L. V. Kirchhoff, S. Hievy, and A. Sher, Molecular mimicry
     of a carbohydrate epitope on a major surface glycoprotein of
     Trypanosoma cruzi by using anti-idiotypic antibodies, J. Immunol.
     135:4155 (1985).
91. J. B. Schilling, B. Clevinger, J. M. Davie, and L. Hood, Amino acid
     sequence of homogeneous antibodies to dextran and DNA rearrange-
     ments in heavy chain V-region gene segments, Nature 283:35 (1980).
92. K. Sege and P. A. Peterson, Use of anti-idiotypic antibodies as cell
     surface receptor probes, Proc. Natl. Acad. Sci. 75:2443 (1978).
93. M. V. Seiden, B. Clevinger, S. McMillan, A. Srouji, R. Lerner, and J.
     M. Davie, Chemical synthesis of idiotopes, J. Exp. Med. 159:1338
     (1984).
94. J. Sharon, E. A. Kabat, and S. L. Morrison, Immunochemical characteri-
     zation of binding sites of hybridoma antibodies specific for
     α(1→6)-linked dextran, Mol. Immunol. 19:389 (1982).
95. J. Sharon, E. A. Kabat, and S. L. Morrison, Association constants of
     hybridoma antibodies specific for α(1→6)-linked dextran determined
     by affinity electrophoresis, Mol. Immunol. 19:389 (1982).
96. J. Sharon, E. A. Kabat, and S. L. Morrison, Studies on mouse hybridomas
     secreting IgM or IgA antibodies to α(1→6)-linked dextran, Mol.
     Immunol. 18:831 (1981).
97. S. K. Sikder, P. N. Akolkar, P. M. Kaladas, S. L. Morrison, and E. A.
     Kabat, Sequences of variable regions of hybridoma antibodies to
     α(1→6)dextran in BALB/c and C57BL/6 mice, J. Immunol.135:4215
     (1985).
98. E. W. Silverton, E. A. Padlan, D. R. Davies, S. Smith-Gill, and M.
     Potter, Crystalline monoclonal antibody Fabs complexed to hen egg
     white lysozyme, J. Mol. Biol. 180:761 (1984).
99. C. A. Slaughter and J. D. Capra, Amino acid sequence diversity within
     the family of antibodies bearing the major antiarsonate cross-
     reactive idiotype of the a strain mouse, J. Exp. Med. 158:1615
     (1983).

100. K. E. Stein, D. A. Zopf, B. M. Johnson, C. B. Miller, and W. E. Paul, Immune response to an isomaltohexosyl-protein conjugate, a thymus-dependent analog of α(1→6)dextran, J. Immunol. 128:1350 (1982).

101. K. E. Stein, D. A. Zopf, C. B. Miller, B. M. Johnson, P.K.A. Mongini, A. Ahmed, and W. E. Paul, Immune response to a thymus-dependent form of B512 dextran requires the presence of Lyb-5⁺ lymphocytes, J. Exp. Med. 157:657 (1983).

102. J. Urbain, Idiotypes, expression of antibody diversity and network concepts, Ann. Immunol. 127:357 (1976).

103. J. L. Winkelhake and E. W. Voss, Jr., Recognition of carrier residues adjacent to hapten by antitrinitrophenyl antibodies, Biochemistry 9:1845 (1970).

104. C. Wood and E. A. Kabat, Immunochemical studies of conjugates of isomaltosyl oligosaccharides to lipid: fractionation of rabbit antibodies to stearylisomaltosyl oligosaccharides and a study of their combining sites by a competitive binding assay, Arch. Biochem. 212:277 (1981).

105. C. Wood and E. A. Kabat, Immunochemical studies on conjugates of isomaltosyl oligosaccharides to lipid. I. Antigenicity of the glycolipids and the production of specific antibodies in rabbits, J. Exp. Med. 154:432 (1981).

106. T. T. Wu and E. A. Kabat, An analysis of the sequences of the variable regions of Bence Jones proteins and myeloma light chains and their implication for antibody complementarity, J. Exp. Med. 132:211 (1970).

107. A. M. Wu, E. A. Kabat, and M. G. Weigert, Immunochemical studies on dextran-specific and levan-specific myeloma proteins from NZB mice, Carbohydrate Res. 66:113 (1978).

108. M. Zanetti, F. T. Liu, J. Rogers, and D. H. Katz, Heavy and light chains of a mouse monoclonal autoantibody express the same idiotype, J. Immunol. 135:1245 (1985).

SECTION II
B CELL DEVELOPMENT, FUNCTION, REPERTOIRE AND ACTIVATION

B Cell Development in Mammals
Max D. Cooper

Control of μ and δ Gene Expression in B Lymphocyte Development
Nicolas Fasel, Michael Briskin, Carla Carter, Herman Govan,
Gary Hermanson, Ronald Law, and Randolph Wall

Functional Maturation of B Cell Repertoire Expression
Barbara G. Froscher and Norman G. Klinman

Receptor Cross-Linkage Stimulates B Cell Activation
Junichiro Mizuguchi, Michael Beaven, Peter Hornbeck,
Wayne Tsang, and William E. Paul

B CELL DEVELOPMENT IN MAMMALS

Max D. Cooper

Cellular Immunobiology Unit, Comprehensive Cancer Center
Departments of Pediatrics and Microbiology
University of Alabama at Birmingham
Birmingham, Alabama

INTRODUCTION

B cells and their antibody-secreting progeny represent one of several differentiation pathways that hemopoietic stem cells (HSC) may enter (8,23). While B cells in birds are generated in the hindgut bursa of Fabricus, mammalian B cells are generated in hemopoietic tissues along with other blood cell lineages (28,29,34). Mammalian B cells appear first in embryonic liver and then the spleen when hemopoiesis is centered in these organs (29). Later in development, they are produced in the bone marrow (28,29,34).

Cells representing important intermediate stages between HSC and B cells have been identified in mammals and studied intensely over the last decade (9,14). This heterogeneous population of early B-lineage cells, termed pre-B, is featured by 1) intensive cellular proliferation, and 2) a cascade of immunoglobulin (Ig) gene rearrangements. This combination of events leads to the generation of clonally diverse B cells.

Ig GENE REARRANGEMENTS IN PRE-B CELLS

The rearrangements begin in the V (variable), D (diversity) and J_H (joining) minigene families which together encode the variable region of Ig heavy chains (1,19,31,37). Pre-B cells undergo sequential rearrangements, first of D and J_H genes and then of a V gene (2) to form a VDJ_H complex encoding the complete heavy chain variable region. This brings upstream V-gene promoter sequences nearer to an enhancer sequence located in the intron between the J_H and μ constant region (C_μ) genes, and effective transcription is initiated (3,11,25). Correct alignment of the VDJ_H rearrangements leads to formation of nuclear transcripts that can be appropriately processed for cytoplasmic μ-chain expression, the primary identifying feature of pre-B cells (6,18,32,35). Subsequent productive rearrangement of light chain V and J_L genes (kappa and lambda) (37) leads to light chain synthesis and formation of complete IgM molecules, which are expressed on the cell surface (18). This event marks the birth of B cells which can then migrate to peripheral lymphoic tissues and undergo clonal selection on the basis of their surface antibody specificity.

GROWTH OF PRE-B CELLS

The kinetics of pre-B cell development have been examined extensively
in mice (13,16,27,38). Progression through the pre-B cell compartment of
differentiation requires an estimated four to five day interval (9). The
doubling time of the pre-B cell population in the 15-day embryonic liver is
approximately 12 hours. (38). Pre-B cells are generated in clusters during
fetal development (13), and discrete pre-B cell colonies can be identified
in the postnatal mouse liver (12,33). The clonal size of these colonies
would suggest that each committed precursor can give rise to daughter pre-B
cells that undergo around six replicative cycles. Thus there is ample
opportunity for the development of intraclonal diversity based on different
VDJ_H and VJ_L rearrangements by sister pre-B cells.

The driving forces for polyclonal pre-B cell growth in hemopoietic
tissues are still poorly understood. Both adherent auxilliary cells and
soluble factors appear to be needed (14). In long-term bone marrow cultures,
pre-B cells are found in close proximity to adherent stromal cells. It has
been suggested (30), but not yet confirmed, that IL-3 may be sufficient for
in vitro growth of pre-B cells.

CELL SURFACE MARKER FOR EARLY B-LINEAGE CELLS

Among other outstanding questions about pre-B cells are the elements
determining their differentiation, regulatory controls for their Ig gene
rearrangements, and the size and location of the graveyard for pre-B cells
undergoing "non-productive" Ig gene rearrangements. Solutions to these
unresolved issues could be more easily reached with a means for precise
identification and isolation of this population of cells from the midst of
other types of hemopoietic cells present in greater numbers.

Consideration of the biological features of pre-B cells led us to predict their expression of novel cell surface molecules. Since pre-B cells
undergo a polyclonal population explosion before acquiring surface immunoglobulin, the presence of cell surface receptors for growth factors could
be expected, as well as receptors for differentiation signals. Cell adhesion
molecules, analogous to those identified for embryonic neural cells, could
also be anticipated since these could serve to prevent pre-B cells from
leaving their birthplace prematurely.

Recently we have identified a cell surface molecule that appears to be
uniquely expressed on the surface of murine pre-B and newly formed B cells
(7). The molecule was identified via an alloantigenic determinant, and the
cells that express it appear to be confined to hemopoietic tissues, namely
the embryonic liver, the neonatal spleen and the bone marrow. The monoclonal
antibody that recognizes this early B lineage marker is called BP-1. It
was made by immunizing a wild mouse (Mus spretus) with the 18.81 pre-B cell
line, and then fusing spleen cells with a non-producer myeloma variant.

The BP-1 antibody identifies pre-B cells and newly-formed B cells but
does not react with cell surface molecules on B cells in peripheral
lymphoid tissues or on any other cell type that we can identify. The BP-1
antibody can be used to purify early B lineage cells from the adult bone
marrow of inbred laboratory mice and Mus 1 strains of wild mice.

The surface molecule identified by the BP-1 antibody is a homodimer
formed by two covalently linked chains of approximately 140,000 M_r. The
function of this molecule is still unknown, but its amplified expression on
neoplastic pre-B and early B cells may suggest a growth regulatory role.
It will also be of interest to determine whether or not this is a highly

conserved molecule which is expressed on early B lineage cells in all
mammals.

B CELL ISOTYPE SWITCHING

Isotype switching, the phenomenon whereby B lymphocytes within a clone
can produce antibodies of different isotypes with identical antigens, is
the last stage in B cell differentiation which involves Ig gene rearrangements. All newly formed B cells express surface IgM molecules (15,17). As
IgM B cells mature they may synthesize and express IgD molecules of the
same antigen specificity (4,22). This is accomplished via processing of an
RNA transcript containing information for both μ- and δ-messages (4,20,24).
When an IgM/IgD B cell switches to the synthesis of IgG, IgA or IgE, the
originally rearranged VDJ_H gene segment is expressed with a $C\gamma$, $C\alpha$ or $C\epsilon$
gene, the C_H genes being located downstream in the order 5' $C\mu$-$C\delta$-$C\gamma_3$-$C\gamma_1$-$\psi\epsilon$
-$C\alpha_1$-$\psi\gamma$-$C\gamma_2$-$C\gamma_4$-$C\epsilon$-$C\alpha_2$ 3' (10,21). Switch (S) regions composed of repetitive DNA sequences are located in the introns 5' to $C\mu$ and each of the other
C_H genes, except $C\delta$ (22,26,36). During the switching process, two S regions
combine allowing the formation of a loop of DNA which is then excised and
deleted. For example, the switch from IgM to IgG_3 involves a recombination
between $S\mu$ and $S\gamma_3$ and deletion of the intervening $C\mu$ and $C\delta$ genes. It has
been proposed that a switch recombinase mediates this event, but such a
postulated nuclear protein has not yet been identified.

For reasons discussed elsewhere (5), we have proposed that the switch
mechanism is initiated early in the life history of B cells as the final
event in a cascade of Ig gene rearrangements. According to this hypothesis,
antigens and T cells exert their influences on the antibody isotypes produced
in an immune response by inducing selective differentiation of $B\gamma$-, $B\alpha$- or
$B\epsilon$-committed B cells. An alternate view is that certain antigens, mitogens
and T cell factors can instruct B cell switching. This issue is discussed
further by other contributors to this volume, who will address the mechanisms
involved in triggering B cell growth and plasma cell differentiation.

REFERENCES

1. F. Alt, N. Rosenberg, S. Lewsi, E. Thomas, and D. Baltimore, Organization and reorganization of immunoglobulin genes in A-MuLV-trans-
   formed cells: Rearrangement of heavy but not light chain genes,
   Cell 27:381 (1981).
2. F. W. Alt, G. D. Yancopoulos, T. K. Blackwell, C. Wood, E. Thomas, M.
   Boss, R. Coffman, and D. Baltimore, Ordered rearrangement of
   immunoglobulin in heavy chain variable region segments, EMBO J.
   3:1209 (1984).
3. J. Banerji, L. Olson, and W. Schaffner, A lymphocyte-specific cellular
   enhancer is located downstream of the joining region in immunoglobulin heavy chain genes, Cell 33:729 (1983).
4. F. R. Blattner and P. W. Tucker, The molecular biology of immunoglobulin D, Nature (London) 307:417 (1984).
5. P. D. Burrows and M. D. Cooper, The immunoglobulin heavy chain class
   switch, Mol. Cell. Biochem. 63:97 (1984).
6. P. D. Burrows, M. LeJeune, and J. F. Kearney, Evidence that murine
   pre-B cells synthesize μ heavy chains but not light chains, Nature
   280:838 (1979).
7. M. D. Cooper, D. Mulvaney, A Coutinho, and P.-A. Cazanave, Identification of a novel cell surface molecule on early B-lineage cells,
   Nature, in press (1986).
8. M. D. Cooper, R.D.A. Peterson, M. A. South, and R. A. Good, The
   functions of the thymus system and the bursa system in the chicken,
   J. Exp. Med. 123:75 (1966).

9. M. D. Cooper, A. Velardi, J. E. Calvert, W. E. Cathings, and H. Kubagawa, Generation of B cell clones during ontogeny, in: "Progress in Immunology," Volume 5, T. Tada, ed., Academic Press Japan, Inc. (1983).

10. J. G. Flanagan and T. H. Rabbitts, Arrangement of human immunoglobulin heavy chain constant regions genes implies evolutionary duplication of a segment containing γ, α and ε genes, Nature (London) 300:709 (1982).

11. S. D. Gillies, S. L. Morrison, V. T. Oi, and S. Tonegawa, A tissue-specific transcription enhancer element is located in the major intron of a rearranged immunoglobulin heavy chain gene, Cell 33:717 (1983).

12. C. E. Grossi, A. Velardi, and M. D. Cooper, Postnatal liver hemopoiesis in mice: generation of pre-B cells, granulocytes, and erythrocytes in discrete colonies, J. Immunol. 135:2302 (1985).

13. W. A. Kamps and M. D. Cooper, Microenvironmental studies of pre-B and B cell development in human and mouse fetuses, J. Immunol. 129:526 (1982).

14. P. W. Kincade, Formation of B lymphocytes in fetal and adult life, Adv. Immunol. 31:177 (1981).

15. P. W. Kincade, A. R. Lawton, D. E. Bockman, and M. D. Cooper, Suppression of immunoglobulin G synthesis as a result of antibody-mediated suppression of immunoglobulin M synthesis in chickens, Proc. Natl. Acad. Sci. U.S.A. 67:1918 (1970).

16. K. S. Landreth, C. Rosse, and J. Clagett, Myelogenous production and maturation of B lymphocytes in the mouse, J. Immunol. 127:2027 (1981).

17. A. Lawton, R. Asofsky, M. B. Hylton, and M. D. Cooper, Suppression of immunoglobulin class synthesis in mice. I. Effects of treatment with antibody to μ chain, J. Exp. Med. 135:277 (1972).

18. D. Levitt and M. D. Cooper, Mouse pre-B cells synthesize and secrete μ heavy chains but not light chains, Cell 19:617 (1980).

19. R. Maki, J. Kearney, C. Paige, and S. Tonegawa, Immunoglobulin gene rearrangement in immature cells, Science 209:1366 (1980).

20. R. Maki, W. Roeder, A. Traunecker, C. Sidman, M. Wabl, W. Raschke, and S. Tonegawa, The role of DNA rearrangement and alternative RNA processing in the expression of immunoglobulin delta genes, Cell 24:353 (1981).

21. N. Migone, S. Oliviero, G. deLange, D. L. Delacroix, D. Boschis, F. Altruda, L. Silengo, M. DeMarchi, and A. O. Carbonara, Multiple gene deletions within the human immunoglobulin heavy-chain cluster, Proc. Natl. Acad. Sci. U.S.A. 81:5811 (1984).

22. G. Möller, ed., Immunoglobulin D: structure, synthesis, membrane representation and function, Immunol. Rev. 37:1 (1977).

23. M.A.S. Moore and J.J.T. Owen, Stem cell migration in developing myeloid and lymphoid system, Lancet ii:658 (1967).

24. K. W. Moore, J. Rogers, T. Hunkapiller, P. Early, C. Nottenburg, I. Weissman, H. Basin, R. Wall, and L. E. Hook, Expression of IgD may use both DNA rearrangement and RNA splicing mechanisms, Proc. Natl. Acad. Sci. U.S.S. 78:1800 (1981).

25. N. S. Neuberger, Expression and regulation of immunoglobulin heavy chain gene transfected into lymphoid cells, EMBO J. 2:1372 (1983).

26. T. Niaido, S. Nakai, and T. Honjo, Switch region of immunoglobulin Cμ gene is composed of simple tandem repetitive sequences, Nature (London) 292:845 (1981).

27. D. G. Osmond, Production and differentiation of B lymphocytes in the bone marrow, in: "Immunoglobulin Genes and B Cell Differentiation," J. Battisto and K. Knight, eds., Elsevier/North Holland, New York (1980).

28. D. G. Osmond and G.J.V. Nossal, Differentition of lymphocytes in mouse bone marrow. I. Quantitative radioautographic studies of anti-

globulin binding by lymphocytes in bone marrow and lymphoid tissues, Cell. Immunol. 13:117 (1974).

29. J.J.T. Owen, M. D. Cooper, and M. C. Raff, In vitro generation of B lymphocytes in mouse fetal liver: a mammalian "bursa equivalent," Nature 249:361 (1974).

30. R. Palacios, M. Gittenson, M. Steinmetz, and J. P. McKearn, Inter-leukin-3 supports growth of mouse pre-B cell clones in vitro, Nature 309:126 (1984).

31. R. P. Perry, D. E. Kelley, C. Coleclough, and J. F. Kearney, Organization and expression of immunoglobulin genes in fetal liver hybridomas, Proc. Natl. Acad. Sci. U.S.A. 78:247 (1981).

32. M. C. Raff, M. Megson, J.J.T. Owen, and M. D. Cooper, Early production of intracellular IgM by B-lymphocyte precursors in mouse, Nature 259:224 (1976).

33. J. Rossant, K. M. Vijh, C. E. Grossi, and M. D. Cooper, Clonal origin of haemopoietic colonies in the post-natal mouse liver, Nature 319:507 (1986).

34. J. E. Ryser and P. Vassalli, Mouse bone marrow lymphocytes and their differentiation, J. Immunol. 113:719 (1974).

35. E. J. Siden, D. Baltimore, D. Clark, and N. E. Rosenberg, Immunoglobulin synthesis by lymphoid cells transformed in vitro by Abelson murine leukemia virus, Cell 16:389 (1979).

36. L. W. Stanton and K. B. Marcu, Nucleotide sequence and properties of the murine γ_3 immunoglobulin heavy chain gene switch region: implications for successive Cγ gene switching, Nuc. Acids Res. 10:2993 (1982).

37. S. Tonegawa, Somatic generation of antibody diversity, Nature 302:575 (1983).

38. A. Velardi and M. D. Cooper, An immunofluorescence analysis of the ontogeny of myeloid, T and B lineage cells in mouse hemopoietic tissues, J. Immunol. 133:672 (1984).

CONTROL OF $\mu + \delta$ GENE EXPRESSION IN B LYMPHOCYTE DEVELOPMENT

Nicolas Fasel, Michael Briskin, Carla Carter, Herman Govan, Gary Hermanson, Ronald Law, and Randolph Wall

Molecular Biology Institute and
Department of Microbiology and Immunology
UCLA School of Medicine, University of California
Los Angeles, California

INTRODUCTION

B lymphocyte development proceeds through an ordered course of immunoglobulin gene rearrangements and expression [reviewed in 3, 24, 42)]. Pre-B cells contain rearranged immunoglobulin μ genes and express intracellular μ heavy chains. Early B lymphocytes express rearranged light chain genes and display monomeric surface IgM. Mature B lymphocytes co-express a new class of immunoglobulin, IgD, along with the IgM on their membranes. Further DNA rearrangements are not involved in the activation of IgD expression. Rather, the μ and δ heavy chains of IgM and IgD are encoded by different heavy chain mRNA species derived from the large $\mu + \delta$ complex transcription unit (Figure 1). Finally, mature plasma cells actively secrete pentameric IgM formed in covalent association with J-chain.

Multiple of μ and δ heavy chain mRNA are generated from the large $\mu + \delta$ transcription unit (15,22,27,28,30,34). Membrane (μ_m) and secreted (μ_s) μ mRNAs are produced by alternative RNA splicing (Figure 1). These two forms of μ mRNA have different 3' sequences coding for secreted or transmembrane COOH-terminal sequences (1,10,38). Based on the universal finding that cleavage and polyadenylation preceded splicing in all eukaryotic genes studied, we previously proposed that cleavage and polyadenylation would determine which μ mRNA would be generated (10,38). This is the simplest model possible, since once polyadenylation of the primary transcripts for μ_s and μ_m mRNA has occurred, RNA splicing would act invariantly on all available exon-intron junctures having complete 5' and 3' splicing signals. Two mechanisms can be envisioned to control the choice of poly(A) sites in the developmentally regulated expression of μ_s and μ_m mRNAs. The first involved the post-transcriptional choice of poly(A) sites at the RNA processing stage. In this case transcription would be equimolar along the entire transcription unit through the μ_m exons at all stages in B cell development. The second model for selective expression of μ_s mRNA late in B cell development involves transcription termination imposed between μ_s and μ_m exons. Transcription through the μ_m exons would be reduced relative to the μ_s region at late stages in B cell maturation.

We have tested these two models for μ mRNA control by analysis of the relative transcription of μ_s and μ_m sequences in cells at different stages in B cell development. Hybridization of labeled RNA from in vitro nuclear transcription assays to excess cloned μ_s and μ_m specific DNA probes, revealed that both μ polyadenylation sites are equally transcribed at all stages in B cell development. Accordingly, we conclude that post-transcriptional events involved in the cleavage and polyadenylation of the μ primary transcripts determine μ_s and μ_m mRNA production.

More complex modes of regulation including transcription termination and post-transcriptional RNA processing choices appear to control δ mRNA production during B cell development (30,45). Mather and associates reported that the δ constant region exons ($C\delta$) were transcribed at 20-50% the level of the μ gene constant region exons (C_μ) in B cell lymphomas (30). In contrast, the C_δ exons in cell lines representative of mature IgM-secreting plasma cells were transcribed at less than 10% the level of the C_μ exons. Similar findings have been reported for resting and activated splenic B cells (44,45). We have now mapped the region of transcription termination between C_μ and C_δ. We observed that ongoing transcription in IgM-secreting hybridoma cells declined 85-95% over a region 500-1000 nucleotides past the μ_m poly(A) site. These findings establish that the developmentally regulated transcription termination sequences which control δ gene expression follow closely after the μ_m poly(A) sequence.

RESULTS

Changes in μ and δ mRNA Levels in B Cell Development

Four heavy chain mRNA species are simultaneously expressed from the μ + δ complex transcription unit in IgM + IgD producing B lymphocytes (15,22,-28,30,34; see also Figure 1). Figure 2 shows the μ and δ cytoplasmic mRNA species and nuclear precursors in the IgM + IgD producing B cell hybridoma line, GCL2.1 (36). In these cells, μ_m RNA (2.35 kb) and μ_s (2.1 kb) mRNA

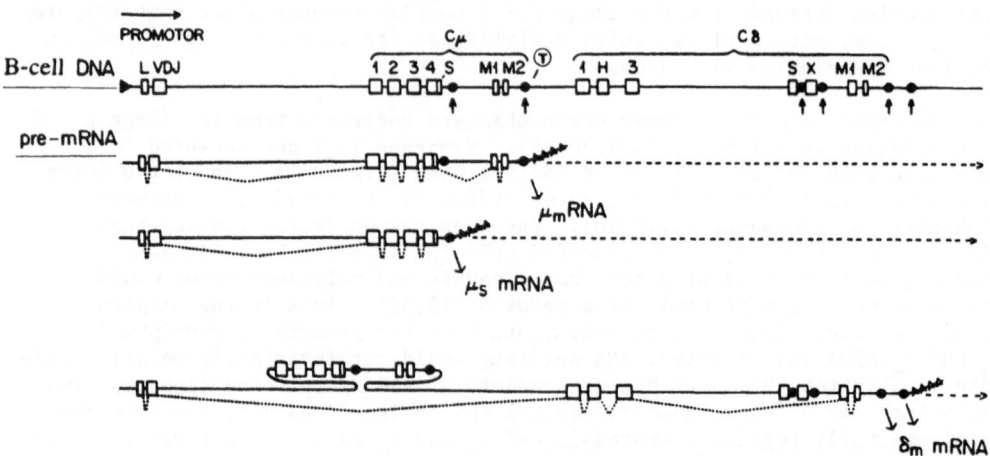

Figure 1. Diagram (to scale) showing the organization of the rearranged and active μ + δ complex transcription unit and the RNA processing events which generate different μ + δ mRNA species. RNA splicing events are shown by small dotted lines. Polyadenylation sites are indicated by ↑ below the DNA. Transcripts continuing past polyadenylation sites are shown by horizontal dotted lines. The region of developmentally regulated transcription termination exerted in IgM secreting cells is denoted by ⓣ.

comprise 70% and 30% respectively of total μ mRNA (Table 1). The sizes of the largest μ-specific nuclear RNA species (12 and 10 kb) correspond to the expected values of μ_m and μ_s primary transcripts in GLC2 cells where the rearranged V_H region is joined to J_H4 (28). The 4.5 kb μ specific nuclear RNA most likely represents a processing intermediate having all exons spliced together except the Cμ4$\rightarrow$M1 exons (35). The two cytoplasmic δ mRNA species (2.35 and 1.6 kb) contain identical coding sequences, with 3'-untranslated region of different lengths (15). These cytoplasmic δ mRNA species are present at approximately 5% the combined level of cytoplasmic μ_m and μ_s mRNA species in GCL2.1 cells (Table 1). Complete transcripts of the μ^s + δ transcription unit in GCL2.1 cells should be approximately 25 kb long (28). The largest δ specific nuclear RNA detectable in GCL2.1 cells ($\sim$10 kb) exactly corresponds to the size expected for a δ mRNA precursor with all sequences between the variable (V_H) region and Cδ1 (including the C exons) spliced out, but with all the δ exons unspliced. Due the correspondence in the size of the μ_s primary transcript and this presumptive δ nuclear RNA processing intermediate, it is not possible to confirm that this species lacks μ gene sequences. Technical limitations may explain the failure to detect the large 25 kb δ primary transcript. Alternatively, splicing of the V_H and C$_\delta$1 exons may occur rapidly to prevent accumulation of detectable δ primary transcripts.

We used a sensitive slot blot assay to determine the ratios of μ and δ mRNA in a number of cell lines representative of different stages in B cell development (Figure 3). A compilation of the results for steady-state levels of μ and δ mRNA is shown in Table 1 along with values for μ_m and μ_s mRNA levels. Only the IgM + IgD producing lymphoma cell line, XT6C (30), and isolated resting mouse splenocytes, contained substantial levels of stable δ mRNA relative to their μ mRNA content. In all early B cells (including pre-B cells) and all IgM-secreting cells, δ mRNA levels were 30- and 100-fold lower than μ mRNA. With the exception of mature unstimulated murine splenocytes, all cell lines representative of early stages in the B cell pathway expressed μ_m mRNA at levels equal to or slightly exceeding μ_s mRNA.

Figure 2. Resolution of μ and δ RNA species in the IgM + IgD-producing cell line, GCL2.1. Isolated poly(A)-containing nuclear and cytoplasmic RNA samples were glyoxyl-treated and electrophoresed in an agarose gel (40). The RNAs were transferred to nitrocellulose and hybridized with ^{32}P-labeled probes as described by Rogers et al. (38). Sizes of hybridized RNA bands were determined in relation to ribosomal RNA standards (39). Sizes shown for μ and δ mRNA species reflect lengths from known sequences. Northern blots of δ RNA (panel A) were exposed approximately 10 longer than those with μ RNA (panel B).

Table 1. Expression of μ_m, μ_s and δ mRNA During B Cell Development

Cell Designation	Immunoglobulin Expression		Ratio of μ_m to μ_s RNA (% μ_s)	Ratio of μ to δ RNA (%δ)
	IgM	IgD		
Pre-B Cells				
JS61-10	μ only	–	50	3
70Z3	μ only	–	40	3
B Cells				
W231	mIgM	–	40	1
GCL2.1	mIgM	mIgD	30	5
X16C	mIgM	mIgD	40	20
Adult splenocytes (unstimulated)	mIgM	mIgD	<10	40
IgM Secreting Cells				
W279	sIgM	–	50	<1
MXW231	sIgM	–	70	2
MXW279	sIgM	–	>90	2
M104E	sIgM	–	>90	<1

Results are summarized from the μ and δ determinations by slot blots on total, poly(A)-containing RNA (Figure 2). The μ and δ RNA values for M104E and X16C are from (30). The ratio of μ_s and μ_m for GCL2.1 cells is from Figure 1. Other values for μ_s and μ_m mRNA levels are compiled from (30) and (25). The immunogloblin proteins expressed by the different cell lines have been previously described (24,30). The pre-B cell line used in these studies, JS61-10, is an Abelson virus transformed spleen cell line obtained from Owen Witte (9). Unstimulated BALB/c spleen cells were isolated by a repeated Percoll gradient procedure reportedly given >90% homogeneous small lymphocytes expressing surface IgM + IgD (8).

Lamson and Koshland reported that μ_s mRNA was at such a low level in unstimulated adult mouse splenocytes that it could not be reliably discriminated from μ_m RNA (25). In IgM-secreting myeloma or hybridoma cells, μ_s mRNA exceeded μ_m mRNA up to ten-fold (1,25,30,35,38).

These collected data document that over the course of B cell development the ratio of μ_s mRNA increased ten-fold over μ_m mRNA, while δ mRNA increases to near μ mRNA and then decreases as much as 100-fold lower than μ mRNA in IgM-secreting cells.

Transcription of μ and δ Gene Segments During B Cell Development

Mather and associates previously reported that transcription of $C\delta$ exons was markedly reduced in IgM-secreting myeloma and hybridoma cells (30). However, this study did not resolve the important issue of whether transcription termination occurred after μ_s or μ_m sequences. We have used a battery of subcloned DNA probes containing most of the $C_\mu \rightarrow C\delta$ region to more precisely map the location of transcription termination between C_μ and $C\delta$ (Figure 4). All of the subcloned probes were experimentally confirmed to lack repetitive sequences which would interfere with transcription mapping (results not shown). RNA from in vitro nuclear transcription reactions was

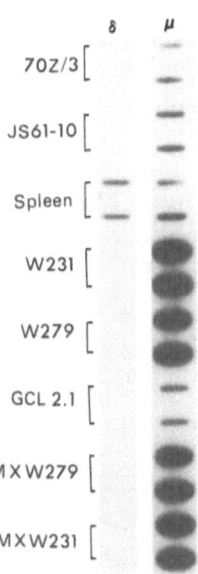

Figure 3. Relative steady state concentrations of μ and δ RNA B cell development. Slot blot hybridizations were carried out as described by Thomas (40). Parallel duplicate 2 μg samples of total poly(A)-containing RNA were hybridized with ^{32}P-labeled μ and δ probes. Equal exposures of hybridized samples were quantitated by integration of densitometer scans.

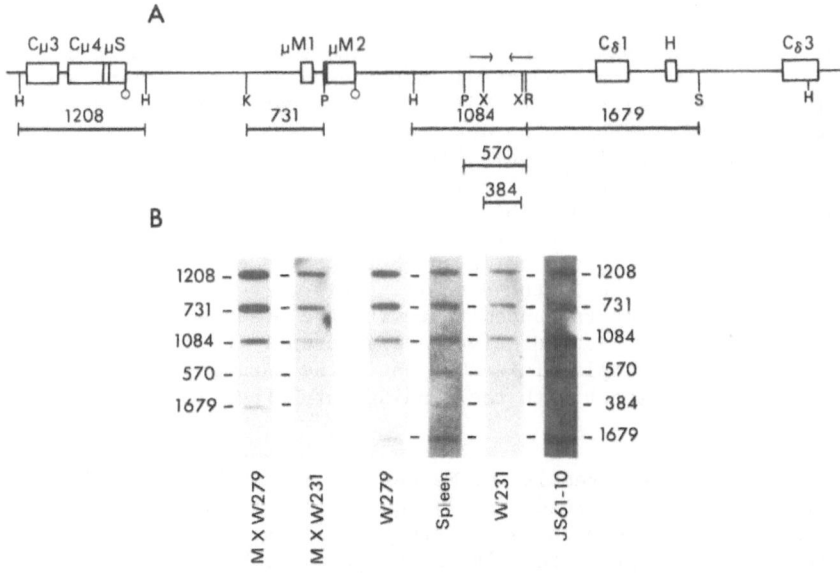

Figure 4. Transcription of $C_\mu \rightarrow C_\delta$ gene segments. A. Subcloned DNA used in the detection of labeled RNA from isolated nuclei transcriptions reactions are shown in location in the gene map (37). The symbols, ⟶⟵, represent large unique inverted repeated sequences (37). B. Panels of exposed autoradiograms from probe DNA slots hybridized with labeled RNA from isolated nuclei transcription reactions (13,30). The numbers refer to specific probes shown in part A and denote the size of the probe (in nucleotides).

53

Table 2. Comparative Transcription of μ and δ Gene Segments at Different Stages in B Cell Development

Cell Designation$^{\mu}$	$C_{\mu} \to C_{\delta}$ Region: Probes:	μS 1208	μM 731	intergenic 1084	intergenic 570	intergenic 384	Cδ 1679
Pre-B Cells							
JS61-10		1.0	0.92	1.1	0.95	–	0.47
B Cells							
W231		1.0	1.3	0.86	0.55	0.47	0.16
Adult splenocytes		1.0	1.2	0.79	0.58	–	0.40
IgM Secreting Cells							
W279		1.0	1.1	0.46	–	–	0.23
MXW231		1.0	1.24	0.36	–	0.05	0.14
MXW279		1.0	1.3	0.27	0.11	–	0.08

Labeled RNA from nuclear transcription reactions hybridized with excess denatured DNA in slots and digested with T1 and RNAse A (13). Hybridized RNA was quantitated by integration of densitometry scans and normalized per kb of probe DNA. Relative transcription refers to the normalized densitometry integration value divided by the μ_s value.

hybridized to an experimentally established excess of probe DNA in slot blots. Under hybridization conditions in DNA excess, the level of hybridized RNA was proportional to input RNA radioactivity. Hybridization intensities with the different probe DNAs were determined by densitometry. Normalized hybridization intensities (i.e., hybridization per kb of probe DNA) showed that the transcription of μ_s and μ_m is essentially equivalent in all cells tested regardless of the μ_s/μ_m mRNA ratio (Table 2). These in vitro transcription assays also showed that the Cδ sequences are transcribed at a level 20-40% that of μ in pre-B cells and B lymphomas even though δ mRNA is 20- to 50-fold lower than μ in these cells. This suggests that transcriptional activation of δ occurs concomitant with the onset of μ transcription in pre-B cells. However, δ transcripts are apparently turned over and not processed into stable cytoplasmic δ mRNA until the mature B cell stage. These results are consistent with the findings of Mather and associates (30).

In agreement with the results of Mather and associates (30) and Yuan and co-workers (44), we observed greatly reduced δ transcription in hybridoma cells representative of terminally differentiated IgM-secreting plasma cells. The decrease in transcription to δ levels occurred within approximately 500-1000 nucleotides past the μ_m poly(A) addition site (Figure 4, Table 2). Transcription normalized over the DNA probe 1084 is reduced 60-80% from the μ_s value. Furthermore, transcription is reduced by 85-95% by DNA probe 570 which lies 1057 nucleotides from the μ_m poly(A) site. Transcription termination in IgM-secreting hybridoma cells is completed prior to the intergenic probes, 570 and 384, since these fragments showed normalized hybridization values equivalent to the Cδ probe.

DISCUSSION

Selective Polyadenylation Controls the Developmentally-Regulated Expression of Membrane or Secreted μ mRNA Species

One of the key findings presented here is that transcription of μ_s and μ_m poly(A) sites is equivalent at all stages in B cell development even though the proportions of μ_m to μ_s heavy chain mRNA vary dramatically (summarized in Tables 1 and 2). This finding eliminates the possibility of transcription termination between the μ_s and μ_m poly(A) sites as a mechanism for controlling the level of μ_s and μ_m mRNA in B cell development. Instead, these findings support the alternative prediction that the differential expression of μ_s and μ_m mRNA in B cell development is regulated through the selective choice of sites for cleavage and polyadenylation of the primary transcript.

Another recent finding further strengthens the selective polyadenylation model. We predicted and have now confirmed a novel RNA processing product, called the amputated transcript (AT), whose 5'-end appears to be generated by cleavage of the heavy chain primary transcript at the μ_s poly(A) site (42). The amputated transcript is polyadenylated at the μ_m site and contains the $\mu_s \rightarrow \mu_m 1$ intron. The M1 and M2 exons in the AT appear to be spliced together as might be expected since the intron separating these exons contains complete 5' and 3' RNA splicing signals. An RNA species such as the AT would not be generated in abundance if appreciable transcription termination occurred between μ_s and μ_m. Other workers (21,35) also have noted an RNA species consistent with the size and sequence content of the AT.

It is now clear that the 3'-ends of most eukaryotic mRNA are produced by cleavage of a larger primary transcript followed by polyadenylation [for review see (2 and 7)]. Studies on the sequences required for polyadenylation now indicate that the AATAAA sequence as well as other sequences located within 50-100 bp 3' of the point of poly(A) addition, are required for correct cleavage and polyadenylation of eukaryotic mRNA [for review see (2,31,-33)]. Danner and Leder have determined that proper cleavage and polyadenylation at the μ_s site required at least 35 nucleotides downstream of the AATAAA signal sequence (6).

The secreted form of heavy chain mRNA strikingly predominates over the membrane mRNA form in mature plasma cells secreting immunoglobulins of all different heavy chain classes [for review see (39)]. We presume that the selective processing at the secreted poly(A) site which produces this predominance of secreted mRNA is imposed by the interaction of sequences in proximity to the secreted poly(A) site of the heavy chain RNA transcript [see (6)] with plasma cell specific trans-acting factors. These could be proteins or as implied by recent evidence, RNA-protein complexes [for review see (2)]. Interestingly, the fusion of non-producing myeloma cells with B lymphocytes expressing membrane immunoglobulin yields hybridoma lines which actively secrete immunoglobulin and whose heavy chain mRNA ratio shifts to predominantly secreted mRNA species [for review see (24)]. This dominant effect suggests that a common cellular processing activity (or complex of activities) may recognize secreted poly(A) sites in all heavy chain classes. In this case, secreted poly(A) sites should contain a conserved sequence recognized by the cleavage enzyme complex involved in polyadenylation. In this regard, Korbin and associates have noted that the sequence, GTCCTGGTTCTTT, is conserved and located within 13-33 nucleotides 3' of the AATAAA sequence in many secreted, but not membrane heavy chain, immunoglobulin gene polyadenylation sites (23). It is intriguing to speculate that this short sequence may direct selective cleavage and polyadenylation at secreted sites in terminally differentiated cells.

The results presented here confirm that δ heavy chain gene expression is subject to both transcriptional and post-transcriptional RNA processing controls [see also (30,44)]. Pre-B cells and B cells at an early stage in B cell development, exhibit the interesting mode of post-transcriptional RNA processing control in which δ gene sequences are transcribed at a level 20-50% that of μ gene segments, but little δ mRNA is processed from these transcripts. In our studies, we have not assayed transcription of the complete δ gene through the δ membrane exons. However, assuming that transcription extends through the membrane δ poly(A) sites to give all the sequences required for δ mRNA processing, δ gene control in pre-B cells and early B cells apparently involves the post-transcriptional decision not to process RNA transcripts. This mode of gene control was originally proposed by Darnell (7). In late stage B lymphocytes actually expressing IgM and IgD (represented by adult mouse splenocytes and lymphoma lines like X16C), RNA processing of δ transcripts generates functional δ mRNA species at levels approximately 30-40% of μ mRNA levels (Table 1; 30,44). As in the choice of membrane and secreted μ mRNAs, the choice of δ poly(A) sites in the exons of μ + δ transcription unit presumably determines the δ mRNA species to be produced. While RNA splicing operates on all available introns in making membrane and secreted μ heavy chain mRNAs, a new mode of control involving selective RNA splicing must occur in making δ mRNA. The splicing apparatus apparently bypasses RNA splice sites in the C_μ exons when splicing the V_H region to the Cδ exons in δ mRNA species (Figure 1; 3,39).

Finally, in IgM-secreting cells (myeloma or hybridoma cells) developmentally regulated transcription termination between μ_m and Cδ imposes the major control on δ expression. The findings reported here locate the region of transcription termination within 500-1000 nucleotides past the μ_m poly(A) addition site. Transcription of δ gene segments in IgM-secreting cells is reduced to 5-10% the level of μ gene segments (Table 2; 30,44). Since the level of stable δ RNA is approximately 1% the level of μ RNA in IgM secreting cells, much of the transcribed δ mRNA is presumably degraded in the nucleus.

Developmentally Regulated Transcription Termination in the μ→δ Intergenic Region

Transcription termination has now been examined in a number of eukaryotic genes [for review see (2)]. These include globin (5,18,19), ovalbumin (26), α-amylase (17), and dihydrofolate reductase (16). In all these cases, transcription proceeds at undiminished levels for some distance (up to 1 kb) beyond the polyadenylation signals. Termination is then reflected by a gradual decline in transcription over some distance up to 1 kb. In the case of the μ→δ intergenic region, we presume that transcription continues at an equimolar level through the μ_m poly(A) addition site. Unfortunately due to directly repeated DNA sequences located in the 500 nucleotide segment following the μ_m poly(A) site (37), it is not possible to unambiguously measure transcription in this region. However, transcription termination is completed within 1000 nucleotides past the μ_m poly(A) addition site. Because transcription termination has already occurred prior to the large inverted repeat sequence located between μ and δ (37), it is unlikely that this interesting structure is involved in the termination process. Clearly, the features of transcription termination in the μ_m→Cδ intergenic region reassemble termination in other eukaryotic genes. However, unlike other genes now studied, termination in the μ + δ gene is developmentally regulated and only exerted in terminally differentiated plasma cells or in their myeloma cell equivalents. Because the formation of hybridomas between myeloma cells and lymphoma cells results in the termination of δ transcription, we infer that dominant, trans-acting regulatory factors (presumably proteins) present in terminally differentiated lymphoid cells interact with μ_m→Cδ intergenic DNA sequences to impose transcription termination.

The mechanisms and signals involved in eukaryotic transcription termin-ation are not yet defined. The activity of transcription termination se-quences must be assayed in transfected cells. One termination transfection experiment has now been reported. In this study Falck-Pederson and associ-ates have determined that an isolated β-globin gene segment containing the polyadenylation site and 1395 nucleotides downstream halted transcription when inserted into the adenovirus E1A gene (12). Termination required the same 5'→3' orientation of the termination fragment as in the globin gene. Interestingly, the flanking gene segment in which termination occurred did not block transcription in either orientation. Falck-Pederson and associates suggested that this may reflect a requirement for the termination sequences to follow cleavage and poly(A) addition signals (12). In this instance, transcription termination would involve recognition of two signals. Computer searches for homologous sequences located in regions showing transcription termination have not been informative. In analogy to yeast genes where terminator sequences are better defined, it has been postulated that termina-tion in higher eukaryotes may occur at short, serially repeated sequences [for review see (2)]. Transcription termination downstream of the ovalbumin gene reportedly does occur in short, serially repeated AT-rich sequences somewhat similar to termination sequences in yeast (26). However, these sequences are not found downstream of other eukaryotic genes.

The termination signals in the μ + δ transcription unit are clearly developmental stage specific and may also be lymphoid cell specific as well. As such, they very likely would bear little resemblance to the termination sequences of other eukaryotic genes. Richards and co-workers postulated that the relatively long, unique inverted sequences immediately

Table 3. Conserved Sequences Flank the Region of Transcription Termination Following the μ_m Poly(A) Addition Site

	μ_m poly(A) site	Sequence 1
Mouse	ACTTTATTGTGAAGGAATTTGTTTTGTTTTTCAAACCTTTCCTGC	
	4274	4318
Human	G----C-G----G--TT------C-----------A----------	
	2789	2832

Sequence 2

Mouse	CCTGATGGAAG AAGGGAAGTAGGGCAG AGAAAATTCCAGGCCT	
	4655	4697
Human	------------G------G-C- -A----G---GGG----------	
	2986	3029

The numbering of the mouse sequences follows the designations in the National Biomedical Research Foundation data base (reference IGCMD). The mouse poly(A) addition site (10,38) occurs 20 nucleotides 3' of the AATAAA sequence. The human μ_m poly(A) addition site has not been reported. However, human μ sequence 1 is located 25 nucleotides 3' of the postulated μ_m AATAAA sequence. The numbering of the human sequences repre-sents the number in Milstein et al. (32). A line indicates that the sequences are identical. The homology searches were performed using a computer program developed by M. Kanehiza (SEQH.EXE, Los Alamos). The final 19 residues of sequence 1 (2813-2832) were previously noted to be very highly conserved (95% homologous) between human and mouse sequences (32).

preceding C_δ may be involved in regulating δ transcription (37). Because transcription terminates well before these inverted sequences, it is unlikely that these structures are involved in the termination process in IgM-secreting cells. This sequence is also not seen in a comparable location in the human $\mu \to \delta$ gene sequence (32). A computer search of the nucleotide sequences of the μ_m poly(A) sites and flanking regions in mice and humans reveals two highly conserved sequences in the region of most active termination following the μ_m poly(A) site (>80% homologous, Table 3). The first is a 44 nucleotide stretch which begins just past the mouse μ_m poly(A) addition site and is in part likely to be involved in cleavage and polyadenylation of μ_m mRNA precursors. The second sequence of 43 nucleotides is located 381 nucleotides 3' of the mouse μ_m poly(A) addition site in the region of most active termination noted in our studies (Table 3). The homology of these flanking sequences is comparable to the most conserved sequences in the mouse and human C_μ exons (32). This striking conservation of non-coding sequences is reminiscent of that noted for C_κ intron sequences later shown to encode the light chain enhancer (11). Because these conserved sequences flank the region of most pronounced transcription decline in IgM secreting cells, these elements may comprise the two signals proposed by Falck-Pederson and associates to be required for termination (12). Gene manipulation studies and analyses of chromatin structure in the region of $\mu \to \delta$ termination are underway to generate further insights into the signals and factors involved in this novel control mechanism.

ACKNOWLEDGEMENTS

We thank R. Deans for his assistance and stimulating advice. We also thank M. Yerington for preparation of this manuscript. This work was supported by research grants from NIH (CA 12800), NSF (PCM 8311332), and by USPHS National Research Awards CA 09056-11 (Gary Hermanson), AI 07126 (Michael Briskin), and GM 07104 (Ronald Law). Nicolas Fasel was supported by a fellowship from the Swiss National Foundation.

REFERENCES

1. F. W. Alt, A.L.M. Bothwell, E. Siden, E. Mather, M. Koshland, and D. Baltimore, Synthesis of secreted and membrane-bound immunoglobulin μ heavy chains is directed by mRNAs that differ at their 3'-ends, Cell 20:293 (1980).
2. M. L. Birnstiel, M. Busslinger, and K. Strub, Transcription termination and 3' processing: the end is in site, Cell 41:349 (1985).
3. F. R. Blattner and P. W. Tucker, The molecular biology of immuno-globulin D, Nature 307:417 (1984).
4. K. Calame, J. Rogers, P. Early, M. Davis, P. Livant, R. Wall, and L. Hood, The mouse C_μ heavy chain immunoglobulin gene segment contains three intervening sequences which separate domains, Nature 284:452 (1980).
5. B. Citron, E. Falck-Pederson, M. Salditt-Georgieff, and J. E. Darnell, Transcription termination occurs within a 1000 bp region downstream of the poly(A) site of the mouse β-globin (major) gene, Nuc. Acids Res. 12:8723 (1984).
6. D. Danner and P. Leder, Role of RNA cleavage/poly(A) addition site in the production of membrane-bound and secreted IgM mRNA, Proc. Natl. Acad. Sci. U.S.A. 82:8658 (1985).
7. J. E. Darnell, Variety in the level of gene control in eukaryotic cells, Nature 297:365 (1982).
8. A. L. DeFranco, E. S. Raveche, R. Asofsky, and W. E. Paul, Frequency of B lymphocytes responsive to anti-immunoglobulin, J. Exp. Med. 155:1523 (1982).

9. K. A. Denis, L. J. Treiman, J. I. St. Claire, and O. N. Witte, Long-term cultures of murine fetal liver retain very early B lymphoid phenotype, J. Exp. Med. 160:1087 (1984).

10. P. Early, J. Rogers, M. Davis, K. Calame, M. Bond, R. Wall, and L. Hood, Two mRNAs can be produced from a single immunoglobulin μ gene by alternative RNA processing pathways, Cell 20:313 (1980).

11. L. Emorine, M. Kuehl, L. Weir, P. Leder, and E. E. Max, A conserved sequence in the immunoglobulin J_k-C_k intron: possible enhancer element, Nature 304:447 (1983).

12. E. Falck-Pederson, J. Logan, T. Shenk, and J. R. Darnell, Transcription termination within the E1A gene of adenovirus induced by insertion of the mouse β-major globin terminator element, Cell 40:897 (1985).

13. N. Fasel, M. Briskin, G. Hermanson, R. Law, and R. Wall, Developmentally regulated transcription termination closely follows the immuno-globulin μ membrane poly(A) site, Nuc. Acids Res., in press (1986).

14. N. Fedoroff, P. K. Wellauer, and R. Wall, Intermolecular duplexes in heterogeneous nuclear RNA from HeLa cells, Cell 10:597 (1977).

15. L. Fitzmaurice, J. Owens, F. R. Blattner, H.-L. Cheng, P. W. Tucker, and J. F. Mushinski, Mouse spleen and IgD-secreting plasmacytomas contain multiple IgD δ chain RNAs, Nature 296:459 (1982).

16. E. G. Frayne, E. J. Leys, G. F. Crouse, A. G. Hook, and R. E. Kellems, Transcription of the mouse dihydrofolate reductase gene proceeds unabated through seven polyadenylation sites and terminates near a region of repeated DNA, Mol. Cell. Biol. 4:2921 (1984).

17. O. Hagenbüchle, P. K. Wellauer, D. L. Cribbs, and U. Schibler, Termina-tion of transcription in the mouse α-amylase gene Amy-2^a occurs at multiple sites downstream of the polyadenylation site, Cell 38:737 (1984).

18. E. Hofer and J. E. Darnell, The primary transcription unit of the mouse β-major globin gene, Cell 23:585 (1981).

19. E. Hofer, R. Hofer-Warbinek, and J. E. Darnell, Globin RNA transcrip-tion: a possible termination site and demonstration of transcrip-tional control correlated with altered chromatin structure, Cell 29:887 (1982).

20. W. M. Holmes, T. Platt, and M. Rosenberg, Termination of transcription in E. coli, Cell 32:1029 (1983).

21. D. J. Kemp, G. Morahan, A. E. Cowman, and A. W. Harris, Production of RNA for secreted immunoglobulin μ chains does not require transcrip-tional termination 5' to the $μ_m$ exons, Nature 301:84 (1983).

22. M. R. Knapp, C.-P. Liu, N. Newell, R. B. Ward, P. W. Tucker, S. Strober, and F. R. Blattner, Simultaneous expression of immunoglobulin μ + δ heavy chains by a cloned B cell lymphoma: a single copy of the V_H gene is shared by two adjacent C_H genes, Proc. Natl. Acad. Sci. U.S.A. 79:2996 (1982).

23. B. Korbin, C. Milcarek, and S. Morrison, Sequences near the 3' secre-tion-specific polyadenylation site influence levels of secretion-specific and membrane-specific IgG2b mRNA in myeloma cells, Mol. Cell. Biol. 6(5):1687 (1986).

24. M. E. Koshland, Molecular aspects of B cell differentiation, J. Immunol. 1:131 (1983).

25. G. Lamson and M. E. Koshland, Changes in J chain and μ chain RNA expression as a function of B cell differentiation, J. Exp. Med. 160:877 (1984).

26. M. A. LeMeur, B. Galliot, and P. Gerlinge, Termination of the ovalbumin gene transcription, EMBO J. 3:2779 (1984).

27. C.-P. Liu, P. W. Tucker, J. F. Mushinski, and F. R. Blattner, Mapping of heavy chain genes for mouse immunoglobulin M and D, Science 209:1348 (1980).

28. R. Maki, W. Roeder, A. Traunecker, C. Sidman, M. Wabl, W. Raschke, and S. Tonegawa, The role of DNA rearrangement and alternative RNA processing in the expression of immunoglobulin delta genes, Cell 24:353 (1981).

29. J. L. Manley, P. A. Sharp, and M. L. Gefter, RNA synthase in isolated nuclei: identification and comparison of adenovirus 2 encoded transcripts synthesized in vitro and in vivo, J. Mol. Biol. 135:171 (1979).

30. E. L. Mather, K. J. Nelson, J. Maimovitch, and R. P. Perry, Mode of regulation of immunoglobulin μ- and δ-chain expression varies during B-lymphocyte maturation, Cell 36:329 (1984).

31. M. A. McDevitt, M. J. Imperiale, H. Ali, and J. R. Nevins, Requirement of a downstream sequence for generation of a Poly(A) addition site, Cell. 37:993 (1984).

32. C. P. Milstein, E. V. Deverson, and R. H. Rabbitts, The sequence of the human immunoglobulin μ-δ intron reveals possible vestigal switch segments, Nuc. Acids Res. 12:6523 (1984).

33. C. Montell, E. F. Fisher, M. H. Caruthers, and A. Berk, Inhibition of RNA cleavage but not polyadenylation by a point mutation in mRNA 3'-consensus sequence AAUAAA, Nature 305:600 (1983).

34. K. W. Moore, J. Rogers, T. Hunkapiller, P. Early, C. Nottenburg, I. Weissman, H. Bazin, R. Wall, and L. E. Hood, Expression of IgD may use both DNA rearrangement and RNA splicing mechanisms, Proc. Natl. Acad. Sci. U.S.A. 78:1800 (1981).

35. K. Nelson, J. Maimovich, and R. P. Perry, Characterization of productive and sterile transcripts from the immunoglobulin heavy chain locus: processing of μ_m and μ_s mRNA, Mol. Cell. Biol. 3:1317 (1983).

36. W. C. Raschke, Expression of murine IgM, IgD and Ia molecules on hybrids of murine LPS blasts with a Syrian hamster B lymphoma, Curr. Top. Microbiol. Immunol. 81:70 (1978).

37. J. E. Richards, A. C. Gilliam, A. Shen, P. W. Tucker, and F. R. Blattner, Unusual sequences in the murine immunoglobulin μ-δ heavy chain region, Nature 306: 483 (1983).

38. J. Rogers, P. Early, C. Carter, K. Calame, M. Bond, L. Hood, and R. Wall, Two mRNAs with different 3'-ends encode membrane and secreted forms of immunoglobulin μ chain, Cell 20:303 (1980).

39. J. Rogers and R. Wall, Immunoglobulin RNA rearrangements in B lymphocyte differentiation, in: " Advances in Immunology," Vol. 35, H. G. Kunkel and F. J. Dixon, eds., Academic Press, New York (1984).

40. P. C. Thomas, Hybridization of denatured RNA, in: "Methods in Enzymology," Vol. 100, K. Moldave and L. Grossman, eds., Academic Press, New York (1983).

41. G. M. Wahl, M. Stern, and G. R. Stark, Efficient transfer of large DNA fragments from agarose gels to diazobenzyloxymethyl-paper and rapid hybridization by using dextran sulfate, Proc. Natl. Acad. Sci. U.S.A. 76:3683 (1979)

42. R. Wall and J. M. Kuehl, Biosynthesis and regulation of immunoglobulins, Ann. Rev. Immunol. 1:393 (1983).

43. B. A. White and F. C. Bancroft, Cytoplasmic dot hybridization, J. Biol. Chem. 257(15):8569 (1982).

44. D. Yuan, A. C. Gilliam, and P. W. Tucker, Regulation of expression of immunoglobulins M and D in murine B cells, Fed. Proc. 44:2652 (1985).

45. D. Yuan and P. W. Tucker, Transcriptional regulation of the μ-δ heavy chain locus in normal murine B lymphocytes, J. Exp. Med. 160:564 (1984).

FUNCTIONAL MATURATION OF B CELL REPERTOIRE EXPRESSION

Barbara G. Froscher and Norman R. Klinman

Department of Immunology
Scripps Clinic and Research Foundation
La Jolla, California

INTRODUCTION

The adult murine primary B cell repertoire is extremely diverse with estimates suggesting that it is comprised of more than 10^7 distinct specificities (4,19,27,30,39). The recognition and specificity of any B cell and its antibody product is determined by the different heavy and light chain gene segments that are selected for rearrangement and expression in that cell. The final mature B cell repertoire of an animal, therefore, is a result of the genetic V region potential of that animal, processes which select from within that genetic potential and environmental influences on the B cells expressing the genetic potential. The extent to which each of these factors functions during the maturation of the B cell repertoire must be evaluated to understand how the immune system of an animal expresses an effective and non-self-detrimental repertoire of B cell recognition specificities.

UTILIZATION OF THE GENETIC POTENTIAL

Since the specificities of mature B cells in the spleen or other tissues reflect the consequences of environmental selection on the potential repertoire as well as the subcellular molecular events responsible for generating variable regions, we have analyzed the pool of possible B cell specificities by studying the immature surface immunoglobulin negative (sIg⁻) generative B cell pool of the bone marrow (21,24,25,43,44). This population should most closely reflect the genetic information available for encoding immunoglobulin molecules and the processes of subcellular selection amongst this genetic material prior to environmental effects.

The Source of B Cell Repertoire Diversity

Numerous strategies for enhancing the diversity in the structure of the variable (V) region of immunoglobulins of primary B cells have been identified including: 1) multiple V gene segments encoded in the germline; 2) association of different combinations of segments during V gene formation (combinatorial diversity); 3) variation in the joining sites of gene segments (junctional diversity); and 4) association of different VH and VL polypeptides during immunoglobulin assembly (2,6,7,9,47). Somatic mutation of rearranged V region genes may also contribute; however, this process may be more relevant after antigenic stimulation and in the generation of secondary B cells (14,16,31). A more extensive discussion of these topics is given elsewhere in this volume. These strategies taken together could easily account for the observed diversity in the B cell repertoire but it is not as yet clear how much of the potential for diversity is actually expressed during the maturation of the B cell repertoire. Are all available sources of diversity utilized randomly in the mouse to generate its B cell repertoire or is there some non-randomness in repertoire generation [reviewed in (22,23,35)]? Numerous lines of evidence suggest that there is in fact marked non-randomness in repertoire generation.

Examples of Non-Random Utilization of V Region Segments

Temporal Acquisition of B Cell Specificities in the Fetal and Neonatal Mouse. The murine antibody repertoire at birth is limited to 10^4-10^5 different specificities and during the first weeks after birth this repertoire undergoes a reproducible and patterned expansion (5,8,20,49,51). The appearance of responses to a given antigen may reflect the acquisition of the ability to process and present that antigen (48,50); however, this does not appear to be the limiting factor in all cases. It has been shown, for example, that although neonatal cells can respond to the hemagglutinin of the influenza virus, trinitrophenyl (TNP) and dinitrophenyl (DNP), the response to these antigens early in neonatal life is reproducibly dominated by a few identifiable clonotypes and there is a notable absence of the vast majority of clonotypes characteristic of the adult response to these antigens (5,8,20,49). For example, while the adult BALB/c mouse expresses between 10^3 and 10^4 distinct DNP responsive clonotypes (19), the early neonatal response to DNA is dominated by very few clonotypes (8,20). A molecular mechanism that contributes to this temporal appearance of clonotypes appears to be the preferential non-random rearrangement of certain VH gene segments as suggested by the finding of a disproportionately high utilization of V gene segments from the VH 7183 and VH 36-60 gene families in fetal and early neonatal B cells (41,45,54,55).

Dominant Clonotype Expression in Adult Animals. Non-randomness in repertoire generation is also a feature in the primary B cells of the adult mouse as demonstrated by the expression of a high frequency of certain clonotypes that are characteristic of all mice of a given genetic background. A good example of this phenomena is the predominant TEPC-15 clonotype in the anti-phosphorylcholine (PC) response of BALB/c mice. TEPC-15 expression requires the use of only a single VH, D, JH, VL and JL combination (40) and it has been shown that the high frequency of TEPC-15 expression is due to a high frequency of occurrence of this clonotype within newly generated precursor cells of the bone marrow pool (21). Therefore, it appears that there is more frequent usage of this combination of gene segments than would be anticipated stochastically. The mechanism of this selective, non-random utilization of V region genes is not known but it obviously plays an important role in the expression of the potential cell repertoire.

Unique V Gene Utilization in Aged Mice. Recently, findings from studies of aged mice have added to our examples of non-randomness in repertoire generation. The frequency of responsive splenic B cells to most antigens is reduced in aged mice (56,58). In contrast to this, the frequency of cells responsive to PC is increased in aged mice. This increased frequency of PC responsive cells is particularly marked in the newly generated sIg⁻ bone marrow precursor cells of aged mice (57). By analyzing the VH genes utilized in hybridomas constructed from bone marrow cells of aged BALB/c mice it was shown that the majority of the hybridomas tested used VH gene segments which hybridize to VH gene family probes other than probes that detect the VH S107 gene family (12). This is in marked contrast to previous findings which consistently demonstrated that essentially all PC-specific hybridomas and myelomas from young adult BALB/c mice use the S107 VH gene segment (40).

Of the ten aged BALB/c hybridomas examined in this study, three contained RNAs which hybridized to the S107 probe (VH S107 family), three contained RNAs which hybridized to the 76 VH gene probe (VH 7183 family), two contained RNAs which hybridized to the J558 probe (VH J558 family) and one contained RNAs which hybridized to the X24 probe (VH X24 family) (12). The RNAs from one of the hybridomas while binding well to the μ probe did not bind any of the VH family probes used (S107,J558, 76, Q52, X24, 36-60, 3609 and J606) and therefore may be using a VH segment from an as yet unidentified family. Not only does this pattern of utilization of VH gene segments in PC-specific immunoglobulin molecules represent unique expression of these gene segments in aged mice as compared with young adult mice, but it should also be noted that it represents a selected rather than a random usage of the various VH gene segment families in that only two are from the much larger VH J558 family. Interestingly, members of the VH 7183 family appear to be most JH proximal and, as mentioned earlier, are frequently utilized in fetal and early neonatal antibodies (18,36) and "autoimmune" antibodies (38).

There are a number of possibilities as to the molecular mechanism underlying the utilization of novel VH gene segments in antibodies specific for PC in the aged mouse. These include: 1) rearrangement and transcription of VH gene segments which are either never or rarely used for encoding any specificity in young mice; 2) recruitment to PC responses of VH gene segments normally used for non-PC specific antibodies in younger mice possibly, for example, by the expression of new light chain variable region genes in aged mice; 3) alteration of some constraints on the functional association of light chain and heavy chain molecules in B cells of aged mice to allow for the atypical association of light and heavy chain molecules to form antibody molecules of new specificities; or 4) accumulation of somatic mutations in V region genes within stem cells of aged mice. Regardless of the underlying mechanism the process is highly reproducible in BALB/c mice over two years of age and clearly represents disparities in V gene utilization in young as opposed to old mice.

Therefore, there are already numerous examples of non-randomness in processes of selection and utilization of the V gene segments which lead to B cell repertoire generation throughout the life span of the mouse. The mechanisms involved and the extent to which patterned V gene segment utilization occurs is as yet unknown; however, it is this very non-randomness which must now be investigated to more completely understand the generation of B cell repertoire diversity.

ENVIRONMENTAL EFFECTS ON B CELL REPERTOIRE EXPRESSION

Numerous studies have shown that many of the characteristics of the mature B cell repertoire, including diversity and the presence of predominant clonotypes, are also present in the sIg⁻ precursor B cell pool (11,18,21,36,-43,44). Thus, these hallmarks of the repertoire exist prior to environmental influences and must be a result of subcellular molecular processes. However, once the animal has generated this potential B cell repertoire, there does appear to be environmentally selective mechanisms which proceed to further refine the repertoire resulting in a lack of fidelity in what is expressed as mature B cells when compared with the potential repertoire. By studying responses of immature B cells in environments which circumvent these environmental selective pressures (i.e., tolerance, idiotypic suppression, etc.) and comparing these responses to those obtained from the mature expressed B cell population of the same animal, it has been possible to delineate numerous examples of environmental modulation of the potential B cell repertoire (11,21,43). In all cases identified to date this modulation takes the form of down regulation but apparently numerous different underlying mechanisms are possible. Three examples demonstrating different phenotypes of down-regulation will be discussed.

Down-Regulation of Specificities Apparently Due to Tolerance

While the abortion of self-reactive clones has long been considered the most likely explanation for self non-discrimination in the immune system, the existence of environmental mechanisms that can suppress mature antigen responsive cells (15) and the demonstration of potentially self-reactive mature B cells (17) have put into question both the necessity and validity of a physiologically relevant clonal abortion mechanism. However, it is clear that one can markedly affect the primary B cell repertoire by experimentally induced tolerance. Furthermore, over the past decade a wealth of studies have demonstrated that maturing neonatal and bone marrow B cells pass through a highly tolerance-susceptible phase (32,33,37) and have defined many of the parameters of the tolerance trigger (52,53). Although the shaping of the mature B cell repertoire by tolerance to environmental and self-antigens has yet to be demonstrated directly, the footprints of such a process are becoming more and more apparent as disparities in the repertoire of sIg^- and mature precursor cells are studied as exemplified in the following two examples.

The mature B cell repertoire of Xid defective (CBA/N X BALB/c)F1 male mice is deficient in responsive mature B cells to PC and a variety of other environmental antigens (52). However, it has been shown that within the sIg^- bone marrow cell pool of Xid defective males there are as many PC specific immune B cells capable of responding to antigenic stimulation in carrier primed BALB/c recipients as there are in the same cell population from BCA/N X BALB/c)F1 non-deficient female mice (21). Thus, it appears that mice bearing the CBA/N immunologic deficit have a normal capacity to generate cells potentially responsive to PC and that the environment present in splenic fragment cultures derived from carrier primed "responder" BALB/c mice permits the maturation and stimulation of these cells. It is apparent that, in situ, these cells would have been eliminated late in their maturation, presumably upon acquisition of their sIg receptors. Since PC is an abundant environmental antigen and B cells of Xid defective mice are unusually tolerance-susceptible (34) of this aspect of the immunologic defect of these mice is likely the result of tolerance to an environmentally abundant antigen.

The response to NP in Igh^b (C.B20) mice is notable because of the paucity of NP responsive mature splenic B cells which produce antibodies homoclitic for NP and bearing the κ light chain. Thus, whereas characteristically a murine response to antigens is dominated by κ homoclitic antibodies the response to NP in IgH^b mice is dominated by λ heteroclitic antibodies (29). Interestingly, however, it was shown that sIg^- bone marrow precursor cells from C.B20 mice contain a predominance of cells whose progeny produce κ light chain-bearing antibodies that are homoclitic for NP and that these cells responded well to stimulation in a carrier primed splenic fragment environment regardless of the Igh haplotype of the recipient mouse (43). Furthermore, it was demonstrated that these κ homoclitic antibody-bearing B cells, which are apparently environmentally eliminated during maturation, produce antibody of higher affinity for NP than do the B cells that are allowed to mature and be expressed in the mature B cell compartment. This finding, and the finding that this environmental down-regulation was not Igh-linked but could be circumvented by carrier primed help in the stimulating environment suggests that tolerance may be the underlying mechanism of this example of down-regulation.

Down-Regulation of Clonotypes Due to Idiotypic Network Effects

A second mechanism that has been demonstrated to markedly affect primary B cell repertoire expression, if experimentally induced, is anti-idiotypic regulation (1,10,26,46). To date, however, most assessments of the relative representation of predominant clonotypes in mature vs immature B cell pools reveal little evidence of an effect on repertoire expression of anti-idiotypic selection (18,21,36,43). However, recent experiments from this laboratory have shown that the response to α(1-3)Dextran (DEX) in the Igh^b C.B20 mouse is subject to an environmental down-regulatory effect which is Igh-linked and therefore potentially a consequence of spontaneously arising anti-idiotypic regulation (11).

The Igh^b mouse has long been considered to be genetically deficient of a V region gene necessary for producing λ bearing α(1-3)DEX specific antibodies which predominate the response to this antigen in mice of the Igh^a haplotype (42). Our recent findings indicate that there are an equal number of λ bearing α(1-3)DEX specific sIg$^-$ bone marrow cells in the C.B20 mouse as in the BALB/c mouse; however, for these cells to functionally respond to DEX they must be stimulated in a carrier-primed non-Igh^b environment (i.e., in a carrier-primed BALB/c mouse) (11). Interestingly the antibodies that are produced by these B cells bear the idiotypic determinants (IdX) which are characteristic of the BALB/c λ bearing α(1-3)DEX specific predominant clonotypes (42). These findings suggest that in this instance the environmental down-regulation of the potential λ DEX specificities in C.B20 mice is by an idiotypic suppressive network which is specific for Igh^b λ bearing α(1-3)DEX-specific antibodies and is present in Igh^b but absent in Igh^a mice.

Other Environmental Effects

Examples of environmental down-regulation apparently linked to non-Igh gene loci have been identified in a few instances. For example, in recombinant inbred murine strains constructed from the progeny of BALB/c X C57BL/6 mice the level of the serum response of TEPC-15 bearing antibodies links to the Igh^a locus (3). However, the overall frequency of PC-specific primary precursor cells appears linked to the MHC locus and the frequency of TEPC-15 bearing precursor cells responsive to PC links to neither Igh nor MHC (3). Another example on non-Igh linked effects is the down-regulation of the κ bearing α(1-3)DEX-specific B cells in the BALB/c mouse (13). Responsive cells of this clonotype are very rare in populations of mature BALB/c spleen cells and immature BALB/c sIg$^-$ bone marrow cells stimulated in the carrier primed syngeneic recipient (H-2^d, Igh^a). The same cell populations stimulated in carrier primed C.B20 mice (H-2^d, Igh^b) also yield very few responsive cells of this clonotype. However, when these cell populations are stimulated in B10.D2 mice (H-2^d, Igh^b) many more cells bearing the κ light chain and specific for α(1-3)DEX linkages respond. This increase in κ DEX responsive cells is most marked in the sIg$^-$ bone marrow cell population and it is clear, therefore, that many of the cells of this specificity are irreversibly silenced when allowed to mature in their native environment. However, some cells of this specificity are present in the mature BALB/c spleen and are potentially stimulatable in the permissive B10.D2 environment. This down-regulatory effect is, apparently, linked to gene loci other than H-2 or Igh as it is present in the C.B20 (H-2^d, Igh^b mouse but absent in the B10.D2 (also H-2^d, Igh^b) mouse which differ only in non-H-2, non-Igh "background" genes.

CONCLUSION

The composition of the mature B cell repertoire of a given murine strain is a consequence of both genetic events leading to the expression of a particular array of VH-VL combinations and clonotype-specific regulatory processes within the environment. It has been demonstrated that even within the sIg⁻ bone marrow precursor cell pool both repertoire diversity and the expression of predominant clonotypes are present, suggesting that these are probably attributable to variable region gene expression. Whereas the extensive diversity at this stage suggests the random usage and association of the large number of variable gene segments, the well-demonstrated patterned acquisition of diversity in neonates, the persistence of dominant clonotypes in adult mice and the appearance of new specificities in aged mice point to marked non-randomness in the selection and expression of V region gene segments. Once the potential repertoire has been selected by random and/or non-random means environmental interactions clearly influence the expression of the B cell repertoire as witnessed by examples of a lack of fidelity in the repertoire as expressed in mature B cell populations when compared to the potential repertoire as expressed in immature sIg⁻ bone marrow precursors. Some of these observed differences appear attributable to tolerance and anti-idiotypic regulation whereas there are now examples of environmental effects on the maturation of the B cell repertoire which may result from as yet undefined mechanisms.

ACKNOWLEDGMENTS

This work has supported by USPHS grants AI 15797 and AG 00080 from the National Institutes of Health.

REFERENCES

1. R. S. Accolla, P. J. Gearhart, N. H. Sigal, M. P. Cancro, and N. R. Klinman, Idiotype-specific neonatal suppression of phosphoryl-choline-responsive B cells, Eur J. Immunol. 7:876 (1977).
2. C. Brack, M. Hirama, R. Lenhard-Schuller, and S. Tonegawa, A complete immunoglobulin gene is created by somatic recombination, Cell 15:1 (1978).
3. M. P. Cancro, N. H. Sigal, and N. R. Klinman, Differential expression of an equivalent clonotype among BALB/c and C57BL/6 mice, J. Exp. Med. 147:1 (1978).
4. M. P. Cancro, W. Gerhard, and N. R. Klinman, The diversity of the influenza specific primary B cell repertoire in BALB/c mice, J. Exp. Med. 147:776 (1978).
5. M. P. Cancro, D. E. Wylie, W. Gerhard, and N. R. Klinman, Patterned acquisition of the antibody repertoire, Proc. Natl. Acad. Sci. U.S.A. 76:6577 (1979).
6. C. Coleclough, D. Cooper, and R. P. Perry, Rearrangement of immuno-globulin heavy chain genes during B lymphocyte development as revealed by studies of mouse plasmacytoma cells, Proc. Natl. Acad. Sci. U.S.A. 77:1422 (1980).
7. S. Cory and J. M. Adams, Delections are associated with somatic rearrangement of immunoglobulin heavy chain genes, Cell 19:37 (1980).
8. K. A. Denis and N. R. Klinman, The genetic and temporal control of neonatal antibody expression, J. Exp. Med. 157:1170 (1983).
9. P. Early, H. Huang, M. David, K. Calame, and L. Hood, An immunoglobulin heavy chain variable region gene is generated from three segments of DNA: V, D, and J, Cell. 19:981 (1980).
10. K. Eichmann, Expression and function of idiotypes on lymphocytes, Adv. Immunol. 26:195 (1978).
11. B. G. Groscher and N. R. Klinman, Strain-specific silencing of a predominant anti-dextran clonotype family, J. Exp. Med. 162:1620 (1985).

12. B. G. Froscher, S. C. Riley, K. B. Marcu, D. Zharhary, and N. R. Klinman, Unique V region gene expression in aged mice, Proc. Natl. Acad. Sci. U.S.A., in press (1986).

13. B. G. Froscher and N. R. Klinman, Non-Igh-linked regulation of a bearing α(1-3)Dextran responsive B cell, in preparation (1986).

14. P. J. Gearhart and D. F. Bogenhagen, Clusters of point mutations are found exclusively around rearranged antibody variable genes, Proc. Natl. Acad. Sci. U.S.A. 80:3439 (1983).

15. R. K. Gershon and K. Kondo, Infectious immunological tolerance, Immunology 21:903 (1971).

16. G. M. Griffiths, C. Berek, M. Kaartinen, and C. Milstein, Somatic mutation and the maturation of immune response to 2-phenyl oxazo-lone, Nature 312:271 (1984).

17. D. E. Harris, L. Cairns, F. S. Rosen, and Y. Borel, A matural model of immunologic tolerance, J. Exp. Med. 156:567 (1982).

18. D. Juy, D. Primi, P. Sanchez, and P.-A. Cazenave, The selection and maintenance of the V region determinant repertoire is germ-line encoded and T cell independent, Eur. J. Immunol. 13:326 (1983).

19. N. R. Klinman and J. L. Press, The B cell specificity repertoires: its relationship to definable subpopulations, Tranplant. Rev. 24:41 (1975).

20. N. R. Klinman and J. L. Press, The characterization of the B cell repertoire specific for the DNP and TNP determinants in neonatal BALB/c mice, J. Exp. Med. 141:1133 (1975).

21. N. R. Klinman and M. R. Stone, The role of variable region gene expres-sion and environmental selection in determining the antiphosphoryl-choline B cell repertoire, J. Exp. Med. 158:1948 (1983).

22. N. R. Klinman, J. L. Press, N. H. Sigal, and P. J. Gearhart, The acquisition of the B cell specificity repertoire. The germ line theory of predetermined permutation of genetic information, in: "The Generation of Diversity: A New Look," A. J. Cunningham, ed., Academic Press, London (1976).

23. N. R. Klinman, N. H. Sigal, E. S. Metcalf, S. K. Pierce, and P. J. Gearhart, The interplay of evolution and environment in B cell diversification, Cold Spring Harbor Symposium on Quant. Biol. 41:165 (1977).

24. N. R. Klinman, D. E. Wylie, and M. P. Cancro, Mechanisms that govern repertoire expression, in: "Immunology 80 - Progress in Immunology. IV." M. Fougereau and J. Dausset, eds., Academic Press, London, (1980).

25. N. R. Klinman, A. F. Schrater, and D. H. Katz, Immature B cells as the target for in vitro tolerance induction, J. Immunol. 126:1970 (1981).

26. H. Kohler, The response to phosphorylcholine: dissecting an immune response, Transplant. Rev. 27:24 (1975).

27. H. W. Kreth and A. R. Williamson, The extent of diversity of antihapten antibodies in inbred mice: anti-NIP (4-hydroxy-5-iodo-3-nitro-phenacetyl) antibodies in CBA/H mice, Eur. J. Immunol. 3:141 (1973).

28. J. T. Kung and W. E. Paul, B lymphocyte subpopulations, Immunol. Today 4:37 (1983).

29. O. Makela and K. Karajalainen, Inherited immunoglobulin idiotypes of the mouse, Immunol. Rev. 34:119 (1977).

30. T. Manser, S. Y. Huang, and M. L. Gefter, Influence of clonal selection on the expression of immunoglobulin variable region genes, Science 226:1283 (1984).

31. D. McKean, K. Huppi, M. Bell, L. Staudt, W. Gerhard, and M. Weigert, Generation of antibody diversity in the immune response of BALB/c mice to influenza virus hemagglutinin, Proc. Natl. Acad. Sci. U.S.A. 81:3180 (1984).

32. E. S. Metcalf and N. R. Klinman, In vitro tolerance induction of neonatal B cells, J. Exp. Med. 143:1327 (1976).

33. E. S. Metcalf and N. R. Klinman, In vitro tolerance induction of neo-
    natal and adult bone marrow cells: a functional marker for B cell
    maturation, J. Immunol. 118:2111 (1977).

34. E. S. Metcalf, I. Scher, and N. R. Klinman, Susceptibility to in vitro
    tolerance induction of adult B cells from mice with an X-linked B
    cell defect, J. Exp. Med. 151:486 (1980).

35. R. I. Near, T. Manser, and M. L. Gefter, The generation of major and
    minor idiotype-bearing families of anti-azophenylarsonate anti-
    bodies: the stochastic utilization of VH gene segments, J. Immunol.
    134:2004 (1985).

36. S. Nishikawa, T. Toshitada, and K. Rajewsky, The expression of a set of
    antibody variable regions in lipopolysaccharide-reactive B cells at
    various states of ontogeny and its control by anti-idiotypic anti-
    body, Eur. J. Immunol. 13:318 (1983).

37. G.J.V. Nossal and B. L. Pike, Ontogeny of B cell precursors responding
    to α(1-3)Dextran in BALB/c mice, J. Exp. Med. 141:904 (1975).

38. M. Onestier, C. Painter, A. Maneheiner-Lory and C. Bona, Restricted set
    of the V genes. An extentive idiotype cross-reactions of auto-
    antibodies, in: "Molecular Basis of B Cell Differentiation and
    Function," M. Ferrarini and B. Pernis, eds., Plenum Publishing
    Corporation, New York, in press (1986).

39. J. A. Owen, N. H. Sigal, and N. R. Klinman, Heterogeneity of the BALB/c
    IgM anti-phosphorylcholine antibody response, Nature 295:347 (1982).

40. R. M. Perlmutter, S. T. Crews, R. Douglas, G. Sorenson, N. Nivera, P.
    J. Gearhart, and L. Hood, The generation of diversity in phosphoryl-
    choline-binding antibodies, Adv. Immunol. 35:1 (1984).

41. R. M. Perlmutter, J. F. Kearney, S. P. Chang, and S. P. Hood,
    Developmentally controlled expression of immunoglobulin VH genes,
    Science 227:1597 (1985).

42. R. Riblet, B. Bloomberg, M. Weigert, R. Lieberman, B. A. Taylor, and M.
    Potter, Genetics of mouse antibodies. I. Linkage of the dextran
    response locus VH-DEX to allotype, Eur. J. Immunol. 5:775 (1975).

43. R. L. Riley and N. R. Klinman, Differences in antibody repertoire for
    (4-hydroxy-3-nitrophenyl)acetyl (NP) in splenic vs immature bone
    marrow precursor cells, J. Immunol. 135:3050 (1985).

44. R. L. Riley, D. E. Wylie, and N. R. Klinman, B cell repertoire diver-
    sification precedes immunoglobulin receptor expression, J. Exp. Med.
    158:1733 (1983).

45. S. R. Riley, S. J. Connors, N. R. Klinman, and R. T. Ogata, Preferential
    expression of VH gene segments by predominant DNP specific BALB/c
    neonatal antibody clonotypes, Proc. Natl. Acad. Sci. U.S.A., in
    press (1986).

46. L. J. Rubenstein, M. Yeh, and C. Bona, Idiotype-anti-idiotype network.
    II. Activation of silent clones by treatment at birth with idiotypes
    is associated with the expansion of idiotype-specific helper T
    cells, J. Exp. Med. 156:506 (1982).

47. J. G. Seidman, A. Leder, M. Nau, B. Norman, and P. Leder, Antibody
    diversity, Science 202:11 (1978).

48. W. K. Sherwin and D. T. Rowlands, Jr., Development of humoral immunity
    in lethally irradiated mice reconstituted with fetal liver, J.
    Immunol. 113:1353 (1974).

49. N. H. Sigal, P. J. Gearhart, J. L. Press, and N. R. Klinman, The late
    acquisition of a "germ line" antibody specificity, Nature 251:51
    (1976).

50. A. Silverstein, J. W. Uhr, K. L. Kraner, and R. J. Lukes, Fetal
    response to antigen stimulus. II. Antibody production by the fetal
    lamb, J. Exp. Med. 117:799 (1963).

51. R. Stohrer and J. F. Kearney, Ontogeny of B cell precursors responding
    to α(1-3)Dextran in BALB/c mice, J. Immunol. 133:2323 (1984).

52. J. M. Teale and N. R. Klinman, Tolerance as an active process, Nature
    288:385 (1980).

53. J. M. Teale and N. R. Klinman, Membrane and metabolic requirements for tolerance of neonatal B cells, J. Immunol. 133:1811 (1984).

54. J. M. Teale and J. F. Kearney, Clonotypic analysis of the expressed fetal B cell repertoire: evidence for the early expression of the 460 idiotype , J. Mol. Cell. Immunol., in press (1986).

55. G. D. Yancopoulos, S. V. Desiderio, M. Paskind, J. F. Kearney, D. Baltimore, and F. W. Alt, Preferential utilization of the most JH-proximal VH gene segments in pre-B cell lines, Nature 311:727 (1984).

56. D. Zharhary and N. R. Klinman, Antigen responsiveness of the mature and generative B cell populations of aged mice, J. Exp. Med. 157:1300 (1983).

57. D. Zharhary and N. R. Klinman, A selective increase in the generation of phosphorylcholine specific B cells associated with aging, J. Immunol. 136:368 (1986).

58. D. Zharhary and N. R. Klinman, The effects of aging on murine B cell responsiveness, in: "Aging and the Immune Response," E. Goidl, ed., Marcel Dekker, New York, in press (1986).

RECEPTOR CROSS-LINKAGE STIMULATES B CELL ACTIVATION

Junichiro Mizuguchi, Michael Beaven, Peter Hornbeck,
Wayne Tsang, and William E. Paul

Laboratory of Immunology, National Institute of Allergy
and Infectious Diseases, and Laboratory of Chemical
Pharmacology, National Heart, Lung, and Blood Institute,
National Institutes of Health, Bethesda, Maryland

INTRODUCTION

The clonal selection theory of the immune response elegantly solves the problem of how it is possible for an individual to make antibodies to virtually any foreign antigen. It does this by postulating that each lymphocyte can only produce antibodies of a single specificity and that a very large number of distinct lymphocytes exist. That may be restated to say that the universe of foreign antigens is matched by an internal universe of lymphocytes. The penalty exacted by this strategy for achieving antibody diversity is that lymphocytes specific for any particular antigenic determinant exist at very low frequency in an unimmunized animal. Since immune responses must be both prompt and of considerable magnitude if they are to protect against pathogenic microorganisms or against newly emerging tumor cells, it is clear that the rare cells specific for any particular antigen must expand in number rapidly. Thus, growth regulation of lymphocytes is a matter of central importance in the physiology of the immune system.

It has been recognized that membrane immunoglobulin (Ig) is the receptor of the B cell (26,35,40); the molecular genetics (4) and chemistry (9) of the T cell receptor are rapidly being elucidated. However, we are only now beginning to understand the mechanisms through which antigen binding to lymphocyte receptors leads to cellular activation. In this communication, we will direct our attention to the mechanisms through which membrane receptors of B cells transmit activation signals.

Membrane Immunoglobulin and Inositol Phospholipid Metabolism

For purposes of simplicity, most work on receptor-mediated B cell activation has relied on the use of anti-Ig antibodies since this ligand binds to the receptors of all B cells. Anti-IgM antibodies activate B cells and cause them to progress through the G1 phase of the cell cycle (5). The first documented step in the process through which receptor cross-linkage by anti-IgM stimulates B cell responses is an increase in the hydrolysis of phosphatidyl inositol bisphosphate (PIP2). We (20,23) and others (3,30), have demonstrated this by labelling the cellular phosphatidyl inositol pool with ^{3}H-myoinositol. Addition of anti-IgM antibodies causes a rapid increase in radioactivity in inositol triphosphate (IP3). Within 30 seconds, striking increases are observed in the 1,4,5 isomer of IP3. This isomer of IP3 is regarded as biologically important since it has been shown to mobilize calcium from intracellular stores in several cell types (12,15,28,36). Levels of the 1,4,5 isomer of IP3 peak at one minute and have returned to basal levels by five minutes after the addition of anti-IgM. The hydrolysis of phosphatidyl inositol bisphosphate is catalyzed by the action of phospholipase C (PLC) (19,34). This strongly suggests that receptor cross-linkage results in activation of PLC, possibly by changing the $[Ca^{++}]$ at which PLC acts to efficiently cleave phosphatidyl inositols. The cleavage of PIP2 by PLC results in a second product, diacylglycerol which, as we discuss below, activates protein kinase C (PKC) (2,37). The rapid appearance of diacylglycerol after addition of anti-IgM antibodies to B cells has been recently demonstrated (3).

A major unsolved question is the nature of the molecules which act as intermediates between membrane Ig and PLC in this signalling pathway. In other systems, receptors transmit signals through the agency of GTP-binding proteins (G proteins) (6,7,25). No evidence for involvement of G proteins in B cell activation through membrane Ig has yet been obtained and, in tumor systems, pertussis toxin, an inhibitor of one type of G protein (the G_i protein), does not appear to influence the signalling which occurs in response to receptor cross-linkage. Jakway and DeFranco (14) have recently shown that pertussis toxin does inhibit responses of macrophage and B cell tumor lines to lipopolysaccharide (LPS), implicating the participation of G_i proteins in this activation pathway; however, LPS appears to stimulate B cell activation by a different mechanism than that used by anti-IgM. Treatment of resting B cells with LPS causes no accumulation of inositol phosphates nor does it lead to an increase in intracellular free calcium concentration $[Ca^{++}]_i$ (21).

The structural elements of immunoglobulins which are critical to signal transmission have not yet been identified, although it appears certain that such signalling depends upon the aggregation of membrane Ig molecules. Monovalent [F(ab)] fragments of anti-Ig do not cause intracellular signalling while divalent [F(ab')$_2$] fragments do. We have demonstrated that anti-IgG2a and anti-IgG2b cause rapid biochemical changes in B lymphocytes bearing IgG2a and IgG2b, respectively (23). This indicates that membrane IgG2a and IgG2b, as well as membrane IgM and IgD, can transmit cellular activation signals when they are cross-linked on B cell membranes. Since the transmembrane domains have the greatest structural homology among different classes of Igs (1,13,31,32), these hydrophobic regions are good candidates to play a major role in the signalling process. The intracytoplasmic portions of membrane Ig are less likely candidates for mediating signal transduction since these regions in IgM and IgD, the two dominant species of membrane Ig, are tripeptides with the sequence lys, val, lys. This seems a rather unlikely signaling entity, although it will require direct tests to rule out its involvement. Indeed, since membrane Ig's of other classes have considerably longer cytoplasmic tails, these regions may prove to have important effects in signalling, perhaps being responsible for any differences in the relative efficacy of different classes of membrane Ig's as signalling entities. Direct testing of the role of the transmembrane and cytoplasmic portions of the Ig molecules in signalling will depend upon derivation of mutant molecules. Site-directed mutagenesis and DNA-mediated gene transfer of the resulting mutant H chain genes would seem to be a direct approach to examine this issue.

In order to determine the feasibility of this approach, we asked whether expression of "new" membrane Ig molecules could be obtained in B lymphomas by DNA-mediated gene transfer and whether such newly expressed membrane Igs would serve as signalling molecules. We obtained from Dr. Sherie Morrison of Columbia University, a genomic clone for an IgG2b heavy chain gene (17). Using spheroplast fusion, we succeeded in obtaining transformants of the

IgM-bearing cell line 6G8. Some of the transformants expressed considerable amounts of the membrane form of the γ2B H chain mRNA. Among these, we identified and cloned a line (6G8.2E10) which expressed surface IgG2b, as detected by flow cytometry using anti-IgG2b specific antibodies. Cross-linkage of the membrane IgG2b of 6G8.2E10 resulted in an intracellular signal as shown by the rapid increase in intracellular free calcium concentration ($[Ca^{++}]_i$) upon addition of anti-IgG2b antibody (23). Incubation of the parental cell line with anti-IgG2b antibodies caused no change in $[Ca^{++}]_i$ within the cell. Both the transformant and the parental cell line expressed membrane IgM and both showed prompt and striking elevations of $[Ca^{++}]_i$ in response to anti-IgM antibodies.

This experiment demonstrates that DNA-mediated gene transfer into B lymphomas is a potentially valuable approach for the analysis of the structural aspects of membrane Ig which play critical roles in the signalling process. We are currently preparing chimeric genes in which various portions of Ig H chains are exchanged with comparable portions of other membrane glycoprotein genes and will test the signalling capacity of the resulting chimeric protein, if they are expressed on the surface of transformants.

Elevation of $[Ca^{++}]_i$ and Induction of Protein Phosphorylation as a Result of Cross-Linking Membrane Immunoglobulin

As noted above, the cross-linkage of membrane Ig by anti-Ig antibodies leads to the rapid appearance of IP3 and diacylglycerol. In association with these events, there is a rapid rise in $[Ca^{++}]_i$. This has been most clearly documented through the use of fluorescent calcium binding dyes (8,38). Almost immediately upon the addition of anti-IgM antibodies, $[Ca^{++}]_i$ rises from a resting level of ~100 nM, reaching concentrations of 300 to 1000 nM (27,29). The initial increase in $[Ca^{++}]_i$ occurs in calcium-free medium, strongly suggesting that it depends upon calcium derived from cellular stores (23). This is consistent with the known action of IP3 in mobilizing calcium from such stores. The maintenance of elevated $[Ca^{++}]_i$ appears to depend on entry of calcium into the cell since calcium levels rapidly return to resting levels in absence of extracellular calcium and the subsequent addition of calcium to the medium causes a rapid increase in $[Ca^{++}]_i$ in such cells. The mechanism of calcium entry has not been established.

A second event associated with the cleavage of PIP2 and the generation of IP3 and diacylglycerol is phosphorylation of a series of proteins. We have undertaken a detailed examination of the pattern of protein phosphorylation in normal B cells and B lymphoma cells as a result of cross-linkage of membrane Ig. Since it is believed that such phosphorylation is catalyzed by PKC activated by diacylglycerol, we have compared the resultant phosphorylation to that which occurs in the same cell types treated with the PKC-activator phorbol myristate acetate (PMA). Normal B cells in which the ATP pool has been labelled by culture in ^{32}P-orthophosphate display rapid phosphorylation of a series of proteins upon stimulation with anti-IgM antibodies or with PMA (11). Many of these proteins are associated with the plasma membrane and/or the cytoskeleton. Three of the membrane-associated induced phosphoproteins bear particular note. They are pp65-70 (pI 5.4-5.6), pp68 (pI 6.4-6.7) and pp62 (pI 6.3-6.8). The wide pI range for each of these proteins reflects the fact that differentially phosphorylated species of these proteins migrate with different isoelectric points. Each of these proteins displays substantial increases in degree of phosphorylation in response to anti-IgM and to PMA, detectable within twenty minutes of stimulation. Two of these membrane-associated phosphoproteins have isomeric phosphorylated forms which are insoluble in NP-40, strongly suggesting that they are bound to cytoskeleton. Phosphopeptide analysis indicates that the pattern of phosphorylation stimulated by anti-IgM is similar to that stimulated by PMA. Furthermore, phosphoamino acid analysis shows that these proteins are phosphorylated at serine and threonine residues; no tyrosine phosphorylation has yet been observed. Both observations strongly support the conclusion that anti-IgM stimulates protein phosphorylation through the action of PKC. Furthermore, overnight treatment of these cells with PMA, which completely depletes immunoreactive PKC, blocks protein phosphorylation in response to anti-IgM or to PMA. This further supports the involvement of PKC in response of B cells to anti-IgM. As we will show below, cells depleted of PKC display normal early events in signal transduction in response to anti-IgM, such as increased inositol phospholipid metabolism and elevation of $[Ca^{++}]_i$. Nevertheless, these cells fail to enter S phase in response to anti-IgM, indicating that protein phosphorylation mediated by PKC is quite important in the proliferation of normal B cells in response to receptor cross-linkage.

Regulation of Signalling Through Membrane Immunoglobulin

Cross-linkage of B cell receptors for antigen may also initiate a potentially important feedback regulatory mechanism which shuts off further signalling by desensitizing the receptor or by changing the state of activation of intermediate molecules involved in signal production. We initially were drawn to study this by an apparently paradoxical set of findings. The action of anti-IgM on resting B cells is mimicked by treatment with PMA and a calcium ionophore (A23187 or ionomycin). Cells treated with PMA and ionophore (24) enter the G2 phase of the cell cycle and will synthesize DNA in the presence of the soluble T cell-derived product B cell stimulatory factor-1 (BSF-1) (22). On the other hand, adding PMA to anti-IgM inhibits the ability of the membrane cross-linking agent to stimulate incorporation of ^{3}H-thymidine in the presence of BSF-1 (10).

Treatment of B cells with anti-IgM or with PMA and a calcium ionophore cause some common cellular biochemical effects but does so through different mechanisms. Thus, anti-IgM leads to enhanced inositol phospholipid metabolism which, in turn, appears to cause elevation in both $[Ca^{++}]_i$ and in PKC-mediated protein phosphorylation. Calcium ionophore and PMA treatment also cause elevated $[Ca^{++}]_i$ and PKC-mediated protein phosphorylation. However, these are direct effects of the added agents, which do not require receptor cross-linkage, PLC-activity, or enhanced inositol phospholipid metabolism. It seemed reasonable to postulate that PMA might act both as a co-factor in B cell stimulation and as an inhibitor of anti-IgM-mediated B cell activation by interfering with the receptor cross-linkage signal transmission process. This appears to be the correct explanation for the PMA-mediated inhibition of anti-IgM stimulation of B cells. Pretreatment of B cells or of several B lymphomas with PMA for periods as short as four minutes inhibits both the increase in inositol phospholipid metabolism in response to anti-IgM antibody and the concomittant increase in $[Ca^{++}]_i$ (20). The inhibition is both concentration and time dependent; as little as 0.1 ng/ml of PMA has a detectable inhibitory effect, but complete inhibition of signalling requires 10 to 100 ng/ml. Furthermore, inhibition is more complete if the cells are pre-incubated in PMA for 1.5 hours. It should be noted, however, that longer periods of inhibition do not block cellular signalling. Rather, 14 to 24 hour pretreatment of B cells with PMA leads to the depletion of PKC; such cells are not inhibited in their signalling in response to anti-IgM, supporting the idea that the inhibitory effect of PMA is due to its action on PKC. A reasonable postulate is that PKC phosphorylates a protein in the signal transmission pathway and this phosphorylated protein either cannot itself transmit a signal or blocks a transmission by some other molecule. Indeed, there are several instances of PMA-stimulated desensitization of cells (16,33,41). PMA causes the phosphorylation of the $alpha_1$-adrenergic receptor, with a consequent diminution in affinity and a diminished signal transmission capability (39). No mechanism for the B cell desensitization in response to PMA has been established, but the effect appears to be largely limited to receptor cross-linkage mediated B cell activation. The response to LPS, which is not dependent on increased inositol phospholipid metabolism, is not blocked by PMA-treatment, nor are some of the effects of BSF-1 on resting B cells.

The desensitization of B cells to receptor cross-linkage stimulated B cell activation by PMA is not likely to be biologically important, unless natural ligands mimic PMA in directly activating PKC. However, a more critical question is whether the physiologic activation of PKC, presumably through the action of diacylglycerol and of elevated $[Ca^{++}]_i$, resulting from receptor cross-linkage, causes a similar desensitization phenomenon. This has not been directly demonstrated, but some results provide strong suggestive evidence that this may be the case. For example, both normal B cells and B lymphoma cells which have been depleted of cellular PKC by extended incubation with PMA display heightened increases in IP1, IP2, and IP3 in response to anti-IgM. The B lymphoma, BAL-17, displays a much more prolonged elevation of $[Ca^{++}]_i$ in response to anti-IgM if its cellular PKC has been depleted. These results strongly suggest that the activation of PKC in response to anti-IgM may also lead to cellular desensitization and the interruption of further signalling. In contrast to the results with PMA, where the interruption in signalling is profound and prolonged, it might be anticipated that anti-IgM-mediated cellular desensitization will be transient. This is so because the natural PKC-activator, diacylglycerol, has a short biological half-life in contrast to PMA and the desensitization blocks not only B cell activation but should also limit the stimulus that causes desensitization. Such receptor-mediated desensitization could have important implications for the tight regulation of cellular activation. Although this is a very attractive concept, there are other explanations of why depletion of cellular PKC might enhance responsiveness to anti-IgM without anti-IgM stimulated PKC-activation being a normal feedback regulator. One approach to examining this point will be to determine the effect of acute inhibition of PKC-mediated phosphorylation using some of the newly derived inhibitors of PKC.

CONCLUSIONS

It is now clear that cross-linking membrane Ig plays a critical role in the B cell activation process. We have reviewed recent work establishing that the inositol phospholipid signalling pathway is induced by receptor cross-linkage. In addition, we have described the increases in $[Ca^{++}]_i$ and the striking protein phosphorylation which occur in such cells. Since elevating $[Ca^{++}]_i$ with ionophores and inducing protein phosphorylation by the action of PMA on PKC also is associated with B cell activation, there is good reason to assume that these events are important in the process which leads to cellular activation. There is suggestive evidence that the signalling process is regulated by an internal feedback control mechanism, which may serve to tightly control the level of activation in response to receptor-mediated signalling.

This work marks an important initial step in understanding the biochemical basis of B lymphocyte activation and growth regulation. However, much remains to be done. B cell activation through receptor cross-linkage is only one mechanism for the stimulation of B cells. It seems clear that LPS activates B cells through a distinct mechanism and it is likely that B cell activation as a result of cognate T cell-B cell interactions does not depend on receptor cross-linkage and the stimulation of the inositol phospholipid pathway. The mechanisms of these biologically important activation systems need to be understood. Equally important is developing an understanding of the biochemical signals involved in tolerance induction and contrasting them to the mechanisms through which cells are activated.

It seems very likely that a detailed understanding of the cellular biochemical mechanisms that underly these activation and tolerance induction pathways will lead to the development of pharmacologic agents which may be valuable clinical tools in regulating immune responses.

ACKNOWLEDGMENTS

We thank Dr. Thomas Chused, Dr. K. P. Huang, and Dr. Sherie Morrison for their help in several aspects of this work. The editorial assistance of Ms. Shirley Starnes is gratefully acknowledged.

REFERENCES

1. K. E. Bernstein, C. B. Alexander, E. P. Reddy, and R. G. Mage, Complete sequence of a cloned cDNA encoding rabbit secreted μ-chain of V_Ha2 allotype: comparisons with $V_H$al and membrane μ sequences, J. Immunol. 132:490 (1984).

2. M. Berridge, Inositol triphosphate and diacylglycerol as second messengers, Biochem. J. 220:345 (1984).

3. M. K. Bijsterbosch, C. J. Meade, G. A. Turner, and G.G.B. Klaus, B lymphocyte receptors and polyphosphoinositide degradation, Cell 41:999 (1985).

4. M. M. Davis, Molecular genetics of the T cell receptor beta chain, Ann. Rev. Immunol. 3:537 (1985).

5. A. L. DeFranco, E. S. Raveche, R. Asofsky, and W. E. Paul, Frequency of B lymphocytes responsive to anti-immunoglobulin, J. Exp. Med. 155:1523 (1982).

6. A. G. Gilman, G proteins and dual control of adenylate cyclase, Cell 36:577 (1984).

7. D. W. Goldman, F. H. Chang, L. A. Gifford, E. J. Goetzl, and H. R. Bourne, Pertussis toxin inhibition of chemotactic factor-induced calcium mobilization and function in human polymorphonuclear leukocytes, J. Exp. Med. 162:145 (1985).

8. G. Grynkiewicz, M. Poenie, and R. Y. Tsien, A new generation of Ca^{2+} indicators with greatly improved fluorescence properties, J. Biol. Chem. 260:3440 (1985).

9. K. Haskins, J. Kappler, and P. Marrack, The major histocompatibility complex-restricted antigen receptor on T cells, Ann. Rev. Immunol. 2:51 (1984).

10. C. M. Hawrylowicz and G.G.B. Klaus, Effects of tumor promoter phorbol myristate acetate on mouse lymphocytes: selective inhibition of B cell activation by mitogens and antigens, Immunology 51:327 (1984).

11. P. Hornbeck and W. E. Paul, Anti-immunoglobulin and phorbol ester induce phosphorylation of proteins associated with the plasma membrane and cytoskeleton in murine B lymphocytes, J. Biol. Chem. in press (1986).

12. J. B. Imboden and J. D. Stobo, Transmembrane signalling by the T cell antigen receptor. Perturbation of the T3-antigen receptor complex generates inositol phosphates and releases calcium ions from intracellular stores, J. Exp. Med. 161:446 (1985).

13. N. Ishida, S. Ueda, H. Hayashida, T. Miyata, and T. Honjo, The nucleotide sequence of the mouse immunoglobulin epsilon gene: comparison with the human epsilon gene sequence, EMBO J. 9:1117 (1982).

14. J. P. Jakway and A. L. DeFranco, Pertussis toxin inhibits responses of B lymphocytes and macrophage cell lines to bacterial lipopolysaccharide, Science, in press (1986).

15. S. K. Joseph, A. P. Thomas, R. J. Williams, R. F. Irvine, and J. R. Williamson, Myo-Inositol 1,4,5-triphosphate. A second messenger for the hormonal mobilization of intracellular Ca^{+4} in liver, J. Biol. Chem. 259:3077 (1984).

16. A. C. King and P. Cuatrecasas, Resolution of high and low affinity epidermal growth factor receptors: inhibition of high affinity component by low temperature, cycloheximide, and phorbol esters, J. Biol. Chem. 257:3053 (1982).

17. B. J. Kobrin, C. Milcarek, and S. L. Morrison, Sequences near the 3' secretion-specific polyadenylation site influence levels of secre-

tion-specific and membrane-specific IgG2b mRNA in myeloma cells, <u>Mol.</u>
<u>Cell. Biol.</u> 6:in press (1986).

18. L.M.F. Leeb-Lundberg, S. Cotecchia, J. W. Lomasney, J. F. DeBernadis, R. J. Lefkowitz, and M. G. Caron, Phorbol esters promote alpha$_1$-adrenergic receptor phosphorylation and receptor uncoupling from inositol phospholipid metabolism, <u>Proc.</u> <u>Natl.</u> <u>Acad.</u> <u>Sci.</u> <u>U.S.A.</u> 82:5651 (1985).

19. P. W. Majerus, D. B. Wilson, T. M. Connolly, T. E. Bross, and E. J. Neufeld, Phosphoinositide turnover provides a link in stimulus-response coupling, <u>Trends</u> <u>in</u> <u>Biochem.</u> <u>Sci.</u> 10:168 (1985).

20. J. Mizuguchi, M. A. Beaven, J. Hu-Li, and W. E. Paul, Phorbol myristate acetate inhibits anti-IgM-mediated signalling in resting B cells, <u>Proc.</u> <u>Natl.</u> <u>Acad.</u> <u>Sci.</u> <u>U.S.A.</u> 83:4474 (1986).

21. J. Mizugushi, M. A. Beaven, J. Ohara, and W. E. Paul, BSF-1 action on resting B cells does not require elevation of inositol phospholipid metabolism or increased $[Ca^{2+}]_i$, <u>J.</u> <u>Immunol.</u> in press (1986).

22. J. Mizuguchi and W. E. Paul, Anti-IgM mediated early and late biochemical events in B lymphocyte activation, <u>Sixth</u> <u>International</u> <u>Congress</u> <u>of</u> <u>Immunology</u> (Abstract) 3(13):9 (1986).

23. J. Mizuguchi, W. Tsang, S. L. Morrison, M. A. Beaven, and W. E. Paul, Membrane IgM, IgD, and IgG act as signal transmission molecules in a series of B lymphomas, <u>J.</u> <u>Immunol.</u> in press (1986).

24. J. G. Monroe and M. J. Kass, Molecular events in B cell activation. I. Signals required to stimulate G_0 to G_1 transition of resting B lymphocytes, <u>J.</u> <u>Immunol.</u> 135:1674 (1985).

25. T. Nakamura and M. Ui, Simultaneous inhibitions of inositol phospholipid breakdown, arachidonic acid release, and histamine secretion in mast cells by islet-activating protein, pertussis toxin. A possible involvement of the toxin-specific substrate in the Ca^{2+}-mobilizing receptor-mediated biosignaling system, <u>J.</u> <u>Biol.</u> <u>Chem.</u> 260:3584 (1985).

26. D. C. Parker, Stimulation of mouse lymphocytes by insoluble anti-mouse immunoglobulins, <u>Nature</u> 258:361 (1975).

27. T. Pozzan, P. Arslan, R. Y. Tsien, and T. J. Rink, Anti-Immunoglobulin, cytoplasmic free calcium, and capping in B lymphocytes, <u>J.</u> <u>Cell</u> <u>Biol.</u> 94:335 (1982).

28. M. Prentki, T. J. Biden, D. Janjic, R. F. Irvine, M. J. Berridge, and C. B. Wollheim, Rapid mobilization of Ca^{2+} from rat insulinoma microsomes by inositol-1,4,5-triphosphate, <u>Nature</u> 309:562 (1984).

29. J. T. Ransom, D. L. DiGiusto, and J. C. Cambier, Single cell analysis of calcium mobilization in anti-immunoglobulin-stimulated B lymphocytes, <u>J.</u> <u>Immunol.</u> 136:54 (1986).

30. J. T. Ransom, L. K. Harris, and J. C. Cambier, Anti-Ig induces release of inositol-1,4,5-triphosphate, which mediates mobilization of intracellular Ca^{++} stores in B lymphocytes, <u>J.</u> <u>Immunol.</u> 137:708 (1986).

31. J. Rogers, E. Choi, L. Souza, C. Carter, C. Word, M. Kuehl, D. Eisenberg, and R. Wall, Gene segments encoding transmembrane carboxyl termini of immunoglobulin gamma chains, <u>Cell</u> 26:19 (1981).

32. J. Rogers, P. Early, C. Carter, K. Calame, M. Bond, L. Hood, and R. Wall, Two mRNAs with different 3' ends encode membrane-bound and secreted forms of immunoglobulin μ chain, <u>Cell</u> 20:303 (1980).

33. R. Sagi-Eisenberg, H. Lieman, and I. Pecht, Protein kinase C regulation of the receptor-coupled calcium signal in histamine-secreting rat basophilic leukemia cells, <u>Nature</u> 313:59 (1985).

34. S. D. Shulka, Phosphatidylinositol specific phospholipase C, <u>Life</u> <u>Sciences</u> 30:1323 (1982).

35. D. G. Sieckmann, R. Asofsky, D. E. Mosier, I. M. Zitron, and W. E. Paul, Activation of mouse lymphocytes by anti-immunoglobulin. I. Parameters of the proliferative response, <u>J.</u> <u>Exp.</u> <u>Med.</u> 147:814 (1978).

36. H. Streb, R. F. Irvine, M. J. Berridge, and I. Schulz, Release of Ca^{2+} from a nonmitochondrial intracellular store in pancreatic acinar cells by inositol-1,4,5-triphosphate, <u>Nature</u> 306:67 (1983).

37. Y. Takai, A. Kishimoto, Y. Iwasa, Y. Kawahara, T. Mori, and Y. Nishi-
zuka, Calcium-dependent activation of a multifunctional protein
kinase by membrane phospholipids, J. Biol. Chem. 254:3692 (1978).
38. R. Y. Tsien, T. Pozzan, and T. J. Rink, Calcium homeostasis in intact
lymphocytes: cytoplasmic free calcium monitored with a new, intra-
cellularly trapped fluorescent indicator, J. Cell. Biol. 94:325
(1982).
39. B. M. Tyler, A. F. Cowman, S. D. Gerondakis, J. M. Adams, and O.
Bernard, mRNA for surface immunoglobulin gamma chains encodes a
highly conserved transmembrane sequence and a 28-residue intracellular domain, Proc. Natl. Acad. Sci. U.S.A. 79:2008 (1982).
40. N. L. Warner, Membrane immunoglobulins and antigen receptors on B and T
lymphocytes, Adv. Immunol. 19:67 (1974).
41. G. B. Zavoico, S. P. Halenda, R. I. Sha'afi, M. B. Feinstein, Phorbol
myristate acetate inhibits thrombin-stimulated Ca^{2+} mobilization and
phosphatidylinositol 4,5-bisphosphate hydrolysis in human platelets,
Proc. Natl. Acad. Sci. U.S.A. 82:3859 (1985).

SECTION III
ANTIBODY IDIOTYPES, ANTI-IDIOTYPES, AND NETWORK REGULATION

Induction of Antibodies to Pseudorabies Virus by Immunization
with Anti-Idiotypic Antibodies
Michael F. Gurish, Tamar Ben-Porat, and Alfred Nisonoff

Network and Regulation of the Idiotypic Repertoire
Carol Victor-Kobrin, Zahava Barak, F. A. Bonilla, and
Constantin Bona

Anti-Hapten Idiotype Models in Studies of Aging and
Idiotype Networks
Gregory W. Siskind, Edmond A. Goidl, Young Tai Kim, Marc E.
Weksler, and G. Jeanette Thorbecke

INDUCTION OF ANTIBODIES TO PSEUDORABIES VIRUS BY IMMUNIZATION WITH ANTI-IDIOTYPIC ANTIBODIES

Michael F. Gurish[1], Tamar Ben-Porat[2], and Alfred Nisonoff[1]

[1]Department of Biology, Rosenstiel Research Center
Brandeis University, Waltham, Massachusetts
[2]Department of Microbiology, School of Medicine
Vanderbilt University, Nashville, Tennessee

INTRODUCTION

In 1974, Niels Jerne (10) proposed that an anti-idiotypic antibody (anti-anti-X) might sometimes express an "internal image" of X; i.e., that the combining region of the anti-idiotypic (anti-Id) antibody could have structural features in common with antigen X (This is consistent with the fact that both can interact with anti-X.) We have suggested the term "related epitope" or anti-Id(RE) to describe the feature held in common by the two substances (19). This term intentionally suggests that the structural relationship might be confined to a single epitope and that the epitopes on X and on anti-anti-X might be serologically cross-reactive but not necessarily identical. Until 1978, Jerne's postulate represented an interesting hypothesis but did not have experimental support. In that year, Sege and Peterson (26) made two observations that are most readily interpreted on the basis of the internal image concept. They prepared antibodies to insulin in rats and affininty-purified them. Anti-Id antibodies were next elicited in rabbits against the purified rat anti-insulin, and adsorbed in the usual way to remove antibodies to non-idiotypic determinants. The absence of anti-insulin was ensured by passage over an insulin-containing column. These anti-Id antibodies mimicked the behavior of insulin in two ways: they inhibited the binding of radiolabeled insulin to rat epididymal fat cells and they stimulated the uptake of α-aminoisobutyric acid by rat thymocytes.

It should be noted that these, and other data to be discussed, have an alternative interpretation: namely, that the insulin receptor shares an epitope with anti-insulin that is recognized by the anti-anti-insulin. This possibility cannot be formally ruled out. It seems to us improbable, however, when one considers the fact that antibodies to a given antigen, prepared in two different rabbits, generally will not share idiotype. [This was the basis for Oudin's original definition of the term (21).] It therefore seems somewhat unlikely that a cell receptor for insulin and anti-insulin antibodies, which must be very distally related on the evolutionary scale, will share conventional idiotypic structures. The presence of structurally related epitopes in insulin and anti-anti-insulin would explain the data without the need to invoke idiotypic similarity between the insulin receptor and anti-insulin antibodies. It should be noted that only a small fraction of the anti-Id might express an internal image of the insulin,

Table 1. Induction of Antibodies to Pathogens by Treatment with Anti-Id

Antigen	Antibody (Ab1)	Anti-Id (Ab2)	Anti-Id Cross-reacts with:	Remarks
Trypanosomes (24)	mouse monoclonal	mouse polyclonal	Ab in immune sera	Ab2 induces protection in 20-30% of mice (syngeneic)
Hepatitis B (13-16) surface Ag (HBs)	human	rabbit	Each of 8 human anti-HBs; anti-HBs from 6 other species (chicken Ab not reactive)	Ab2 induces anti-HBs in mice
Reovirus (2,11,20,27) type 3 (reo)	mouse polyclonal	rabbit; mouse polyclonal	Polyclonal anti-reo (types 1 and 3); several monoclonal anti-reo antibodies; reo receptors on lymphocytes and neuronal cells	Ab2 primes for type 3 reo-specific delayed type hypersensitivity
Sendai virus (3,4) (SV)	SV-specific T cell clone (in place of Ab)	mouse monoclonal	T cells or T cell clones from SV-immune mice	Ab2 confers protection against SV; primes for SV-specific delayed hyper-sensitivity
Rabies virus (22) glycoprotein	mouse monoclonal	rabbit	Only homologous Id	Ab2 induces viral-neutralizing antibodies
E. coli K13 (28) polysaccharide	mouse monoclonal	mouse monoclonal	Ab in preimmune and immune sera of mice and in immune sera of rats	Ab2 given neonatally primes for protection against lethal dose of E. coli K13

Table 1. (continued)

Antigen	Antibody (Ab1)	Anti-Id (Ab2)	Anti-Id Cross-reacts with:	Remarks
Strep. (17) pneumoniae	mouse anti-phosphocholine (myeloma protein)	mouse monoclonal coupled to KLH		Ab2 induces and antiphospho-choline AB and protection in syngeneic mice
Herpes simplex (6) type 1 (HSV-1)	mouse monoclonal	rabbit		Ab2 induces delayed type hypersensitivity to HSV-1
Listeria [12] monocytogenes (LM)	LM-specific, T-hybridoma (in place of Ab)	syngeneic mouse polyclonal		Ab2 induces protection against subsequent LM infection
Poliovirus [30] type II	mouse monodonal	mouse monoclonal (syngeneic with Ab1	Ab1 from rats, mice, guinea pigs, humans	Ab2 induces anti-polio neutralizing antibody in syngeneic mice. Protection not observed.
Schistosoma [7] mansoni (SM)	rat monoclonal (protective)	rat monoclonal		AB2 induces cytotoxic anti-SM antibodies. Some recip-ients protected against SM (syngeneic).

83

since the amounts of anti-Id used in the experiments of Sege and Peterson were probably in great stoichiometric excess over the insulin receptors. Despite these arguments, which we find rather convincing, the alternative interpretation, that insulin receptors and anti-insulin antibodies share "conventional" idiotypic determinants, cannot be excluded.

In the same paper (26), Sege and Peterson showed that anti-Id directed against antibodies to rat retinol-binding protein were bound by rat intestinal epithelial cells, and that anti-Id competed with retinol-binding protein for access to combining sites on the epithelial cells. Again the data were taken as evidence for the presence of an internal image of retinol-binding protein in the anti-Id.

Following the studies of Sege and Peterson, anti-Id (anti-anti-X) has been shown to interact with cell receptors for X in several other systems; the relevant antigens include a chemotactic factor (18), alprenolol (β-adrenergic receptor) (9,25), thyroid stimulating hormone (5), an agonist of the acetylcholine receptor (1,31), reovirus (2,11,20,27). A novel feature of such experiments is that antibodies are induced that interact with receptors without using the receptor for immunization; a ligand of the receptor is used instead. In view of the difficulty of collecting substantial quantities of most cell receptors, this approach can be of great value, particularly if monoclonal anti-Id with the desired properties can be induced.

Another area of interest, to which the concept of internal image is relevant, is the use of anti-Id to induce the formation of antibodies specific for pathogens. In 1981, it was suggested that anti-Id bearing an internal image of a virus or bacterium could have potential use as a vaccine (19,23). The induction of antibodies to pathogens by this technique has now been demonstrated in several systems. In a few instances, varying degrees of protection against the infectious agent have also been achieved. Much of the relevant published data is summarized in Table 1.

Induction of Antibodies to Pseudorabies Virus (PRV) by Inoculation of Anti-Id

We have been engaged in studies designed to induce antibodies, and possibly protection, against PRV through the use of anti-idiotypic reagents. PRV is a herpes virus that infects many mammalian species and is of commercial importance in swine. The virus can be neutralized by antibodies to a 98 kilodalton envelop protein, and this protein can be precipitated from solution by certain BALB/c monoclonal neutralizing antibodies (8). The studies described here made use of two of these monoclonal antibodies (mAb) designated M1 and M7.

Preparation of Anti-Id Antibodies

Rabbit anti-Id antibodies were prepared against mAb M1 by multiple inoculations of 1 mg quantities subcutaneously in complete Freund's adjuvant (CFA). The resulting antiserum was thoroughly adsorbed with normal mouse globulins coupled to Sepharose 4B, and the remaining antibodies were affinity-purified on mAb M1, conjugated to Sepharose; the bound antibodies were eluted with 3 M NaSCN and dialyzed immediately.

Polyclonal mouse anti-Id was prepared against mAb M7. To enhance its immunogenicity in the mouse, the mAb was conjugated to keyhold limpet hemocyanin (KLH) with glutaraldehyde prior to inoculation. 200 μg quantities of the conjugate were inoculated i.p. in CFA into A/J mice, using a 1:9 ratio of antigen solution to CFA in order to induce ascites (29). An immunoglobulin fraction of the ascites was adsorbed by passage over Sepharose coupled to BALB/c immunoglobulins. The anti-Id was then purified by adsorption to, and elution from mAb M7 conjugated to Sepharose.

84

Table 2. Induction of Anti-PRV Titers by Immunization with A/J Anti-Id Directed to a Monoclonal Anti-PRV Antibody (M7)[a]

Strain Immunized	Antigen	Anti-PRV titers[b]	
		cpm	μg/ml[d]
A/J	anti-M7(Id)[a]	14,500[c]	228
		13,700	196
		15,700	276
		10,000	92
	anti-arsonate (mean of 5 mice)	2,700[e]	control
BALB/c	anti-M7(Id)	16,200[c]	311
		6,600	29
		14,300	227
		14,000	212
		4,400	20
	anti-arsonate (mean of 5 mice)	1,500[e]	control
C57BL/6	anti-M7(Id)	8,500[c]	62
		2,400	0
		2,800	1
		8,400	61
		1,900	0
		2,200	0
	anti-arsonate (mean of 5 mice)	2,700[e]	control

[a] 0.2 to 0.4 mg of anti-Id conjugated to KLH was inoculated 3X at monthly intervals as an emulsion in CFA. Mice were bled 26 days later.
[b] Data are for individual mice expect as indicated.
[c] cpm ^{125}I-labeled purified rabbit antimouse Fab bound, corrected for binding by serum from normal mice.
[d] Using protein M7 to obtain a standard curve. Values are corrected by subtracting the average value for the control mice. These values are: A/J = 12 μg/ml; BALB/c = 5 μg/ml; C57BL/6 = 12 μg/ml.
[e] Control

Idiotypic specificity of each of the two anti-Id antibody preparations was demonstrated by their capacity to completely inhibit the binding of the corresponding antibody (M1 or M7) to the wells of polyvinylchloride microtiter plates previously exposed to lysates of PRV-infected rabbit kidney cells. The inhibition by each anti-Id preparation was specific for its respective ligand (M1 or M7). Idiotypic specificity was further demonstrated by direct, specific binding of radiolabeled, purified M1 or M7 by the corresponding anti-Id.

Induction of Anti-PRV Antibodies by Rabbit Anti-Id

Induction of anti-PRV antibodies in syngeneic (BALB/c) mice and allogeneic (A/J) mice was first demonstrated by immunization with rabbit anti-M1 (Id). After three i.p. inoculations of 200 μg quantities of anti-Id emulsi-

Table 3. Inhibition of Binding of ^{125}I-labeled M7 (Monoclonal Anti–PRV) to PRV-coated Wells by Antibody Induced by Challenge with Anti-M7(Id)[a]

Strain Immunized	Antigen	Percent Inhibition of binding of ^{125}I–M7 [b]
A/J	anti-M7(Id)	70
		62
		78
		60
	anti-arsonate (mean of 5 mice)	5
BALB/c	anti-M7(Id)	80
		46
		77
		78
		32
	anti-arsonate (mean of 5 mice)	1
C57BL/6	anti-M7(Id)	61
		6
		1
		64
		0
		3
	anti-arsonate (mean of 5 mice)	0

[a] Anti-M7(Id) was conjugated to KLH prior to inoculation.
[b] 10 ng of ^{125}I-labeled M7 was used in each test. Sera were diluted 1:125. Six, 24, 96 ng of unlabeled M7 caused 47%, 64%, and 78% inhibition, respectively. 1500 ng of unlabeled M1 caused 3% inhibition.

fied in CFA, the mice were bled, their sera pooled and adsorbed by passage over rabbit-Ig-Sepharose to remove antirabbit antibodies. The sera were then tested for anti-PRV binding activity, using antigen-coated microtiter trays. Binding was detected by developing the wells with affinity-purified ^{125}I-rabbit antimouse Fab (RAMFab) and quantified by comparison of the data with a standard curve constructed using M1 or M7 purified with protein-A Sepharose. Sera of mice immunized with normal rabbit immunoglobulin contained no detectable anti-PRV antibodies. The pooled serum of A/J mice immunized with rabbit anti-M1 (Id) contained approximately 15 µg/ml of anti-PRV and the BALB/c pool approximately 9 µg/ml. When subsequently challenged with ten LD_{50} units of PRV, all control mice died within five to seven days. One of five of the A/J mice and three of six of the BALB/c mice immunized with rabbit anti-M1 (Id) survived. Because of the small numbers of animals, we are currently repeating and expanding this experiment to verify the results.

Induction of Anti-PRV by Murine Anti-Id

More impressive titers of anti-PRV antibodies have recently been obtained by immunizing mice with affinity-purified A/J anti-M7(Id) coupled to

KLH. The antibodies were conjugated to KLH (with glutaraldehyde) to enhance
their immunogenicity. Control mice were injected with purified A/J anti-
arsonate antibodies conjugated to KLH. In each case the antigen was emulsified with CFA and inoculated i.p. After three inoculations of 200 µg into
A/J, BALB/c, and C57BL/6 mice, the mice were bled and individually titered.
The results of the assays for direct binding are presented in Table 2 as
counts per minute (CPM) of radioiodinated RAMFab bound; these data were
converted to µg/ml on the basis of a standard curve constructed using pure
M7. The dilution of serum tested in each case was 1:625. All of the A/J
and BALB/c mice and two of five of the C57BL/6 mice responded to
immunization with the anti-M7(Id) by producing good titers of anti-PRV
antibodies (Table 2). In contrast, none of the mice immunized with
anti-arsonate antibodies produced significant titers of anti-PRV.

The same sera were also tested for their ability to inhibit the binding
of radiolabeled M7 to PRV-coated trays. The results are presented in Table
3. The data for inhibition of binding of M7 are in complete accord with the
direct binding results of Table 2. All of the sera which contained anti-PRV
antibodies, as measured by uptake of ^{125}I-RAMFab, also inhibited the binding
of ^{125}I-labeled M7.

These data demonstrate that immunization with anti-M7(Id) induced the
formation of anti-PRV antibodies. They further indicate that some of these
antibodies are directed to the same viral epitope that is recognized by mAb
M7. The latter result is consistent with the presence of an internal image
of PRV in the mouse anti-M7(Id); it is further supported by the fact that
anti-PRV was induced in three strains of mice that differ in Igh allotype.

Another observation was also consistent with this conclusion. We found
that unlabeled M7 can cause a maximum of ∿35 inhibition of the binding of
radiolabeled M1 to PRV-coated wells. Virtually the same result was obtained
with each anti-PRV antiserum induced by anti-M7(Id); a maximum of 36%
inhibition was observed, with an average of approximately 25% inhibition.

Collectively, the results indicate that by immunization with anti-Id,
we have induced antibodies in three different strains of mice that are specific for the epitope recognized by M7 on the 98 kilodalton envelope
protein. Experiments are in progress to evaluate the protective effects of
such immunization.

ACKNOWLEDGEMENTS

This work was supported by Grants AI-22068 and AI-10947 from the
National Institutes of Health. Dr. Gurish is supported by a post-doctoral
fellowship from The Arthritis Foundation.

REFERENCES

1. W. L. Cleveland, N. H. Wassermann, R. Sarangarajan, A. S. Penn, and B.
   F. Erlanger, Monoclonal antibodies to the acetylcholine receptor by a
   normally functioning auto-anti-idiotypic mechanism, Nature 305:56
   (1983).
2. M. S. Co, G. N. Gaulton, K. K. McDade, B. N. Fields, and M. I. Greene,
   Isolation and biochemical characterization of the mammalian reovirus
   type 3 cell-surface receptor, J. Exp. Med. 160:1195 (1984).
3. H.C.J. Ertl and R. W. Finberg, Sendai virus-specific T cell clones:
   Induction of cytolytic T cells by an anti-idiotypic antibody directed
   against a helper T cell clone, Proc. Natl. Acad. Sci. U.S.A. 81:2850
   (1984).
4. H.C.J. Ertl, E. Homas, S. Tournas, and R. W. Finberg, Sendai virus-

specific T cell clones. V. Induction of a virus specific response by anti-idiotypic antibodies directed against a T helper cell clone, J. Exp. Med. 159:1778 (1984).

5. N. R. Farid, R. Briones-Urbina, and M. Nazrul-Islam, Biologic activity of anti-thyrotropin anti-idiotypic antibody, J. Cell. Biochem. 19:305 (1982).

6. P.G.H. Gell and P.A.H. Moss, Production of cell-mediated immune response to herpes simplex by immunization with anti-idiotypic hetero-antisera, J. Gen. Virol. 66:1801 (1985).

7. J. M. Grzych, M. Capron, P. H. Lambert, C. Dissous, S. Torres, and A. Capron, An anti-idiotypic vaccine against experimental schistosomiasis, Nature 316:74 (1985).

8. H. Hampl, T. Ben-Porat, L. Ehrlicher, K. Habermehl, and A. S. Kaplan, Characterization of the envelope proteins of pseudorabies virus, J. Virol. 52:583 (1984).

9. C. J. Homcy, S. G. Rockson, and E. Haber, An anti-idiotypic antibody that recognizes the beta-adrenergic receptor, J. Clin. Invest. 69:1147 (1982).

10. N. K. Jerne, Towards a network theory of the immune system, Ann. Immunol. 125C:373 (1974).

11. R. S. Kauffman, J. H. Noseworthy, J. T. Nepom, R. Finberg, B. N. Fields, and M. I. Greene, Cell receptors for mammalian reovirus II. Monoclonal anti-idiotypic antibody blocks viral binding to cells, J. Immunol. 131:2539 (1983).

12. S.H.E. Kaufmann, K. Eichmann, I. Muller, and L. J. Wrazel, Vaccination against the intracellular becterium Listeria monocytogenes with a clonotypic antiserum, J. Immunol. 134:4123 (1985).

13. R. C. Kennedy, K. Adker-Storthz, R. D. Henkel, Y. Sanchez, J. L. Melnick, and G. R. Dreesman, Immune response to hepatitis B surface antigen: enhancement by prior injection of antibodies to the idiotype, Science 221:853 (1983).

14. R. C. Kennedy and G. R. Dreesman, Enhancement of the immune response to hepatitis B surface antigen: in vivo administration of anti-idiotype induced anti-HBs that expresses a similar idiotype, J. Exp. Med. 159:655 (1984).

15. R. C. Kennedy, I. Ionescu-Matiu, Y. Sanchez, and G. R. Dreesman, Detection of interspecies idiotypic cross-reactions associated with antibodies to hepatitis B surface antigen, Eur. J. Immunol. 13:232 (1983).

16. R. C. Kennedy, J. L. Melnick, and G. R. Dreesman, Antibody to hepatitis B virus induced by injecting antibodies to the idiotype, Science 223:930 (1984).

17. M. K. McNamara, R. E. Ward, and H. Kohler, Monoclonal idiotype vaccine against Streptococcus pneumoniae infection, Science 226:1325 (1984).

18. W. A. Marasco and E. L. Becker, Anti-idiotype as antibody against the formyl peptide chemotaxis receptor of the neutrophil, J. Immunol. 128:963 (1982).

19. A. Nisonoff and E. Lamoyi, Implications of the presence of an internal image of the antigen in anti-idiotypic antibodies: possible application to vaccine production, Clin. Immunol. Immunopathol. 21:397 (1981).

20. J. H. Noseworthy, B. N. Fields, M. A. Dichter, C. Sobotka, E. Pizer, L. L. Perry, J. T. Nepom, and M. I. Green, Cell receptors for mammalian reovirus I. Syngeneic monoclonal anti-idiotypic antibody identifies a cell surface receptor for reovirus, J. Immunol. 131:2533 (1983).

21. J. Oudin and M. Michel, Une nouvelle forme d'allotypie des globulins du sérum du lapin, apparement lieé a la fonction et à la specificité anticorps, C.R. Acad. Sci. (Paris) 257:805 (1963).

22. K. J. Reagan, W. H. Wunner, T. J. Wiktor, and H. Koprowski, Anti-idiotypic antibodies induce neutralizing antibodies to rabies virus glycoprotein, J. Virology 48:660 (1983).

23. I. M. Roitt, D. K. Male, G. Guarnotta, L. P. de Carvalho, A. Cooke, F. C. Hay, P. M. Lydyard, Y. Thanavala, and J. Ivanyi, Idiotypic networks and their possible exploitation for manipulation of the immune response, Lancet i:1041 (1981).

24. D. L. Sacks, K. M. Esser, and A. Sher, Immunization of mice against African trypanosomiasis using anti-idiotypic antibodies, J. Exp. Med. 155:1108 (1982).

25. A. B. Schreiber, P. O. Couraud, C. Andre, B. Vray, and A. D. Strosberg, Anti-alprenolol anti-idiotypic antibodies bind to beta-adrenergic receptors and modulate catecholamine-sensitive adenylate cyclase, Proc. Natl. Acad. Sci. U.S.A. 77:7385 (1980).

26. K. Sege and P. A. Peterson, Use of anti-idiotypic antibodies as cell surface receptor probes, Proc. Natl. Acad. Sci. U.S.A. 75:2443 (1978).

27. A. H. Sharpe, G. N. Gaulton, K. K. McDade, B. N. Fields, and M. I. Greene, Syngenic monoclonal anti-idiotype can induce cellular immunity to reovirus, J. Exp. Med. 160:1195 (1984).

28. K. E. Stein and T. Soderstrom, Neonatal administration of idiotype or anti-idiotype primes for protection against Escherichia coli K13 infection in mice, J. Exp. Med. 100:1001 (1984).

29. A. S. Tung, S. Sato, and A. Nisonoff, Production of large amounts of antibodies in individual mice, J. Immunol. 116:676 (1976).

30. F.G.C.M. Uytdehaag and A.D.M.E. Osterhaus, Induction of neutralizing antibody in mice against Poliovirus type II with monoclonal anti-idiotypic antibody, J. Immunol. 134:1225 (1985).

31. N. H. Wasserman, A. S. Penn, P. I. Freimuth, N. Treptow, S. Wentzel, W. L. Cleveland, and B. F. Erlanger, Anti-idiotypic route to anti-acetylcholine receptor antibodies and experimental myasthenia gravis, Proc. Natl. Acad. Sci. U.S.A. 79:4810 (1982).

NETWORK AND REGULATION OF THE IDIOTYPIC REPERTOIRE

Carol Victor-Kobrin, Zahava Barak, F. A. Bonilla, and
Constantin Bona

Department of Microbiology
Mount Sinai School of Medicine
New York, New York

The emergence and evolution of the immune and idiotypic repertoires of
the immune system are closely intertwined, given that idiotypes are after
all the antigenic markers of the antibody molecule's variable region. Those
factors which can affect the expression of these two repertoires will differ
according to the maturity of the immune system. At this point we would like
to distinguish between those forces affecting the primary or early repertoire
versus those influencing the expression of the later secondary repertoire.

The primary immune and idiotypic repertoires are present at birth and
are established during the early stages of B cell differentiation (i.e., the
pre-B cell stage) when these cells lack any membrane associated idiotype
bearing immunoglobulin receptors which can interact with any external antigens
or anti-idiotypic molecules. Therefore, at this early stage, the repertoire
is determined solely by the genetic programming which is executed to generate
the functional immunoglobulin variable regions. Those molecular mechanisms
which can influence this programming process will exert the largest influence
on the development of the primary immune and idiotypic repertoire.

An examination of the molecular processes involved in the generation of
functional variable regions for immunoglobulin heavy and light chains, reveals
several potential points where changes can be introduced into the germline
encoded repertoire. The variable regions of the immunoglobulin heavy and
light chains are encoded by three discrete genomic segments which through a
series of recombinational processes are juxtaposed to create the intact variable region. The V_H, D and J_H segments, and the V_L and J_L segments encode
the variable regions for the heavy and light chains, respectively. Each of
these five types of segments occur in multiple copies in the genome, with
each copy encoding a different amino acid structure. Therefore, even though
restrictions might exist in the pairing of different heavy and light chain
variable regions, a tremendous source of variable region diversity can result
from the random combinatorial association of the different genomic segments
which encode the respective heavy and light chain variable regions. Furthermore, additional somatic diversity can be introduced as a result of the recombination events which juxtapose the various variable region genomic segments. The recombination junctions between these various genomic segments
exhibit great nucleotide diversity as a result of both the flexibility allowed
in this system as to the choice of the exact point at which the recombination

will occur in order to maintain the correct reading frame as well as the "de novo" addition of nucleotides which has been frequently observed in this region. Both of these factors which contribute to the "junctional diversity" seen in this system, play an important role in determining the coding region of the third hypervariable regions (CDRIII) of the heavy and light chains. Because it is in CDRIII where these recombinational junctions occur in the antibody molecule, this region not only plays a pivotal role in forming the antibody combining site but also has been shown to be important in the expression of idiotypes in several systems.

Another potential source of diversity for the primary immune and idiotypic repertoires might be the occurrence of somatic mutations in those genomic sequences encoding the hypervariable regions of the immunoglobulin heavy and light chains. Although the exact extent to which this mechanism does play a role at this stage of B cell maturity is quite unclear because few mutations are generally observed in the variable regions of IgM antibodies when their sequences were compared to the germline gene sequences from which they were derived.

Finally, it should be mentioned that because the antigen binding sites and the expression of idiotypic determinants are both generated from the interactions of the variable regions of the heavy and light chains, whatever limited combinatorial association of heavy and light chain variable regions is permitted to occur, will still increase the diversity of the primary immune and idiotypic repertoire.

In contrast to the primary repertoire, the secondary repertoire is established after birth at a later stage of B cell differentiation when membrane associated, idiotype-bearing immunoglobulin receptors are already displayed by these cells. Hence, the B cell can now interact with external environmental factors now rendering the secondary repertoire susceptible to the modulating influence of immunogenic or tolerogenic stimuli elicited by antigens, idiotypes and anti-idiotypes. These three factors can act to stably fix the immune and idiotypic repertoire for the duration of an individual's life. The effects of these three factors are best illustrated by the following three examples.

A) Effect of antigen. A study of the clonotypic pattern of the PR8 influenza virus immune response showed that certain clones present at birth, disappear and are replaced by others during adult life. However, Cancro and associates (4) observed that the administration after birth of the PR8 virus resulted in the persistence of some of the "young" clonotypes throughout adult life.

B) Effect of idiotypes. Immunization of adult mice with the $\beta 2,6$, $\beta 1,2$ linked polyfructosan bacterial levan, activates B cell clones specific for these linkages which express the dominant IdX A, B, and G idiotype system shared by various inulin binding myeloma proteins. By contrast, clones specific for only the $\beta 2,6$ fructosan linkage bearing the A48-UPC10 idiotype represent a minor component of this response. Rubinstein and co-workers (13) showed that the administration of UPC10 myeloma protein (IgG2a) to pregnant females, which successfully crossed the placenta into fetal circulation, led to the dominance of these $\beta 2,6$ fructosan binding A48-UPC10 Id$^+$ clones in the anti-bacterial levan immune response for several months after birth in the progeny of these treated females.

C) Effect of anti-idiotype. Working the same A48-UPC10 model idiotype system described in the preceding section, it was observed that the neonatal administration of minute amounts of anti-A48-UPC Id antibodies (10 ng) caused a long lasting activation of the A48-UPC10 Id$^+$ $\beta 2,6$ fructosan binding clones, which otherwise represent a minor component of the bacterial levan

immune response (8). However, experiments performed on the T15 model idiotype system of phosphocholine binding antibodies showed that anti-idiotype
could exert a negative effect on clones expressing the complementary idiotype.
Immunization of adult mice with phosphocholine leads to the activation of
antigen-specific clones expressing the dominant cross-reactive T15 IdX idiotype. Administration at birth of high amounts of anti-T15 IdX antibodies
causes a long lasting suppression of the T15 IdX bearing clones with the
emergence of phosphocholine binding T15 IdX⁻ clones (14) which represent a
minor component of the primary phosphocholine specific repertoire.

A major emphasis of our laboratory over the past few years has been to
study the role of idiotype mediated regulatory processes in shaping the secondary repertoire. In particular, we sought to identify those particular idiotopes which participate in these regulatory processes under relatively physiological conditions which we uphold by working only in a strictly autologous
system.

Anti-idiotypic antibodies will define two basic types of idiotopes, the
cross-reactive and individual idiotope. Whereas the individual idiotope
represents the phenotypic marker of a unique somatic event which occurred in
a single clone, the cross-reactive idiotope is shared by several clones utilizing similar immunoglobulin variable region genomic segments. Working
again in the A48-UPC10 idiotype system of β2,6 fructosan binding clones we
described a subset of cross reactive idiotopes which were borne by these
clones and were singled out and designated as regulatory idiotopes because
they appeared to be the major target of regulatory forces within the immune
system (2).

Regulatory idiotopes are defined by three criteria (2). A) They are
autoimmunogenic. B) They are shared by antibodies exhibiting different antigen specificities. C) They are recognized by regulatory T cells which could
contribute to their dominant expression.

In order to fully appreciate the implications of immunoregulation through
regulatory idiotopes, we proceeded to perform a complete immunochemical and
molecular characterization of antibody molecules bearing the A48-UPC10 regulatory idiotopes. Our studies were specifically directed at addressing the
following three issues: A) whether or not expression of the A48-UPC10 regulatory idiotopes could be correlated with expression of a germline V_H gene
derived from the V_H X24 germline gene family. Earlier studies (15) had suggested that these regulatory idiotopes were phenotypic markers of germline
V_H genes. The V_H X24 family is the smallest murine V_H family identified,
located at the 5' terminus of the murine V_H locus and consisting only of two
highly homologous (>93% nucleotide homology) V_H genes, the V_H X24 and V_H441-4
germline genes (3). The V_H441-4 germline gene is utilized by A48 and UPC10
to encode their respective V_H regions. B) To establish the degree of heterogeneity if any of the antigen binding specificities exhibited by antibodies
expressing A48-UPC10 regulatory idiotopes and utilizing germline V_H genes
deriving from the V_H X24 germline gene family. C) To investigate the role
which the bacterial levan antigen played in the activation of B cell clones
bearing A48-UPC10 regulatory idiotopes.

The experimental strategy devised to carry out these goals was to activate A48-UPC10 regulatory idiotope bearing clones using syngeneic reagents
and then immortalize those clones as hybridomas. By using syngeneic reagents
to effect this activation, we are assured that this activation is being
achieved only through regulatory processes involving the recognition of regulatory idiotopes. Therefore, these hybridomas are truly the experimental
subjects needed for this study, namely the clonal products resulting from
immunoregulation through regulatory idiotopes.

Previous studies had shown that the activation of A48-UPC10 Id[+] clones could be achieved in several ways. They include: administration at birth of 10 ng of the A48 monoclonal protein; in utero exposure to UPC10 monoclonal protein; neonatal injection of syngeneic polyclonal anti-A48 Id antibodies; immunization of adult mice with a syngeneic polyclonal anti-A48 Id-KLH conjugate followed by an immunogenic challenge with bacterial levan; or the immunization of adult animals with syngeneic monoclonal anti-A48-UPC10 Id-KLH conjugates followed by an immunogenic challenge with bacterial levan (2,6,8,13). Based on these studies, hybridomas used in this study were prepared from BALB/c mice treated in the following ways:

A) Untreated one month old mice; B) injected at birth with 10 µg of A48 monoclonal protein, and followed in only some of the animals by an immunogenic challenge of bacterial levan at one month of age; C) injected at birth with 10 ng of syngeneic polyclonal anti-A48 Id antibodies, and followed in some of the animals by an immunogenic challenge of bacterial levan at one month of age; D) adult mice immunized with a polyclonal syngeneic anti-A48 Id antibody-KLH conjugate, and followed in some animals by an immunogenic challenge with bacterial levan.

The hybridomas generated from these seven groups of animals will be selected according to two separate criteria: A) expression of antibody bearing the A48-UPC10 regulatory idiotopes which is based on the ability of the monoclonal antibody to inhibit the binding of radioactively tagged A48 or UPC10 to syngeneic polyclonal anti-A48-UPC10 Id antibodies in a competitive inhibition radioimmunoassay; B) demonstration of m-RNA in cytoplasmic lysates of the hybridomas which can hybridize to a V_H441-4 germline gene probe using RNA slot blotting techniques.

DESCRIPTION OF THE REAGENTS AND RADIOIMMUNOASSAY TECHNIQUES USED TO ANALYZE IDIOTYPE EXPRESSION AND ANTIGEN SPECIFICITY BY THE MONOCLONAL ANTIBODIES SECRETED BY THE HYBRIDOMAS UNDER STUDY

The fructosan linkage specificity of the test monoclonal antibodies was determined by studying their binding to three polyfructosans: bacterial levan, a branched homosaccharide consisting of a backbone of β2,6 linked fructosan residues with β2,1 linkages occurring at the branch points, rye levan (100% β2,6 linked fructosan residues), and inulin (100% β2,1 linked fructosan residues). As can be seen in Table 1, A48 and UPC10 must be specific for the β2,6 linkage since they bind bacterial and rye levan. J606 is specific for the β2,1 linkage since it binds to bacterial levan and inulin.

Table 1. Pattern of Binding to Polyfructosans of Monoclonal Proteins Bearing A48 Idiotopes

Monoclonal Protein	Rye Levan β2,6 fructosan	Bacterial Levan β2,6, β2,1 fructosan	Inulin β2,1 fructosan
A48	5,659 ± 275*	12,819 ± 945	91 ± 5
UPC10	1,353 ± 95	19,233 ± 723	188 ± 30
J606	360 ± 87	4,265 ± 833	5,875 ± 419
2-11-3	102 ± 3	12,354 ± 697	151 ± 26
MOPC-460	225 ± 79	376 ± 116	44 ± 2

*cpm average of triplicates ± SD

Table 2. Specificity of Binding of Monoclonal. Anti-Id Antibodies

Microtiter Plates Coated with 10 µg Monoclonal Proteins	Binding of ^{125}I-labeled Anti-Id Antibodies		
	IDA10 (Anti-A48 Id)	10-1 (Anti-UPC10 Id)	HyX24-14 (Anti-X24 Id)
BSA	220 ± 15*	94 ± 10	34 ± 2
A48	24,406 ± 1,175	185 ± 8	71 ± 4
UPC10	10,944 ± 139	3,322 ± 29	50 ± 4
X44	262 ± 15	179 ± 6	11,546 ± 143
PY102	429 ± 13	195 ± 25	45 ± 8

*cpm mean of triplicates ± SD

Monoclonal antibody 2-11-3 would be interpreted as being specific for a branch point determinant in bacterial levan since it binds only to that polysaccharide.

The test monoclonal antibodies were also assayed for binding to lysozyme, streptococcal group A polysaccharide, β1,6D galactans and PR8 influenza virus since antibodies which are specific for these substances have been observed to also derive their V_H genes from the V_H X24 germline gene family (7). The radioimmunoassays were carried out as previously described (15) by binding the various antigens to the wells of polyvinyl chloride plates, incubating the test monoclonal antibodies with the antigen-coated plates and detecting any bound antibody with an ^{125}I labeled monoclonal anti-kappa light chain reagent.

Idiotype expression by the test monoclonal antibodies was studied using a large panel of monoclonal anti-idiotopes. The specificities of the three most intensively used reagents are shown in Table 2. IDA10 (kindly given to us by Dr. Pierre Legrain, Pasteur Institute) is a syngeneic (BALB/c) anti-idiotope generated against the A48 myeloma protein (10). 10-1 (also given to us by Dr. Pierre Legrain) is a semi-syngeneic [(BALBxA/J)F1] anti-idiotope generated against the UPC10 monoclonal protein (15). HyX24-14 idiotope (kindly given to us by Dr. Michael Potter, NIH) is an allogeneic (A/J) anti-idiotope generated against the α1,6 D galactan binding myeloma protein XRPC24 which derives its V_H gene from the V_H X24 germline gene (12). IDA10 recognizes a cross-reactive idiotope which is present on both A48 and UPC10 since it specifically binds to both proteins. 10-1 and HyX24-14 recognize idiotopes present only on UPC10 and XRPC24 respectively, since they bind only to these proteins.

All idiotype radioimmunoassays were carried out by coating the wells of polyvinyl chloride microtiter plates with the test monoclonal proteins and incubating the coated plates with the ^{125}I labeled monoclonal anti-idiotopes.

ANALYSIS OF ANTIGEN SPECIFICITY AND EXPRESSION OF REGULATORY IDIOTOPES ON MONOCLONAL ANTIBODIES SELECTED FOR EXPRESSION OF A48 IDIOTOPES

The results described in this section pertain to the A48 Id bearing monoclonal antibodies secreted by hybridomas isolated from BALB/c mice in whom the A48 Id bearing B cell precursors were activated using four previously described protocols (Table 3). These hybridomas were selected for this analysis for their ability to secrete a monoclonal antibody which could inhibit

Table 3. Proportion of Monoclonal Antibodies Selected for Expression of A48
Idiotopes Which Bind to Syngeneic Polyclonal Anti-Id Antibodies

Origin of Antibodies	Binding to	
	Anti-A48 Id	Anti-UPC10 Id
BALB/c mice injected after birth with 10 µg A48 and one month later with bacterial levan	1/1	0/1
BALB/c mice injected after birth with 10 ng anti-A48 Id antibodies and one month later with bacterial levan	6/6	2/6
Adult BALB/c mice immunized with anti-A48 Id-KLH conjugate and then with bacterial levan	5/5	1/5
Adult BALB/c mice immunized with monoclonal anti-A48 Id KLH conjugate	4/4	0/4

the binding of ^{3}H labeled A48 to syngeneic polyclonal anti-A48 Id antibodies
(6) as can be seen in Table 3. While all of these monoclonal antibodies
bind to the syngeneic polyclonal anti-A48 Id antibodies relatively few bind
to the syngeneic polyclonal anti-UPC10 Id antibodies.

The binding of these monoclonal antibodies to the monoclonal anti-idiotopes is shown in Table 4 and shows a similar pattern of binding as was observed with the polyclonal anti-idiotypes. All the antibodies except for
one bound to IDA10, the monoclonal anti-A48 Id reagent. By contrast, relatively few bound to the 10-1 anti-UPC10 Id reagent, and those which did bind

Table 4. Proportion of Monoclonal Antibodies Selected for Expression of A48
Idiotopes Which Bind to Monoclonal Anti-Idiotopes

Origin of Antibodies	Binding to		
	IDA 10	10-1	HyX24-14
BALB/c mice injected after birth with 10 µg A48 and one month later with bacterial levan	1/1	0/1	0/1
BALB/c mice injected after birth with 10 ng anti-A48 Id antibodies and one month later with bacterial levan	4/5	1/5	0/5
Adult BALB/c mice immunized with anti-A48 Id-KLH conjugate and then with bacterial levan	6/6	0/6	0/6
Adult BALB/c mice immunized with mono-clonal anti-A48 Id-KLH conjugate	4/4	2/4	0/4

Table 5. Antigen Specificities of Antibodies Selected for
the Expression of A48-Idiotype

Origin of Antibodies	Rye levan (2,6 fructosan)	Binding to β2,6, β2-1 branch point determinants of bacterial levan	Galactan (β6,1-galactan)	IDA10 (only)
A48, UPC10, MOPC173 myeloma protein	A48, UPC10	-	MOPC173	
BALB/c mice injected at birth with 10 μg A48 and one month later immune bacterial levan	1/1	0/1	0/1	0/1
BALB/c mice injected at birth with 10 ng anti-A48 Id antibodies and one month later immunized with bacterial levan	4/8	4/8	0/8	0/8
Adult BALB/c mice immunized with anti-A48 Id-KLH conjugate and then with bacterial levan	3/5	0/5	0/5	2/5
Adult BALB/c mice immunized with monoclonal anti-A48-KLH conjugate	0/4	1/4	2/4	1/4

were not necessarily the same antibodies which bound to the polyclonal anti-UPC10 Id antibodies. None of the antibodies bound to HyX24-14, the monoclonal anti-X24 Id, in spite of the fact that its V_H derives from the V_H X24 germline which shows 93% nucleotide homology to the V_H441-4 germline which A48 and UPC10 utilize.

These data collectively suggest that idiotopes present on UPC10, such as that defined by 10-1, represent a minor idiotope among these monoclonal antibodies.

An analysis of the antigen binding specificities of these monoclonal antibodies is shown in Table 5.

The vast majority are specific for the β2,6 fructosan linkage as is found in rye levan. The fact that some of these A48 Id bearing clones demonstrate binding specificities for branch point determinants in the bacterial levan polysaccharide and β1,6 D-galactans, was completely unanticipated because these two antigenic specificities have never been observed among the A48 Id$^+$ myeloma repertoire. The galactan specificity by these monoclonal antibodies is not too surprising since several galactan binding myeloma and hybridomas derive their V_H from the V_H441-4 as well as the V_H X24 germline V_H genes. Interestingly, the occurrence of these galactan binding clones as well as the true Ab$_3$ clones (those binding only to IDA10 and to none of the foreign antigens tested, including lysozyme and the PR8 influenza virus) was

Table 6. Proportion of Antibodies Selected for the Expression of A48 Id Which Use V_H X24 Derived Genes

Origin of Antibodies	V_H X24 Derived Gene
BALB/c mice injected after birth with 10 µg A48 and one month later with bacterial levan	1/1
BALB/c mice injected after birth with 10 ng anti-A48 Id antibodies and one month later with bacterial levan	5/7
Adult BALB/c mice immunized with anti-A48 Id-KLH conjugate and then immunized with bacterial levan	4/4
Adult BALB/c mice immunized with monoclonal anti-A48 Id-KLH conjugate	4/4

more prevalent among the treated adult animals than among those administered the A48 Id or anti-A48 Id at birth.

In addition, these hybridomas were examined for usage of a germline V_H gene deriving from the V_H X24 germline gene family by Northern blotting experiments. The vast majority of these hybridomas produced an immunoglobulin heavy chain mRNA which did hybridize under highly stringent conditions to a V_H441-4 germline gene probe (Table 6). The most striking observation to emerge from these experiments was the extremely high correlation which existed between IDA10 idiotope expression and usage of a germline V_H gene deriving from the V_H X24 germline gene family. Of the 16 hybridomas studied only two derived from mice administered anti-Id antibodies at birth did not show this correlation.

ANALYSIS OF ANTIGEN SPECIFICITY AND EXPRESSION OF REGULATORY IDIOTOPES ON MONOCLONAL ANTIBODIES SELECTED FOR USAGE OF A V_H X24 DERIVED GERMLINE V_H GENE

The results presented in this section pertain to those monoclonal antibodies secreted by hybridomas which were selected for their production of an immunoglobulin heavy chain mRNA which hybridizes to the V_H441-4 probe. The data presented in the previous section showed that clones expressing A48 idiotopes and exhibiting fructosan binding specificities were preferentially activated in idiotypically manipulated mice who were subsequently challenged with bacterial levan. In order to fairly assess the impact which this challenge has on this clonal activation process, the hybridomas studied in this section were generated from manipulated mice who did not receive a bacterial levan antigenic challenge (Table 8). In the absence of this antigenic challenge, splenic lymphocytes of these mice were mitogenically activated for 48 hours prior to the fusion event such that the yield of hybrids would be maximized in this protocol which favors the activated blast cell. Lipopolysaccharide and nocardia water soluble mitogen were chosen since they collectively activate non-overlapping B cell subsets corresponding to 80% of the repertoire.

As shown in Table 7, of 534 hybridomas generated in this fashion from the various groups of mice, 12 were selected based on slot blotting analysis

Table 7. Frequency of Hybridomas Utilizing V_H X24 Derived Germline V_H Sequences

Origin of Antibodies	In Vitro Stimulation LPS	NWSM	Total
One month old BALB/c	2/95 (2.1%)	4/73 (5.5%)	6/168 (3.6%)
One month old BALB/c injected at birth with 10 µg A48	1/99 (1.0%)	1/95 (1.1%)	2/194 (1.0%)
One month old BALB/c injected at birth with 10 ng IDA10	1/114 (0.9%)	3/58 (5.2%)	4/172 (2.3%)
Total	4/308 (1.3%)	8/226 (3.5%)	12/534 (2.2%)

and later confirmed by Northern blotting experiments which produced heavy chain mRNA encoding V_H sequences complementary to the V_H441-4 germline gene probe.

The results of the binding of the 12 monoclonal antibodies secreted by these V_H441-4[+] hybridomas to syngeneic polyclonal anti-A48 Id or UPC10 Id antibodies are presented in Table 8. Only four of them bound to the anti-A48 Id antibodies, with a different four binding to the anti-UPC10 Id antibodies.

An analysis of the idiotope expression by these 12 V_H X24 expressing hybridomas by monoclonal anti-idiotopes is presented in Table 9. Seven of these bound to IDA10, three to HyX24-14 and one to 10-1. This pattern of expression is quite different from that observed among hybridomas which were selected for A48 Id expression as described in Section II. Consistent with their selection by an anti-A48 Id antibody, virtually all bound to the monoclonal anti-A48 Id, IDA10 but none to HyX24-14.

Table 8. Proportion of Antibodies Selected with V_H441-4 Germline Gene Probe Which Bind to Polyclonal Anti-Id Antibodies

Origin of Antibodies	Binding to Anti-A48 Id	Anti-UPC10 Id
One month old BALB/c	2/6	2/6
One month old BALB/c injected with 10 µg A48	1/2	1/2
One month old BALB/c injected at birth with 10 ng anti-A48 Id	1/4	1/4
Total	4/12	4/12

Table 9. Proportion of Antibodies Selected with V_H441-4 Germline Gene
Probe Which Binds to Monoclonal Anti-Id Antibodies

Origin of Antibodies	IDA10	Binding to 10-1	HyX24-14
One month old BALB/c	2/6	1/6	1/6
One month old BALB/c injected at birth with 10 μg A48	2/2	0/2	1/2
One month old BALB/c injected at birth with 10 ng anti-A48 Id	3/4	0/4	1/4
Total	7/12	1/12	3/12

The antigen specificity of these 12 V_H441-4[+] monoclonal antibodies was investigated using a panel of antigens which are known to elicit specific antibodies which derive their V_H from the V_H X24 germline gene family (Table 10).

Antigenic specificities were found for four of these antibodies; two were galactan specific, one was influenza virus PR8 specific and one was termed multispecific because it bound to bacterial levan, lysozyme, influenza virus PR8 and galactan. In this latter instance, only the binding to the PR8 virus and galactan was respectively inhibited by both PR8 virus as well as galactan (Bonilla et al., manuscript in preparation).

V_H SEQUENCE ANALYSIS OF MONOCLONAL ANTIBODIES BEARING A48 REGULATORY IDIOTOPES

Legrain and associates recently published partial nucleotide sequences of six V_H genes expressed by six A48 Id[+] hybridomas derived from adult BALB/c hyperimmunized with monoclonal anti-A48 Id antibody-KLH conjugates (11). These sequences showed that all these antibodies used V_H genes derived from the V_H441-4 germline gene which were expressed in the context of all four J_H segments and with D genes originating from the three major D segment families (DQ52, Dsp2, DF116). However, because of several unresolved sequence ambiguities as well as the incompleteness of the sequences, this study could not adequately address the issue of somatic mutation in these antibodies and its effect on the idiotype expression. To this end we established in our laboratory the technique of cloning duplex cDNA molecules corresponding to the full length rearranged and expressed V_H gene, and unambiguously sequencing through this region using Maxam Gilbert nucleotide modification reaction. The sequences of two of these antibodies are presented in Figure 1. 1-5-1 is a hybridoma generated from a BALB/c mouse injected at birth with 10 μg A48 and challenged one month later with bacterial levan. 3-14-9 was obtained from an adult BALB/c mouse which was hyperimmunized with a syngeneic poly-clonal anti-A48 Id-KLH conjugate and challenged after completion of the immu-nization schedule with bacterial levan. Both these hybridomas express the same J_H4 segment as well as identical 12 nucleotide long D-segments. This D-segment is completely different from that used by A48 and UPC10, or any of those utilized by Legrain's six A48 Id[+] hybridomas. With respect to the V_H region of these two hybridomas, several nucleotide differences are noted between their expressed V-gene and the consensus V_H441-4 germline gene uti-lized by A48 and UPC10. However, we do not interpret all these differences in

Table 10. Antigen Specificity of Monoclonal Antibodies Selected with V_H441-4 Germline Gene Probe

Origin of Antibodies	Bacterial Levan	Galactan	Lysozyme	Streptococcus Group A Polysaccharide	Influenza Virus PR8	Multi-specific	Unknown
One month old BALB/c	0/6	0/6	0/6	0/6	0/6	0/6	5/6
One month old BALB/c injected at birth with 10 μg A48	0/2	0/2	0/2	0/2	1/2	0/2	1/2
One month old BALB/c injected at birth with 10 ng anti-A48 Id antibodies	0/4	2/4	0/4	0/4	0/4	0/4	2/4

```
                                                          10                                      20
                      Glu Val Lys Leu Leu Glu Ser Gly Gly Gly Leu Val Gln Pro Gly Gly Ser Leu Lys Leu Ser Cys Ala Ala Ser
VH441-4(VHGal39.1)    GAG GTG AAG CTT CTC GAG TCT GGA GGT GGC CTG GTG CAG CCT GGA GGA TCC CTG AAA CTC TCC TGT GCA GCC TCA
                                                                                      Asn
VH X24 (VHGal55.1)    ... ... ... ... ... ... ... ... ... ... ... ... ... ... ... ... ... ... ..T ... ... ... ... ... ...
           A48
           U10        ... ... ... ... ... ... ... ... ... ... ... ... ... ... ... ... ... ... ... ... ... ... ... ... ...
           1.5.1                                                                              Asn
           3.14.9     ... ... ... ... ... ... ... ... ... ... ... ... ... ... ... ... ... ... ..T ... ... ... ... ... ...

                                      30  <---CDR1--->                  40                                    <-50
                      Gly Phe Asp Phe Ser Arg Tyr Trp Met Ser Trp Val Arg Gln Ala Pro Gly Lys Gly Leu Glu Trp Ile Gly Glu
VH441-4(VHGal39.1)    GGA TTC GAT TTT AGT AGA TAC TGG ATG AGT TGG GTC CGG CAG GCT CCA GGG AAA GGG CTA GAA TGG ATT GGA GAA
                                                                  Ala                             Gln
VH X24 (VHGal55.1)    ... ... ... ... ... ... ... ... ... ... ... .CT ... ... ... ... ... ... ... .AG ... ... ... ... ...
                                                                                      Arg
           A48        ... ... ... ... ... ... ... ... ... ... ... ... ... ... ... ... ... .G. ... ... ... ... ... ... ...
                                          Gly
           U10        ... ... ... ... ... G.. ... ... ... ... ... ... ... ... ... ... ... ... ... ... ... ... ... ... ...
                                                                                                  Gln
           1.5.1                                                                      ... ... .AG ... ... ..C ... ...
                                                                  Ala                 Leu         Gln
           3.14.9     ... ... ... ... ... ... ... ... ... ... ... .CT ... ... ... .T. ... ... ... .AG ... ... ... ... ...

                      -----a------------------------CDR2-----60------------------>                70
                      Ile Asn Pro Asp Ser Ser Thr Ile Asn Tyr Thr Pro Ser Leu Lys Asp Lys Phe Ile Ile Ser Arg Asp Asn Ala
VH441-4(VHGal39.1)    ATT AAT CCA GAT AGC AGT ACT ATA AAC TAT ACG CCA TCT CTA AAG GAT AAA TTC ATC ATC TCC AGA GAC AAC GCC
                                  Gly
VH X24 (VHGal55.1)    ... ... ... .GA ... ... ... ... ... ... ... ... ... ... ... ... ... ... ... ... ... ... ... ... ...
           A48        ... ... ... ... ... ... ... ... ... ... ... ... ... ... ... ... ... ... ... ... ... ... ... ... ...
           U10        ... ... ... ... ... ... ... ... ... ... ... ... ... ... ... ... ... ... ... ... ... ... ... ... ...
                              Leu Gly
           1.5.1      ..C ... .T. .GA ... ... ... ... ... ... ... ... ... ... ... ... ... ... ... ... ... ... ... ... ...
                                  Gly
           3.14.9     ... ... ... .GA ... ... ... ... ... ... ... ... ... ... ... ... ... ... ... ... ... ... ... ... ...

                                          80          a   b   c                           90
                      Lys Asn Thr Leu Tyr Leu Gln Met Ser Lys Val Arg Ser Glu Asp Thr Ala Leu Tyr Tyr Cys Ala Arg <--------D-------->
VH441-4 (VHGal39.1)   AAA AAT ACT CTG TAC CTG CAA ATG AGC AAA GTG AGA TCT GAG GAC ACA GCC CTT TAT TAC TGT GCA AGA
VH X24 (VHGal55.1)    ... ... ... ... ... ... ... ... ... ... ... ... ... ... ... ... ... ... ... ... ... ... ...
                                                                                                              Asn Trp Asp Arg Gly
           A48        ... ... ... ... ... ... ... ... ... ... ... ... ... ... ... ... ... ... ... ... ... ... ... AAC TGG GAC AGG GGG   JH3
                                                                                                                          Val
           U10        ... ... ... ... ... ... ... ... ... ... ... ... ... ... ... ... ... ... ... ... ... ... ... ... ... ... GT. ..C   JH2
                                                                                                              Lev Lev Ala Lys
           1.5.1      ... ... ... ... ... ... ... ... ... ... ... ... ... ... ... ... ... ... ... ... ... ... ... CTA TT. .C. .A.       JH4
                                                                                                              Lev Lev Ala Lys
           3.14.9     ... ... ... ... ... ... ... ... ... ... ... ... ... ... ... ... ... ... ... ... ... ... ... CTA TT. .C. .A.       JH4
```

Figure 1

mutations b   for the most part, they correspond to the nucleotide differences wh_   lineate the V_H441-4 gene from its closely related family
member, the V_H ℓ4 gene. Hence, these differences are in fact indicative of
these two V_H genes as deriving from the closely related V_H X24 germline gene,
and not the V_H441-4 gene. Overall, the 1-5-1 and 3-14-9 V_H sequences show
few nucleotide changes from the V_H X24 germline gene sequence which is consistent with their being IgM antibodies which generally show relatively
little somatic mutation.

CONCLUSIONS

The observations reported in this communication on monoclonal antibodies
deriving their V_H gene from the V_H X24 germline gene family constitute an
essential element in our quest to further our understanding of idiotype driven
events by elucidating a molecular basis for regulatory idiotype expression.
The overall frequency of hybridomas utilizing V_H X24 derived germline V_H
genes from the LPS and NWSM responsive B cell populations derived from all
our groups of normal and idiotype manipulated animals was approximately 2%
(12 out of 534 hybridomas analyzed). Considering that the proportional representation of the V_H X24 germline gene family among all murine germline V_H
genes is in fact two genes out of a postulated total repertoire of 100 such
V_H genes (3), the frequency of V_H X24 utilizing hybridomas is directly proportional to this family's representation in the murine V_H repertoire. These
results differ from those of Rajewsky and co-workers (5) who, working in a
slightly different system with a much smaller sample size, reported that
among 51 hybridomas derived from LPS blasts of adult C57BL/6 splenic B cells,
three expressed V_H genes derived from the V_H X24 family, which is three times
as many as they would have anticipated from the family size. Nevertheless,
among our hybridomas utilizing V_H X24 derived V_H genes, a very large proportion of them also expressed A48 idiotopes (defined by syngeneic polyclonal
or monoclonal reagents), regardless of whether or not the animals from which
they were derived were immunized with bacterial levan. These results strongly
suggest that the A48 regulatory idiotopes may function as a phenotypic marker
for germline genes deriving from this family.

The antigen binding analysis of these V_H X24 expressing hybridomas did
reveal major differences in the specificities which depended on whether or
not the mice from which they were derived were immunized with bacterial levan
or not. Among the levan-immunized mice, the majority of the hybridomas derived from them were specific for polyfructosans, whereas the non-levan
immunized mice yielded none. These results suggest that antigen does play
an important role in selecting for expression a particular subset of clones
among all those which use V_H X24 derived V_H genes, express the A48 regulatory
idiotopes and, of course, were activated and expanded by treatment with anti-
idiotype or idiotype. This may be related to a restricted pairing between
V_H X24 derived V_H genes and a particular V_K light chain gene in order to
create a suitable combining site for bacterial levan binding. Indeed, it is
known that V_H genes derived from the V_H X24 family are utilized by a variety
of antibodies binding many different antigenic substances. However, when
these V_H genes are paired with light chains deriving from the V_K10 family as
is the case with UPC10 and A48, the antibodies generally manifest a fructosan
specificity (9).

Interesting differences were also noted between the types of clones
activated in the neonatal versus the adult animal. Injection at birth of
A48 or anti-A48 Id antibodies followed by an antigenic challenge of bacterial
levan activated a group of Ab_1 type clones which exhibited various specificities for polyfructosans. Some like A48 or UPC10 were specific for the β2,6
fructosan linkage while others showed a specificity for branch point determinants in the bacterial levan polysaccharide. By contrast, by hyperimmuniz-

ing adult animals with anti-A48 Id-KLH conjugates and re   s of whether
or not they received an antigenic challenge of bacterial   ı, a wider spectrum of clones were activated including those of the Ab$_3$ ι _ (bind only to
the anti-A48 Id antibody or IDA10), and those binding other antigens such as
galactan. The activation of those galactan binding clones is in perfect
concordance with our previous observations that XRPC44, a galactan-binding
myeloma protein, shares a family of idiotopes with UPC10, which are defined
by a syngeneic polyclonal anti-UPC10 Id reagent (15).

Recent data generated in our laboratory as well as those reported by
Auffrey (1) and Legrain (11) point to the germline V_H gene as the most plau-
sible region encoding the structural correlate for the A48-UPC10 regulatory
idiotopes. The data collectively demonstrate that monoclonal antibodies
bearing these idiotopes express a variety of different J_H and D segments and
our preliminary sequence data show very few nucleotide changes from the germline V_H gene in two such antibodies of the IgM class. However, it should be
emphasized that the molecular investigation of the basis of idiotype expression in this system is really only in its infancy, and only further V_H sequence analyses coupled with studies on the V_K structures manifested by A48-
UPC10 Id bearing antibodies will definitely clarify this issue.

ACKNOWLEDGMENTS

This work was supported by National Science Foundation Grant
#PCM-8408660. F. A. Bonilla is a trainee of the Medical Scientist Training
Grant #GrO-7280.

REFERENCES

1. C. Auffrey, J. L. Sikorav, R. Ollo, and F. Rougeon, Correlation between
    D region structure and antigen-binding specificity: evidence from the
    comparison of closely related immunoglobulin V_H sequences, Ann. Immunol.
    (Inst. Pasteur) 132d:77 (1981).
2. C. A. Bona, E. Heber-Katz, and W. G. Paul, Idiotype-anti-idiotype
    regulation. I. Immunization with a levan-binding myeloma protein leads
    to the appearance of auto-anti(anti-idiotype) antibodies and to activa-
    tion of silent clones, J. Exp. Med. 153:951 (1981).
3. P. H. Brodeur and R. Riblet, The immunoglobulin heavy chain variable
    region (Igh-V) locus in mouse. I. One hundred Igh-V genes comprise seven
    families of homologous genes, Eur. J. Immunol. 14:922 (1984).
4. M. P. Cancro, M. A. Thompson, S. Raychandhuri, and D. Hibbert, Ontogeny
    of the HA-responsive B cell repertoire. Interaction of heritable and
    inducible mechanisms in the establishment of phenotype in idiotype in
    biology and medicine, H. Kohler, J. Urbain, and P. A. Cazenave, eds.,
    Academic Press, New York (1984).
5. R. Dildrop, V. Krawinkel, E. Winter, and K. Rajewsky, V_H gene expression
    in murine lipopolysaccharide blasts distributes over the nine known V_H
    gene groups and may be random, Eur. J. Immunol. 15:1154 (1985).
6. B. Goldberg, W. E. Paul, and C. A. Bona, Idiotype anti-idiotype regula-
    tion. IV. Expression of common regulatory idiotopes on fructosan-binding
    and non-fructosan binding monoclonal immunoglobulin, J. Exp. Med.
    158:515 (1983).
7. A. B. Hartman and S. Rudikoff, J_H genes encoding the immune response to
    β(1,6)-galactan: somatic mutation in IgM molecules, EMBO J. 3:3023
    (1984).
8. J. Hiernaux, C. Bona, and P. J. Baker, Neonatal treatment with low doses
    of anti-idiotypic antibody leads to the expression of a silent clone, J.
    Exp. Med. 153:1004 (1981).

9. E. A. Kabat, T. T. Wu, H. Bilofsky, M. Reid-Miller, and H. Perry, Sequences of proteins of immunological interest, U.S. Department of Health and Human Services, National Institutes of Health, Bethesda, Maryland (1983).

10. P. Legrain, D. Noegtle, G. Buttin, and P. A. Cazenave, Idiotype anti-idiotype interactions and the control of the anti-2,6 polyfructosan response in the mouse: specificity and idiotypy of anti-ABPC48 anti-idiotypic monoclonal antibodies, Eur. J. Immunol. 11:678 (1981).

11. P. Legrain, J. Rocca-Serra, A. Moulin, M. Fougereau, and G. Buttin, A single V_H gene associated with a variety of D- and J-segments encodes for a large family of ABPC48 related antibodies induced by anti-idiotypic immunization, Mol. Immunol. 22:437 (1985).

12. M. Pawlita, E. Mushinsky, R. J. Feldman, and M. Potter, A monoclonal antibody that defines an idiotype with two subsites in galactan-binding myeloma patients, J. Exp. Med. 154:1946 (1981).

13. L. J. Rubinstein, C. B. Victor-Kobrin, and C. A. Bona, The function of idiotypes and anti-idiotypes on the development of the immune repertoire, Devel. Comp. Immunol. Suppl. 3:109 (1984).

14. D. S. Strayer, W.M.F. Lee, D. A. Rowley, and H. Kohler, Anti-receptor antibody. II. Induction of long-term unresponsiveness in neonatal mice, J. Immunol. 114:728 (1985).

15. C. Victor-Kobrin, F. A. Bonilla, B. Bellon, and C. A. Bona, Immunochemical and molecular characterization of regulatory idiotopes expressed by monoclonal antibodies exhibiting or lacking β2,6 fructosan binding activity, J. Exp. Med. 162:697 (1985).

ANTI-HAPTEN IDIOTYPE MODELS IN STUDIES OF

AGING AND IDIOTYPE NETWORKS

Gregory W. Siskind, Edmond A. Goidl, Young Tai Kim,
Marc E. Weksler, and G. Jeanette Thorbecke

Department of Medicine, Cornell University Medical College
New York, New York; Department of Microbiology, University
of Maryland School of Medicine, Baltimore, Maryland; and
Department of Pathology, New York University School of
Medicine, New York, New York

There now are considerable data which are consistent with the view,
originally formalized by Jerne (1) that the immune system is self-regulated
through the existence of a network of idiotypes (ids) and anti-ids. The
elements in this network (B cells, T cells, and serum antibodies) normally
exist in a steady state. Introduction of antigen results in expansion of
specific clones thereby perturbing the steady state. Subsequent shifts in
the distribution of ids and anti-ids occur which constitute the cellular
basis of the immune response and immunologic memory.

A number of laboratories have demonstrated that following presentation
of a hapten-carrier conjugate both anti-hapten and anti-anti-hapten (anti-id)
antibodies are produced (2,13-16,18). In our laboratory anti-id specific
for anti-2,4,6-trinitrophenyl (TNP) antibody has been demonstrated by two
techniques. First an enzyme-linked immunoadsorbent assay (ELISA) in which
we measure the binding of purified, enzyme-labeled, anti-TNP antibody to
microwells coated with the sample to be assayed (3). The second technique
is hapten-augmentation of plaque formation (4,8,16,19). We have observed
that in some situations the number of plaque forming cells (PFC) detected in
a Jerne (11) hemolysis-in-gel assay is greater in the presence of low concentrations of hapten than in the absence of hapten. Evidence was obtained
that such hapten-augmentable PFC are cells whose secretion of antibody had
been reversibly down-regulated by the binding of auto-anti-id to cell surface
id. When hapten is added to the agar, the hapten and anti-id in effect compete for binding to cell surface id. Thus, in the presence of appropriate
concentrations of hapten the anti-id is displaced, the cell resumes secreting
antibody and a plaque is generated. Evidence supporting this view includes:
a) elution of anti-id from hapten-immune spleen cells by incubation with
hapten (4); and b) observation that treatment of antibody secreting cells
with a known anti-id inhibits antibody secretion and that this inhibition is
reversible by hapten (4,8). Using these methods we have shown that, following immunization of mice, rabbits or chickens with either T-dependent or
relatively T-independent TNP conjugates, auto-anti-id specific for anti-TNP
antibody is spontaneously produced (1,5,9,16). The auto-anti-id response
was shown to be T-cell dependent (17) and to exhibit distinct kinetics in
primary and secondary responses (5).

Table 1. Effect of Age on the Hapten-Augmentable PFC Response
of C57BL/6 Mice Immunized with TNP-F*

| Days After Antigen | Mean Percentage Augmentation (Incidence > 10%) | |
	6 - 8 Weeks Old (%)	78 Weeks Old (%)
4	1 ± 1 (0/4)	49 ± 18 (5/5)
7	39 ± 15 (3/4)	532 ± 256 (5/5)
11	20 ± 7 (3/5)	369 ± 157 (3/4)

*C57BL/6 mice were injected with 10 μg TNP-F iv and sacrificed at the day
indicated for PFC assay. The data are presented as mean ± standard error
for the percentage hapten-augmentable PFC, that is the percentage increase
in the number of anti-TNP PFC detected in the presence of a low-concentra-
tion (approximately 10^{-7} M) of TNP-epsilon-amino-n-caproic acid, as compared with the number of anti-TNP PFC detected in the absence of hapten.
The number of mice having more than 10% hapten-augmentable PFC/total
number of mice studied are indicated in parentheses. Data are adapted
from Goidl et al. (6).

Of particular interest is the finding (6,7) that, when assayed either
by hapten-augmentable PFC or by ELISA, there is an age-associated increase
in auto-anti-id production (Table 1). This suggests that at least part of
the well-documented decreased immune responsiveness of aged animals may be
due to excessive down-regulation by auto-anti-id. The remainder of this
chapter will be devoted to a discussion of the cellular mechanisms underlying
this increased auto-anti-id response of aged mice.

In order to determine if the increased auto-anti-id response of aged
mice is an intrinsic property of the lymphoid cell population or is a consequence of the "internal milieu" of aged animals we have carried out cell

Table 2. Hapten-Augmentable PFC Following Immunization with TNP-F of
Lethally Irradiated Recipients of Spleen or Bone Marrow
Cells from Old or Young Donors*

Cells Transferred	Age of Cell Donors (months)	Mean Percentage Hapten-Augmentable PFC (%)
Spleen	4	6 ± 5
Spleen	18	109 ± 25
Spleen + Thymus	Spleen 18; Thymus 2	79 ± 13
Bone Marrow	2-3	13 ± 3
Bone Marrow	18	7 ± 5

*Lethally irradiated mice are injected with the indicated cells from normal,
naive donors of the ages indicated. Recipients are immunized with 10 μg
TNP-F iv on the day of cell transfer and are assayed for anti-TNP PFC seven
days after antigen injection. Data, for groups of four or five mice, are
calculated as indicated in the footnote to Table 1. Data adapted from
Goidl et al. (7).

Table 3. Influence of Splenic T Cells on the Hapten-Augmentable
PFC Response Following Immunization with TNP-F*

| Age of Cell Donors | | Mean Percentage |
Bone Marrow Donors (months)	Splenic T Cell Donors (months)	Hapten-Augmentable PFC (%)
2-3	2-3	12 ± 4 (6)
2-3	18	55 ± 12 (9)
18	2-3	16 ± 5 (10)
18	18	38 ± 12 (7)

*Lethally irradiated mice are reconstituted with a mixture of syngeneic
BM cells and syngeneic nylon wool purified splenic T cells from naive
donors of the ages indicated. Recipients are immunized with 10 μg TNP-F
iv five days after cell transfer and are assayed for anti-TNP PFC seven
days after antigen injection. Data are calculated as indicated in the
footnote to Table 1. Data have been adapted from Goidl et al. (7).

transfer experiments in which lethally irradiated young mice are reconstituted with spleen cells from either young or old syngeneic donors (7). The
tendency of old mice to produce high levels of auto-anti-id is transferred
with spleen cells from old donors (Table 2), suggesting that it is an intrinsic property of the lymphoid cell population. In contrast, irradiated mice
reconstituted with bone marrow (BM) from old or young donors behave indis-
tinguishably with respect to their auto-anti-id response: both producing
low levels of anti-id (Table 2). Thus it appears that the marked auto-anti-
id response of aged mice is a property of their peripheral lymphoid cell
population and does not reflect the distribution of ids generated from the
BM which is probably comparable in old and young animals in this system.

To determine the cell type in the peripheral lymphoid cell population
which is responsible for influencing the magnitude of the auto-anti-id response mixed cell transfer studies have been performed (7). Lethally irradiated mice are reconstituted with BM from either old or young donors together
with nylon wool purified splenic T cells from old or young donors. The
results indicate that the magnitude of the auto-anti-id response of the recipients is determined by the age of the T cell donors irrespective of the
age of the BM donors (Table 3). Thus the increased auto-anti-id response of
aged mice appears to be determined by the peripheral T cell population.
This could be due either to an id-specific "helper" effect of the T cell
population brought into effect after antigen challenge, or to the T cell
population inducing a shift in the distribution of ids maintained in the B
cell population as a consequence of id-anti-id interactions which occur in
the absence of antigen. These possibilities may be distinguished by serial
cell transfer experiments. Lethally irradiated young mice are reconstituted
with BM from young donors together with nylon wool purified splenic T cells
from either young or old donors. Six weeks later the mice are sacrificed;
their spleen cells are collected and are treated with anti-Thy 1 and complement; the surviving cells are transferred, together with thymus cells from
young donors, into lethally irradiated recipients which are then immunized
with TNP-Ficoll (F). As indicated in Table 4 secondary recipients of B cells
which have resided in the primary recipient with T cells from young donors
produce low levels of hapten-augmentable PFC, while recipients of B cells
which have resided with T cells from old donors have a relatively high incidence of hapten-augmentable PFC. The results are thus consistent with the

Table 4. Modification of the B Cell Population by T Cells from
Donors of Different Ages*

Age of T Cell Donor to Primary Host (months)	Number of Mice Studied	Incidence of Mice Having >20% Hapten-Augmentable PFC (%)
2	15	7
24	13	54

*Lethally irradiated mice are reconstituted with BM from young donors and splenic T cells from young or old mice. Six weeks later the mice are sacrificed and their anti-Thy 1 plus complement treated splenic cells (B cells) are transferred, together with 2×10^7 thymocytes from young donors into lethally irradiated mice which are immunized with 10 μg TNP-F iv five days later. Mice are assayed for anti-TNP PFC six days after antigen injection. Data are calculated as indicated in the footnote to Table 1.

hypothesis that the T cells from aged donors induce a shift in id distribution among the B cells such that a higher incidence of hapten-augmentable PFC is generated.

The data described above suggest that the distribution of ids produced by the BM of old and young mice is similar (in the TNP system) and that the increased production of auto-anti-id by old mice is a consequence of shifts in id distribution induced by peripheral T cells. If this hypothesis were correct one would expect that if old mice were able to repopulate their peripheral lymphoid system with cells from their own BM they would then produce a low incidence of hapten-augmentable PFC in their response to TNP-F. To test this hypothesis, mice were given a usually lethal dose of irradiation while a portion of their BM was partially protected by a lead shield (12). One week after irradiation their spleens contain fewer than 10% of the number of nucleated cells present in spleens of control mice. The number of nucleated cells in their spleen increases progressively with time to achieve control levels at six to seven weeks after irradiation. Similarly when spleen cells from such irradiated mice are cultured with TNP-polyacrylamide beads (PAA) one week after irradiation they generate less than 5% the number of anti-TNP PFC as do spleen cells from control mice. Recovery of responsiveness occurs progressively with time after irradiation to reach control levels in six to seven weeks. Thus, mice given a normally lethal dose of radiation while their BM is shielded survive and repopulate their peripheral immune system, presumably from their own BM, within six to seven weeks. Based upon these observations we have immunized mice with TNP-F six to seven weeks after irradiation with BM shielding (12). As predicted, old mice, following recovery from radiation with their BM shielded, produce a low incidence of hapten augmentable PFC (Table 5). Based upon the hypothesis offered above we would predict that the auto-anti-id response could be modified by peripheral T cells. That is, if mice irradiated while their BM is shielded are given T cells from old donors they would subsequently respond like old mice after recovery and produce a relatively high incidence of hapten-augmentable PFC. On the other hand, irradiated mice which receive T cells from young donors would be expected to behave like young mice and produce relatively few hapten-augmentable PFC when immunized after recovery from radiation. The results of such experiments (12) are consistent with these predictions (Table 6). Again the question arises as to whether the T cells act by inducing a shift in id distribution among the B cell population or by a type of id-specific helper effect. To distinguish between these possibilities trans-

Table 5. Hapten-Augmentable PFC and Serum Auto-Anti-id in C57BL/6 Mice Immunized with TNP-F After Recovery from Irradiation with Their BM Shielded*

Age (months)	Irradiation	Number of Mice Studied	Incidence of Mice Having >20% Hapten-Augmentable PFC (%)	Mean Percentage Hapten-Augmentable (%)	Binding of Anti-TNP** (A450 nm)
2-3	-	49	31	19 ± 2	0.28 ± 0.04
2-3	+	43	40	25 ± 5	0.28 ± 0.04
18-24	-	43	70	45 ± 5	0.40 ± 0.07
18-24	+	48	23	21 ± 4	0.29 ± 0.04

*Mice are irradiated while their BM is partially shielded by lead. Six weeks after irradiation they are immunized with 10µg TNP-F iv and are assayed for anti-TNP PFC six days after antigen injection. Data are calculated as indicated in footnote to Table 1. Data are adapted from Kim et al. (12)
**Serum auto-anti-id assayed by ELISA (see Methods).

Table 6. Splenic T Cells Influence the Incidence of Hapten-Augmentable PFC and Serum Auto-anti-id in Mice Which Have Recovered from Irradiation with Their BM Shielded*

Irradiated Mice (months)	Age of T Cell Donor (months)	Number of Mice Studied	Incidence of Mice Having >20% Hapten-Augmentable PFC (%)	Mean Percentage Hapten-Augmentable PFC (%)	Binding of Anti-TNP** (A405 nm)
2-3	none	12	25	17 ± 5	–
2-3	2	18	28	16 ± 3	0.17 ± 0.04 (6)
2-3	24	16	75	31 ± 5	0.31 ± 0.09 (5)
18-24	none	11	27	16 ± 3	–
18-24	2	12	17	10 ± 4	–
18-24	24	14	71	36 ± 6	–

*Mice are irradiated while their BM is partially shielded by lead. One wek later they receive nylon wool purified splenic T cells from donors of the indicated age (or no T cells). Six weeks after cell transfer they are immunized with 10 μg TNP-F iv and are assayed for anti-TNP PFC six days after antigen injection. Data calculated as indicated in the footnote to Table 1. Data are adapted from Kim et al. (12).

Table 7. Modification of the B Cell Population by T Cells Present During
Recovery from Irradiation with BM Shielding*

Group	Number of Mice Studied	Incidence of Mice Having >20% Hapten-Augmentable PFC (%)	Mean Percentage Hapten-Augmentable PFC (%)
Reconstituted with B cells from donors given T cells from 2-3 month old mice	17	29	10 ± 2
Reconstituted with B cells from donors given T cells from 18-24 month old mice	22	77	29 ± 2

*Nylon wool purified splenic T cells from old or young donors are injected into mice five days after they are irradiated with their BM shielded. Six weeks later the mice are sacrificed and their anti-Thy 1 plus complement treated splenic cells (B cells) are injected, together with 2×10^7 thymocytes from young donors, into lethally irradiated mice which are immunized with 10 µg TNP-F iv one day later. The mice are assayed for anti-TNP PFC six days after antigen injection. Data are calculated as indicated in footnote to Table 1.

fer experiments have been carried out using, as the B cell source, anti-Thy-1 treated spleen cells either from mice which have recovered from radiation in the presence of T cells from old donors or from mice which have recovered from radiation in the presence of T cells from young donors. All recipients receive thymus cells from young mice and are immunized with TNP-F. The results in Table 7 show that the incidence of hapten-augmentable PFC in recipients is greater when the B cells have recovered from irradiation in the presence of T cells from old donors than when they have recovered in the presence of T cells from young donors. The results are thus consistent with the hypothesis that peripheral T cells bring about a shift in id distribution among the B cell population.

We suggest that the long-lived peripheral T cell population serves as a repository of information about life-long interactions with self and environmental antigens. As a consequence of id-anti-id interactions, it shapes the clonal distribution of the peripheral B cell population, stimulating or inhibiting B cells as they arise from the BM on the basis of the id they bear. This provides a powerful adoptive mechanism for host defense in that it fine tunes the B cell population to the precise challenges faced by the host in its particular microenvironment. The T cell population, because of its long lifespan, is ideally suited for this type of memory function.

ACKNOWLEDGMENTS

This work is supported in part by grants from the National Institutes of Health, U.S.P.H.S. numbers: AI-11694, AG-00541, AG-00842 and AG-04860.

REFERENCES

1. B. S. Bhogal, A. J. Edelman, J. J. Gibbons, E. B. Jacobson, G. W. Siskind, and G. J. Thorbecke, Production of auto-anti-idiotypic antibody during the normal immune response. 10. Response to TNP-Ficoll in the chicken, Cell. Immunol. 91:159 (1985).

2. H. Cosenza, Detection of anti-idiotype reactive cells in response to phosphorylcholine, Eur. J. Immunol. 6:114 (1976).

3. J. J. Gibbons, E. A. Goidl, G. M. Shepherd, G. J. Thorbecke, and G. W. Siskind, Production of auto-anti-idiotypic antibody during the normal immune response. 12. An enzyme-liked immunosorbent assay for auto-anti-idiotype antibody, J. Immunol. Meth. 79:231 (1985).

4. E. A. Goidl, A. F. Schrater, G. W. Siskind, and G. J. Thorbecke, Production of auto-anti-idiotypic antibody during the normal immune response to TNP-Ficoll. 2. Hapten-reversible inhibition of anti-TNP plaque forming cells by immune serum as an assay for auto anti-idiotypic antibody, J. Exp. Med. 150:154 (1979).

5. E. A. Goidl, A. F. Schrater, G. J. Thorbecke, and G. W. Siskind, Production of auto-anti-idiotypic antibody during the normal immune response. 4. Studies of the primary and secondary responses to thymus-dependent and thymus-independent antigens, Eur. J. Immunol. 10:810 (1980).

6. E. A. Goidl, G. J. Thorbecke, M. E. Weksler, and G. W. Siskind, Production of auto-anti-idiotypic antibody during the normal immune response: changes in the auto-anti-idiotypic antibody response and the idiotype repertoire associated with aging, Proc. Natl. Acad. Sci. U.S.A. 77:6788 (1980).

7. E. A. Goidl, J. W. Choy, J. J. Gibbons, M. E. Weksler, G. J. Thorbecke, and G. W. Siskind, Production of auto-anti-idiotypic antibody during the normal immune response. 7. Analysis of the cellular basis for the increased auto-anti-idiotypic antibody production by aged mice, J. Exp. Med. 157:1635 (1983).

8. E. A. Goidl, T. Hayama, G. M. Shepherd, G. W. Siskind, and G. J. Thorbecke, Production of auto-anti-idiotypic antibody during the normal immune response. 6. Hapten augmentation of plaque formation and hapten- reversible inhibition of plaque formation as assays for anti-idiotype antibody, J. Immunol. Meth. 58:1 (1983).

9. E. A. Goidl, C. Samarut, A. Schneider-Gadicke, N. Hochwald, G. J. Thorbecke, and G. W. Siskind, Production of auto-anti-idiotypic antibody during the normal immune response. 9. Characteristics of the auto-anti-idiotype antibody and its production, Cell Immunol. 85:25 (1984).

10. N. K. Jerne, Towards a network theory of the immune system, Ann. Immunol. (Inst. Pasteur) 125c:373 (1974).

11. N. K. Jerne, A. A. Nordin, and C. Henry, in: "Cell-Bound Antibody," B. Amos and H. Koprowski, eds., Wistar Institute Press, Philadelphia (1963).

12. Y. T. Kim, E. A. Goidl, C. Samarut, M. E. Weksler, G. J. Thorbecke, and G. W. Siskind, Bone marrow function. 1. Peripheral T cells are responsible for the increased auto-anti-idiotype response of older mice, J. Exp. Med. 161:1237 (1985).

13. L. Kluskens and H. Kohler, Regulation of immune response by autogenous antibody against receptor, Proc. Natl. Acad. Sci. U.S.A. 71:5083 (1974).

14. T. J. McKearn, F. P. Stuart, and F. W. Fitch, Anti-idiotypic antibody in rat transplantation immunity. I. Production of anti-idiotypic antibody in animals repeatedly immunized with alloantigens, J. Immunol. 113:1876 (1974).

15. L. S. Rodkey, Studies of idiotypic antibodies - production and characterization of auto-anti-idiotypic antisera, J. Exp. Med. 139:712 (1974).

16. A. F. Schrater, E. A. Goidl, G. J. Thorbecke, and G. W. Siskind, Auto-anti-idiotypic antibody during the normal immune response to TNP-Ficoll. 1. Occurrence in AKR-J and BALB/c mice of hapten-augment-able, anti-TNP plaque forming cells and their accelerated appearance in recipients of immune spleen cells, J. Exp. Med. 150:138 (1979).

17. A. F. Schrater, E. A. Goidl, G. J. Thorbecke, and G. W. Siskind, Production of auto-anti-idiotypic antibody during the normal immune response to TNP-Ficoll. 3. Absence in nu/nu mice - evidence for T cell dependence of the anti-idiotypic antibody response, J. Exp. Med. 150:808 (1979).

18. N. Tasiaux, R. Leuwenkroon, C. Bruyns, and J. Urbain, Occurrence and meaning of lymphocytes bearing auto-anti-idiotypic receptors during immune response, Eur. J. Immunol. 8:464 (1978).

19. G. J. Thorbecke and G. W. Siskind, in: "The Biology of Idiotypes," M. I. Green and A. Nisonoff, eds., Plenum Publishing Corporation, New York (1984).

SECTION IV
IMMUNOLOGIC INTERVENTION WITH ANTI-IDIOTYPE ANTIBODIES

Antibodies to Acetylcholine, Adenosine and Glucocorticoid
Receptors by an Auto Anti-Idiotypic Route
B. F. Erlanger, W. L. Cleveland, N. H. Wasserman, H. H. Ku,
B. L. Hill, R. Sarangarajan, R. Rajagopalan, E. Cayanis,
I. S. Edelman, A. S. Penn, and K. K. Wan

Idiotypic Interactions in the Treatment of Human Diseases
Raif S. Geha

Regulation of Autoimmune Diseases
Norman Talal

ANTIBODIES TO ACETYLCHOLINE, ADENOSINE AND GLUCOCORTICOID

RECEPTORS BY AN AUTO-ANTI-IDIOTYPIC ROUTE

B. F. Erlanger[1], W. L. Cleveland[1], N. H. Wasserman[1], H. H.
Ku[1], B. L. Hill[1], R. Sarangarajan[1], R. Rajagopalan[1], E.
Cayanis[2], I. S. Edelman[2], A. S. Penn[3], and K. K. Wan[4]

Departments of Microbiology[1], Biochemistry[2], and
Neurology[3], Columbia University, Cancer Center, College
of Physicians and Surgeons, New York, New York
Department of Biochemistry[4], University of Toronto,
Toronto, Canada

INTRODUCTION

We will present data in support of the view that products of a functioning anti-idiotype network can cause an autoimmune disease, specifically the
experimental form of myasthenia gravis (MG). It will be demonstrated that
the disease can be induced in the rabbit by active immunization with an anti-
ligand (19,20,52) and in the mouse by passive administration of hybridoma
cells that secrete a monoclonal anti-idiotypic antibody specific for the
binding site of the nicotinic acetylcholine receptor (AChR). We will also
describe how an auto-anti-idiotypic procedure can produce monoclonal antibodies to receptors other than AChR, in particular the glucocorticoid receptor of rat liver cytosol and the adenosine receptors. With respect to the
former, we will report on a monoclonal antibody that cross-reacts with the
B-chain of insulin.

Early Experiments in Rabbits

Our experiments began with the synthesis of a potent agonist of AChR,
trans-3,3'-bis[α-(trimethylammonio)methyl] azobenzene (Bis Q) (1). This
compound is constrained in structure (51) and because of its potency as an
agonist it can be concluded that its molecular "topography" is complementary
to that of the combining site of AChR.

A derivative of Bis Q was prepared which could be linked to a protein
carrier (Figure 1) to produce antibodies specific for Bis Q. We predicted
that the specificity of these antibodies would resemble the specificity of
AChR when the latter is in its activated state (26), i.e., that the antibodies would bind agonists but not antagonists and that the hierarchical
order of binding to agonists would be like that of AChR. This is precisely
what was found (19,20,52).

Specifically purified anti-Bis Q was then prepared by affinity chromatography and used to immunize rabbits. Because anti-Bis Q mimicked AChR, we
speculated that anti-anti Bis Q might mimic anti-AChR. If so, the rabbits

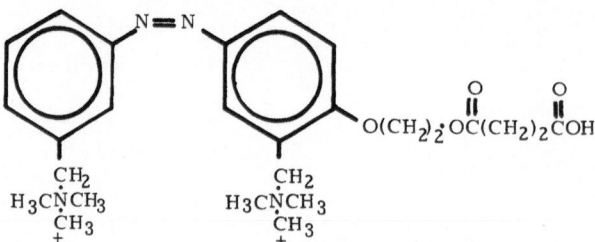

Figure 1. Compound linked to bovine serum albumin (BSA) for immunization:
4-(succinoyloxy)-3,3'-bis[α-(trimethylammonio)methyl]azobenzene

should show signs of experimental MG, since it was shown (40) that experimental MG was produced in rabbits immunized with purified Torpedo AChR.

Of five rabbits immunized with anti-Bis Q, four showed signs of experimental MG after the first booster injection. The signs were severe to mild and, in all cases, the signs disappeared after subsequent booster injections. In one case, severe signs were seen when the rabbit was re-immunized after a "rest" of several months.

The same transient phenomenon was observed when sera of the rabbits were examined for the presence of antibodies to AChR (Figure 2), i.e., after

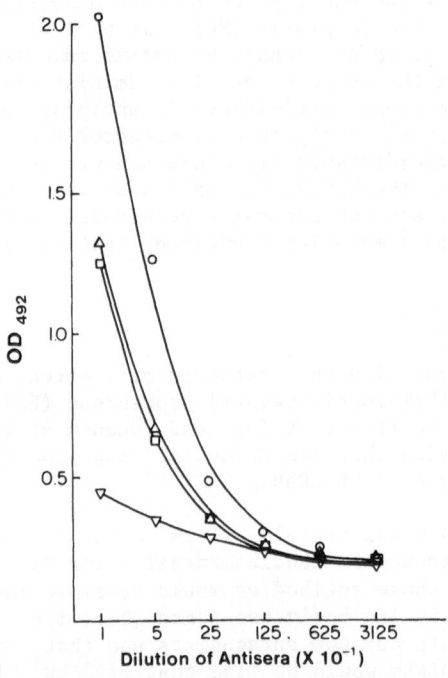

Figure 2. Transient response of rabbit 522 to immunization with Bis Q
immunogen as seen by an ELISA in which plastic wells were
coated with AChR. 0-0, 21 days after first boost (animal shows
severe muscle weakness); Δ-Δ, 7 days after second boost (mini-
mal signs of muscle weakness); □-□ , 32 days after second
boost (animal appears normal); ∇-∇ , 6 days after fourth
boost (animal appears normal).

120

the first booster immunization an elevated titer of anti-receptor was seen; after subsequent boosters the titer fell.

In order to be sure that the signs of MG in the rabbits were induced by an anti-idiotypic response directed at the combining site of anti-Bis Q, we examined several samples of sera taken from a rabbit when it was showing signs of experimental MG, to determine whether they inhibited the binding of [^{3}H]-Bis Q to anti-Bis Q. Inhibition was seen with three sera. One sample of serum, however, caused enhanced binding. Indeed, this serum, itself, could bind [^{3}H]-Bis Q. We reasoned that an auto-anti-idiotypic response had been stimulated in this rabbit, resulting in the expression of anti-anti-anti-Bis Q, which would resemble anti-Bis Q in its binding specificity (39).

Experiments in Mice

As we had concluded that an auto-anti-idiotypic response had been induced in the rabbits (yielding anti-anti-anti-Bis Q), we reasoned that it would be feasible to obtain anti-anti-Bis Q antibodies (= anti-AChR) in a one-step procedure by immunizing with Bis Q-BSA and allowing the idiotypic network of the immunized animal to produce anti-anti-Bis Q, i.e., we would rely upon the naturally occurring auto-anti-idiotypic response (29). We chose the monoclonal route for these experiments because we could then avoid the complicating factor of idiotype-anti-idiotype interactions that would occur in sera.

Upon immunization of BALB/c mice with Bis Q-BSA, fusion with a non-secreting myeloma cell line and screening for anti-anti-Bis Q antibodies in hybridoma cell supernatants using rabbit anti-Bis Q, we found a very substantial auto-anti-idiotypic response (11). We were able to isolate three hybridomas that secreted anti-anti-Bis Q that cross reacted with AChR from Torpedo, Electrophorus electricus and rat muscle. One of these monoclonal antibodies (F8-D5 an IgM, kappa) was examined in detail.

It had the following properties:

1) Binding to AChR from rat muscle, Electrophorus electricus and Torpedo was inhibited by decamethonium (I_{50} = 5 x 10^{-5}M) and by α-bungarotoxin (I_{50} = 0.7 x 10^{-6}M).

2) When tested in J. Lindstrom's laboratory in a reconstituted vesicle system containing Torpedo AChR (49), it inhibited ^{134}Cs flux in the presence of 10^{-3}M carbamylcholine (Figure 3).

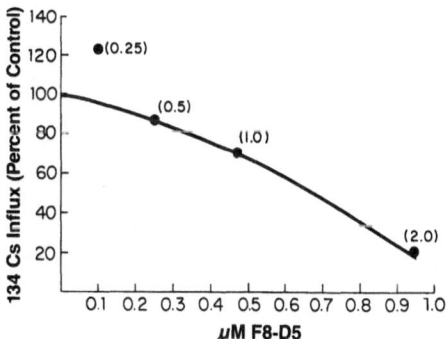

Figure 3. Effect of F8-Df on ^{134}Cs flux in reconstituted liposomes with purified Torpedo AChR. Carbachol at 10^{-3}M. Numbers in parenthesis represent ratio of antibody to receptor. At an equimolar ratio about 30% inhibition was seen.

3) Immunofluorescence experiments showed binding to Torpedo electric tissue (Figure 4), the pattern of binding being identical to that seen with rabbit antibody raised by immunization with Torpedo AChR.

4) When hybridoma cells producing F8D5 were allowed to multiply intra-peritoneally in three male and three female BALB/c mice, all of the females showed signs of experimental MG, which could be temporarily alleviated by injection of neostigmine (Figure 5).

The last experimental finding is a most significant one. We had shown earlier (above) that experimental MG could be produced actively in rabbits by an anti-idiotypic route. We have now shown that a monoclonal product of an auto-anti-idiotypic response can also produce experimental MG by passive transfer. Taken together, we conclude that it is time to take seriously the possibility of an anti-idiotypic etiology for MG and other autoimmune dis-eases. Questions that must be answered, however, include the nature of the

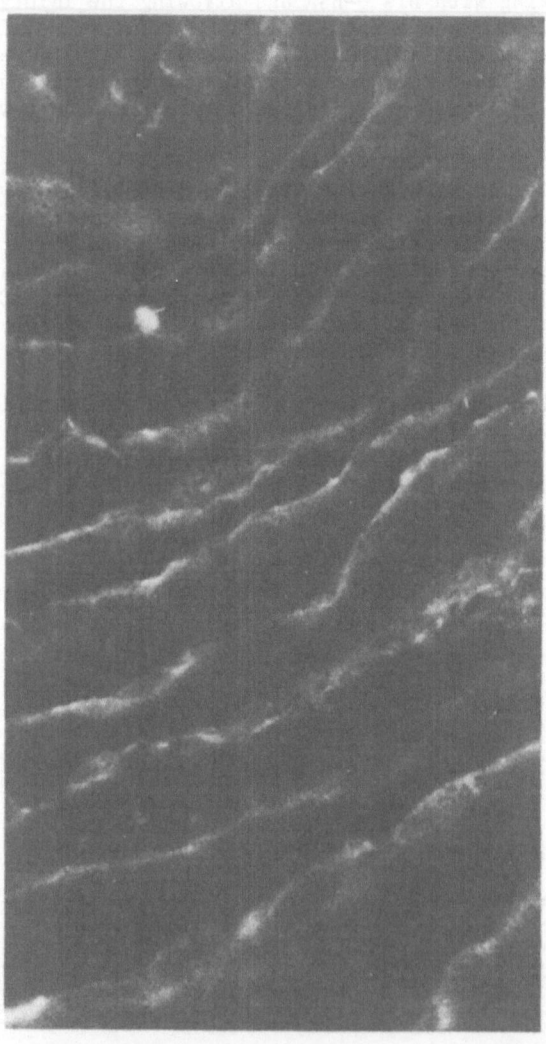

Figure 4.   Immunofluorescence of sectioned tissue of the electric organ of
            Torpedo californica using F8-D5 and fluorescein-tagged rabbit
            anti-mouse globulin.

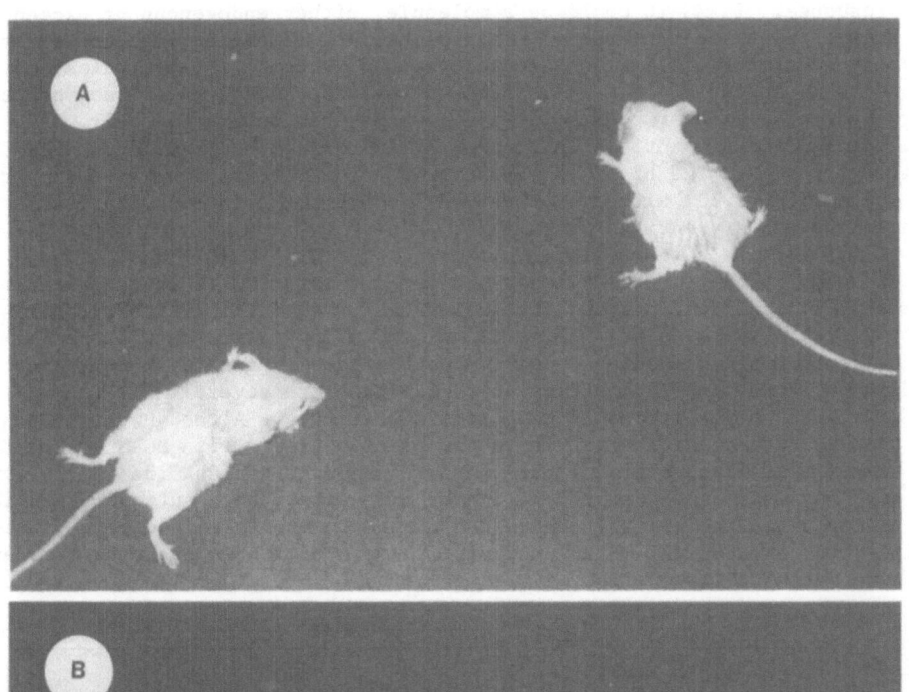

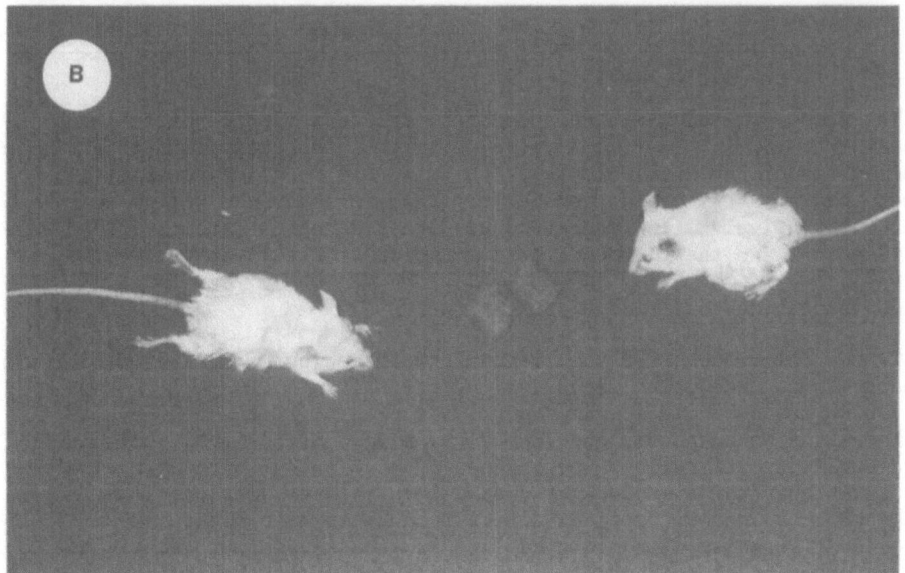

Figure 5. (A) Six 37 day old BALB/c mice (3 males, 3 females) were pristane-treated. Seven days later they were irradiated with 500 rads and on the next day 10^6 cells of F8-D5 were administered i.p. Ascites fluid appeared in the abdomens of both sexes by the 12th day and was collected. By the 14th day the female mice showed signs of severe muscle weakness. Two are shown in the figure. (B) The mice in (A) were treated as follows: one on the right was given neostigmine (66 µg/kg) i.p. and one on the left was injected i.p. with an equal volume of water. After an interval of 30 minutes, the mice appeared as shown, i.e., the mouse on the right showed sufficient strength to stand and to attempt to approach food. The mouse on the left showed no improvement. After about an additional 40 minutes the mouse on the right weakened and resembled the other one.

primary antigen responsible for the subsequent pathological auto-anti-idiotypic response. In MG it could be a molecule, either endogenous or exogenous,
that shares idiotypic features with acetylcholine. Examples might be other
naturally occurring choline-containing compounds such as the lecithins, or
components of bacterial cell walls such as the phosphocholine of pneumococcal
C carbohydrate. Another possibility is a virus that enters the cell via
AChR. Anti-idiotypic antibodies to the anti-viral antibody would then be
specific for AChR. The highly interesting studies with rabies virus support
this suggestion (8,30) although of course, we are not proposing that rabies
virus is the primary antigen in MG.

Finally, if the auto-anti-idiotypic mechanism for MG is to be taken
seriously, it is most important that evidence for anti-idiotypic antibodies
reactive with AChR be seen in patients with MG. In this respect there is
good evidence that antibodies specific for the combining site of AChR are
found in patients with MG, particularly when they are severely ill (22).
Anti-idiotypic antibodies would have this specificity. Although, it is true
that the majority of antibodies in the serum of patients with MG are directed
at a "main immunogenic region (MIR)" on the α subunit of AChR (32), a region
that does not include the acetylcholine binding site, these antibodies could
have arisen after the primary damage was caused by the anti-idiotypic (anti-
binding site) antibodies, with subsequent release of AChR-containing membrane
fragments into the circulation.

The Universality of the Auto-Anti-Idiotypic Strategy for the Production of Monoclonal Anti-Receptor Antibodies

The auto-anti-idiotypic approach has yielded a monoclonal anti-AChR
antibody that in many functional aspects, mimics the activities of anti-AChR
raised by immunizing with receptor. An important question to answer is
whether this strategy can be applied to other receptors as well. We can
answer affirmatively with respect to two other receptor systems, the adenosine receptors and the glucocorticoid receptor of rat liver cytosol.

The Adenosine Receptors

We have also succeeded in extending the monoclonal auto-anti-idiotypic
procedure to the adenosine receptors (4,7,12,21,50,55).

Adenosine is a potent, endogenous pharmacologically active regulatory
molecule. Among its reported activities are: a) modulation of the release
of transmitters from a variety of neuronal cell types, including cells of
the electric organs of Torpedo and Electrophoresis electricus (58). ATP is
co-stored in granules with acetylcholine in about equimolar quantities (15,57).
There is evidence that the co-release of ATP and acetylcholine into the synaptic cleft is followed by hydrolysis of ATP to adenosine, which, by interaction with an adenosine receptor on the presynaptic surface, inhibits further
release of acetylcholine and ATP. b) Adenosine has a role in the regulation
of blood flow to the heart (2), brain (3), skeletal muscle (5), and other
tissues, by causing vasodilation. c) There is evidence that adenosine functions as a neurotransmitter (35), particularly in the hypothalamus and in
the striatum (54).

Most of the effects of adenosine are inhibited by caffeine and other
xanthine derivatives which act as antagonists for receptors of adenosine.

Two types of adenosine receptors have been identified on the outer surface of cytoplasmic membranes: A_1 or Ri, which, by interaction with adenosine, causes a decrease in adenylate cyclase activity, and A_2 (or Ra) which,
when bound to adenosine, leads to an increase in adenylate cyclase activity.
The specificities of the two types of receptors require that the 2' and 3'

hydroxyl groups of the ribose moiety of adenosine and other agonists be intact. The receptors differ in their affinities for effector molecules. The A_1 receptor is a high affinity (nanomolar concentrations) receptor for adenosine. N^6-(L-phenyl-isopropyl) adenosine (L-PIA) and N^6-cyclohexyladenosine (CHA) bind to A_1 with a higher affinity than adenosine (6,47); 5'-N-ethyl-carboxamidoadenosine (NECA) binds to the A_1 receptor with a lower affinity than that of adenosine. The binding affinity of L-PIA is 100 times greater than that of the D-isomer.

The A_2 receptor has a lower affininty for adenosine (micro-molar concentrations) and the potency of various adenosine analogues is NECA > adenosine L-PIA. The stereospecificity of the A_2 receptor for L-PIA is much less than that of the A_1 receptor (37), i.e., the D-isomer also binds well.

There are, as yet, no reports of success in the isolation of an adenosine receptor in a pure or highly purified state. Binding studies have all been done on very crude membrane or detergent solubilized preparations. Apparently there have been some unsuccessful attempts using affinity chromatography. Two laboratories have recently reported the successful labeling of the A_1 receptor with photoaffinity reagents (10,48). In one case, chick cerebellum tissues were the source of the receptor and a protein of a M_r-36,000 was labeled. In the other case, cerebral cortex tissue and adipocyte membranes were the targets of the photoaffinity label; a protein of M_r-38,000 was labeled. We have made considerable progress with the anti-idiotypic strategy.

Our strategy in preparing anti-idiotypic antibodies that react with adenosine receptors called for immunization of BALB/c mice with a bovine serum albumin (BSA) conjugate of adenosine N^6-caproic acid (ACA-BSA) which was prepared by an adaptation of a procedure of Zemlicki and Sorm (56). The protocol we then followed was essentially identical to the one we used for the AChR system, except that screening for anti-anti-adenosine (by ELISA) was for binding to a specifically purified rabbit anti-adenosine produced by immunization with ACA-BSA. Two clones were isolated, A218 and A221 which bound to a partially purified adenosine receptor preparation (34), the binding of which could be inhibited by L-phenylisopropyladenosine (L-PIA), an adenosine receptor agonist.

When the membrane proteins were solubilized with 1% cholic acid and analyzed by SDS-PAGE and Western blotting, both A2 18 and A2 21 recognized a 62kD band under non-reducing conditions. Under reducing conditions, binding to 53kD and 36kD bands occurred. The latter band has also been seen by photoaffinity labeling (10,48).

The Glucocorticoid Receptor of Rat Liver Cytosol

The ligand we chose to use in these studies (9) is a derivative of triamcinolone (TA), a potent synthetic glucocorticoid. It was converted to a 5-ketohexanoic N-hydroxysuccinimide ester (TKH) which, in turn, can be coupled to the amino groups of proteins (Figure 6). The steroid-protein conjugates (18) are then suitable immunogens to elicit anti-steroid antibodies and, presumably, via the idiotypic network to yield anti-anti-steroid.

Immunization of BALB/c mice with a thyroglobulin conjugate of TA, TKH-thyroglobulin, following our usual protocol (11), resulted in five hybridoma lines that secreted antibody, that bound to Fab fragments of a specifically purified polyclonal rabbit anti-TA. Antibody from one of these clones, 8G11-C6, depleted rat liver cytosol of glucocorticoid receptor. This was determined by passing a rat liver cytosol preparation over a column of anti-mouse IgM beads to which 8G11-6, an IgM was adsorbed.

The binding of 8G11-C6 antibody to Fab fragments of rabbit anti-TA was not inhibited by TA, but was inhibited by rabbit serum albumin (RSA) conjugates of TA (TKH-RSA) and deoxycorticosterone-RSA (Figure 7). Less inhibition was seen with RSA conjugates of cortisone, testosterone and essentially none with an RSA conjugate of 17-B estradiol. This pattern is in accord with what was found to be the binding affinities to rabbit anti-TA (not shown).

Binding of 8G11-C6 to anti-steroid was completely inhibited by rat liver cytosol preparations, crude and partially purified (9), indicating homology in their respective combining sites. To characterize 8G11-C6 antibody further, Western blotting experiments were carried out. A major reactive band with a molecular weight of about 87,000 was seen (Figure 7). This is consistent with the observations of others that purified transformed glucocorticoid receptor has a molecular weight anywhere from 78,000 to 90,000 (9). Moreover, it agrees with the results of a recent report of the sequence of the gene for the human glucocorticoid receptor (27). As noted above, neither the binding of 8G11-C6 to anti-TA nor to receptor was inhibited by TA. Thus in neither case did the antibody appear to be directed at the respective combining sites. In order to "map" the antibody's target site, inhibition studies were carried out with protein and oligopeptide derivatives of TA (TKH proteins and peptides). The results appear in Table 1. Binding of 8G11-C6 antibody to anti-TA was inhibited by the appropriate TKH conjugates and by molecules as small as TKH lysine. Binding to the receptor on the other hand, although inhibited by the appropriate TKH protein conjugates, was not inhibited by peptides as large as TKH-hexapeptide.

Thus the anti-idiotypic antibody, 8G11-C6, is specific for an epitope in or in close vicinity to the combining site of anti-TA but at a further distance from the binding site of the glucocorticoid receptor (see next section).

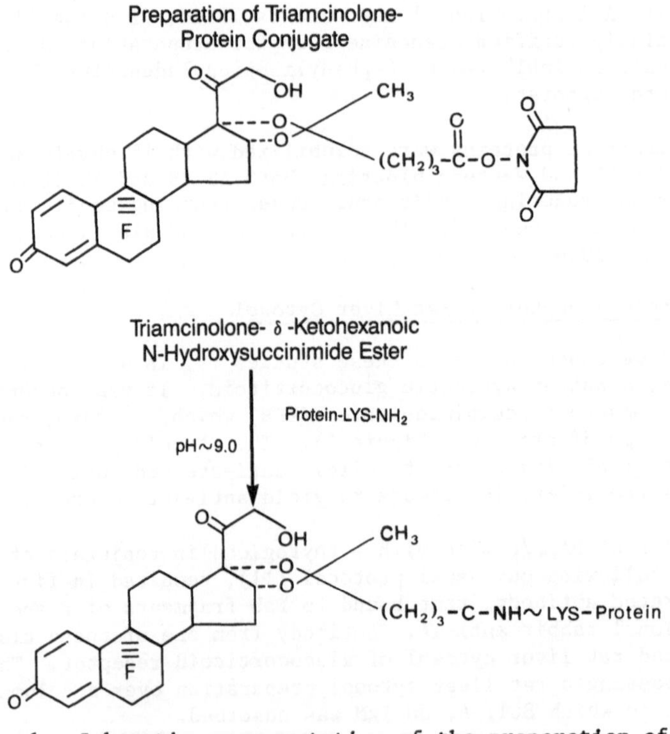

Figure 6. Schematic representation of the preparation of the triamcinolone-protein conjugates.

In an attempt to estimate the distance of the target epitope of 8G11-C6 from the binding site of the receptor, a TA derivative of the B chain of insulin was prepared and tested as an inhibitor. Inhibition of binding was seen, although the pattern was too complex to be consistent with a classical competitive process. Surprisingly, insulin, which was used as a control, was a competitive inhibitor with an apparent K_I of 0.7×10^{-5} M. When the reaction was examined in detail, it was found that the glucocorticoid receptor and insulin shared an epitope recognizable by 8G11-C6.

The glucocorticoid receptor has recently been cloned and sequenced (27, 33). It was of interest, therefore, to examine its sequence for homology with the B chain of insulin. This was done by a computer search employing the program, ALIGN, which uses a version of the Needleman and Wunsch algorithm (36) and a mutation data matrix (14,46) for detecting relationships between protein sequences. The results are shown in Figure 8.

Regions in the glucocorticoid receptor and in the B-chain of insulin that could be cross-reactive epitopes include amino acids 105-108 of the receptor and 1-4 of the B-chain. In this case, two of four amino acids are identical and a third pair, Asn and Gln, are highly homologous structures.

Homologies can also be seen upon comparison of residues 5-14 of B-chain and 285-294 of the glucocorticoid receptor. The match of the Cys residues should be noted. Moreover, rat insulin B-chain has a Pro at position 9,

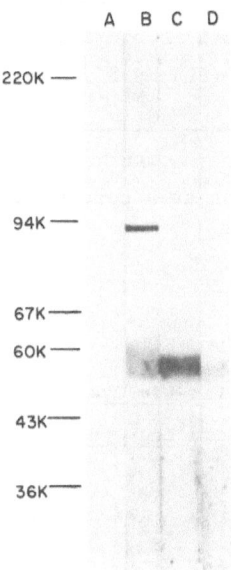

Figure 7. Western blots of rat liver glucocorticoid receptor using the anti-idiotype, 8G11-C6. The glucocorticoid receptor was partially purified by ammonium sulfate precipitation, resolved on SDS-polyacrylamide gels, electroblotted onto introcellulose and immunostained alkaline phosphate-labeled rabbit anti-mouse Ig. Lane A: Control - no antibody. Lane B: Anti-idiotype (8G11-C6) to the glucocorticoid receptor. Lane C: Anti-idiotype (A²-21), to the adenosine receptor. Lane D: Anti-idiotype (D-2), to TSH receptor. Standard proteins employed as molecular weight markers included Ferritin (subunit), phosphorylase b, Albumin, Catalase, and ovalbumin, the MW value of these proteins is indicated to the left of the gel.

Table 1. A Comparison of the Inhibition of Binding of the Anti-Idiotype of 8G11-C$_6$ to Either the Antisteroid or to the Glucocorticoid Receptor

	I_{50}(M) Antisteroid	I_{50}(M) Glucocorticoid Receptor
Steroid-RSA Conjugate		
TKH-RSA	7×10^{-7}	7×10^{-7}
Deoxycorticosterone	7×10^{-7}	7×10^{-7}
Cortisone-RSA	7×10^{-6}	ND
Testosterone-RSA	2×10^{-4}	2.9×10^{-4} (30%)
Estradiol-17B-RSA	2.5×10^{-4} (30%)	NI
TKH-Peptide Conjugate		
TKH Lysine	4.8×10^{-4}	ND
TKH Gly-Lys OH	3.8×10^{-4}	NI
TKH Gly-Lys-Gly OH	2.3×10^{-4}	NI
TKH Lys-Lys-Lys OH	6.7×10^{-4}	ND
TKH Ala-Lys-Ala-Ala-Ala OH (5L)	3.5×10^{-4}	NI
TKH Ala-Lys-Ala-Ala-Ala OH (LDLLL)	3.3×10^{-4}	NI
TKH Ala-Ala-Ala-Ala-Ala-Ala OH (6L)	9.5×10^{-4}	NI

ND – not done; NI = no inhibition at a concentration > 2.5×10^{-4} M

```
            1             4    5              10            14
Hu B-Chain  Phe Val Asn  Gln  ──  His Leu Cys Gly Ser* His Leu Val Glu Ala ──
                                           x          x   x   x   x
Hu-Gluc.    Phe Pro Gln  Gln  /  Glu Leu Cys Thr Pro  Gly Val Ile Lys Glu /
            105         108    285                                        294

            15            21         22            25
Hu-B Chain  Leu Tyr Leu Val Cys Gly Glu**  ──  Arg Gly Phe Phe ──
                x               x             x
Hu-Gluc.    Leu Cys Leu Val Cys Ser Asp  /  Lys Val Phe Phe /
            420                 426         442         445

            26            30
Hu B-Chain  Tyr Thr Pro Lys Ala·
                x   x
Hu-Gluc.    Phe Ala Pro Asp Leu·
            623             627
```

*Pro in Rat Insulin
**Asp in Fish and Guinea Pig Insulins
ˣOne base change in the triplet yields identity.

Figure 8. Structural homologies between insulin B-chain and the glucocorticoid receptor.

instead of Ser (45), an identical match with position of 289 of the glucocorticoid receptor.

A more striking comparison is between sequence 15-21 of insulin and
420-426 of the glucocorticoid receptor, part of its DNA binding domain (27).
In this case, four out of seven (including Cys) are identical, with others,
Gly-Glu, residues 20 and 21, respectively, in the B-chain, and Ser-Asp,
residues 425 and 426 in the receptor, having structural homology. It should
also be noted that both fish and guinea pig insulin B-chains have Asp
instead of Glu at position 21 (45).

Sequence 22 to 25 of the B-chain on insulin and 442-445 of the receptor,
also in its DNA-binding domain (27) are also likely candidates as cross-reactive epitopes. The sequence Phe-Phe is shared by both and Arg in the B-
chain matches with Lys in the receptor.

At this time, the data are insufficient to identify the cross-reacting
epitope. This question can be approached by synthesizing the homologous
peptide sequences, and determining their ability to inhibit the reaction of
antibody with glucocorticoid receptor.

Can we attach any biological significance to the various regions of
homology in insulin and the glucocorticoid receptor? According to the alignment score of the computer program (ALIGN), the homologies found have no
significance beyond what would be found in 100 random run comparisons, in
particular because of penalties accorded the many sequence gaps in the glucocorticoid receptor. On the other hand, identity is seen in 37% of the matched
residues, with the Cys residues in phase. If we equate Arg with Lys, Glu
with Asp, Gln with Asn, Phe with Tyr and Ileu and Leu and Val, then we have
identity and homology in 17 of 30 residues, or 57%. The same comparative
analysis of bovine and guinea pig insulins yields only a 70% homology (21 of
30 amino acids). Moreover, it is interesting to note that single base changes
in triplet codons would make sequences 442-445 of the glucocorticoid receptor
and to 22-25 of the B chain of insulin identical with respect to three out
of four amino acids. Six out of seven amino acid residues in 420-426 of the
receptor would match sequence 15-21 of insulin, i.e., Cys would become Tyr
and Asp would be Glu; and seven out of ten residues of 285-294 of the receptor
would match 5-14 of the B-chain of insulin. There is also the aforementioned
sequence homology around the Cys residues of the B-chain of insulin and the
glucocorticoid receptor.

The relationships discussed above are, to a considerable degree, specula-
tive. Nevertheless, they stem from a clear observation, namely that a monoclonal antibody specific for glucocorticoid receptor binds the B-chain of
insulin. Future studies will be aimed at identifying the cross-reactive
epitope and at examining cross-specificities of other receptor-specific and
insulin-specific antibodies.

What Does an Anti-Idiotypic Antibody Recognize?

We have raised antibodies to the combining sites of anti-ligand antibodies by exploiting a normally functioning idiotypic network. Subsets of
the anti-idiotypic network have been found to bind to receptors of the ligand.
In two cases, when adenosine or Bis Q were the ligands, binding of the anti-
idiotypic antibody to the receptor was competitively inhibited by ligand.
In the case of the glucocorticoid receptor, this was not true. On the other
hand, in all cases, binding of the anti-idiotype to idiotype was inhibited
by ligand or low molecular weight derivatives of the ligand.

There are idiotype-anti-idiotype interactions that are not inhibited by
the specific ligand. These have been explained as being "non-combining site

specific" (16), i.e., interactions with epitopes not directly involved in
the binding interaction. This designation could also apply to our anti-glucocorticoid receptor antibody, 8G11-C6, with respect to its reaction with
receptor. On the other hand, it is difficult to imagine why an epitope not
associated with the binding site of the receptor would share homology with
an epitope in or very near to the binding site of the anti-steroid, the idiotypic antibody. In fact, the rationale of the auto-anti-idiotypic strategy
would tend to eliminate this interpretation.

The conceptual difficulties arise as a result of the simplistic way in
which antibody-combining sites, and binding sites, in general, are customarily
represented, i.e., as a cleft or groove in a solid form. The use of this
archaic representation is misleading and not in accord with our present understanding of the structure of ligand-binding proteins, of which the immunoglobulin molecule is only one example. In reality, the amino acids that directly
participate in the binding interactions also provide idiotopes that can yield
reactions with anti-idiotypic antibodies that need not be inhibited by specific ligands.

As seen in Figure 9, which represents the Fab fragment of mouse myeloma
protein specific for phosphorylcholine (13), most of the complementarity-
determining amino acid residues which function in binding are, on their
"reverse" aspects (i.e., the surfaces not directly involved in binding),
exposed to solution and available as antigenic determinants. Moreover, the
reverse aspects, which are as idiotypic and, in their own way, as reflective
of specificity as the obverse, could very well share determinants with reverse
surfaces of the binding site of a receptor specific for the same ligand.
Anti-idiotypic antibodies directed at these determinants of the antibody,
therefore, could cross-react with receptors specific for the same ligand.
Their reactions might or might not be inhibited by specific ligands, depending
upon the effect of the binding interaction on the integrity of the combining
site. Our anti-glucocorticoid antibody (8G11-C6) may fall into this class.

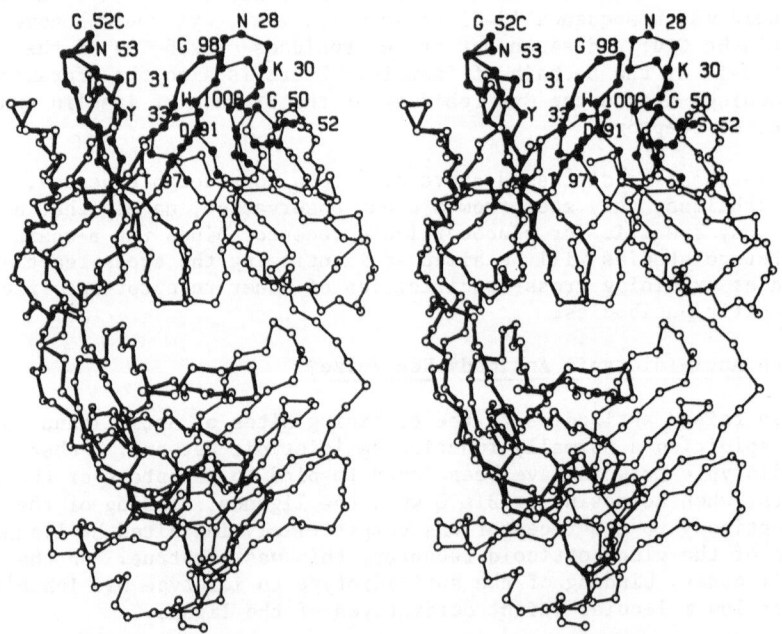

Figure 9. Stereo drawing of α-carbon backbone of McPC603 Fab.
Complementarity-determining residues are shown as filled
circles (14 with permission).

Further studies on the inhibition of the reaction of 8G11-C6 with receptor by ligand derivatives could be fruitful in this regard.

There are anti-idiotypic antibodies that have been designated as "internal images" or homobodies (31,38). They can be identified operationally as antibodies that mimic the ligand in that, for example, they will bind to "all" antibodies that bind that ligand. Our anti-AChR and anti-adenosine receptor antibodies fulfill this requirement in that they bind to their respective receptors and to polyclonal rabbit and monoclonal mouse antibodies, and binding can be completely inhibited by ligand.

Because of the aforementioned "cleft or groove" representation, reservations have been raised about the internal image concept because of the implied requirement that an antibody must insert itself into the "cleft" of another antibody or receptor (41). In fact, an "internal image" antibody could just as well bind by reacting partially with determinants on reverse aspects of the binding site of the receptor or the anti-ligand antibody. For another, but similar, viewpoint on this matter, see Roitt et al. (42).

Among internal images that have been described are anti-idiotypic antibodies that mimic insulin (43) and alprenolol (28,44). It might seem surprising that a protein can mimic a low molecular weight, non-peptide organic compound like alprenolol. On the other hand, antibody specificity is governed by the same physicochemical principles that influence the specificity of other ligand-binding proteins such as enzymes and receptors. With respect to the latter, the endorphins, which are polypeptides, bind to the same receptor as does morphine (25), an alkaloid, i.e., the polypeptide is an image of the alkaloid. Moreover, since proteins can assume complementary conformations that allow binding of an almost infinite variety of molecules and macromolecules, it is not illogical that they can also assume regional conformations which, like the endorphins, act as images of these molecules. Therefore, it should not be surprising if internal image antibodies were to be found that can mimic components of polysaccharides and nucleic acids as well and thereby be recognized by their respective specific binding proteins. As such, they should be extremely useful biological reagents. Moreover, if they are normally present in vivo, there must be consequences with respect to immune regulation and autoimmunity.

ACKNOWLEDGMENTS

This chapter represents research supported by grants from the National Institutes of Health (NS-15581 to B. F. Erlanger and AM 25536 to I. S. Edelman); the Muscular Dystrophy Association (to B. F. Erlanger and A. S. Penn); the New York Heart Association; and a postdoctoral fellowship in the Laboratory of J. Lindstrom to K. K. Wan from the Canadian Medical Research Council.

REFERENCES

1. E. Bartels, N. H. Wassermann, and B. F. Erlanger, Photochromic activators of the acetylcholine receptor, Proc. Natl. Acad. Sic. U.S.A. 68:1820 (1971).
2. R. M. Berne, The role of adenosine in the regulation of coronary blood flow, Circ. Res. 47:807 (1980).
3. R. M. Berne, R. Rubio, and R. R. Curnish, Release of adenosine from ischemic brain effect on cerebral vascular resistance and incorporation into cerebral adenine nucleotides, Circ. Res. 35:262 (1974).
4. R. M. Berne and R. M. Knabb, Adenosine in the local regulation of blood flow - a brief overview, Fed. Proc. 42:3136 (1983).
5. E. L. Bockman, R. M. Berne, and R. Rubio, Adenosine and active hyperemia - dog skeletal muscle, Am. J. Physiol. 230:1531 (1976).

6. R. J. Bruns, J. W. Daly, and S. H. Snyder, Adenosine receptors in brain membranes: binding of N^6-cyclohexyl[^{3}H]adenosine and 1,3-diethyl-8-[^{3}H]phenylxanthine, Proc. Natl. Acad. Sci. U.S.A. 77:5547 (1980).

7. G. Burnstock, Purinergic receptors, J. Theoret. Biol. 62:491 (1976).

8. T. G. Burrage, G. H. Tignor, and A. L. Smith, Rabies virus binding at neuromuscular junctions, Virus. Res. 2:273 (1985).

9. E. Cayanis, R. Rajagopalan, W. L. Cleveland, and I. S. Edelman, Generation of an auto anti-idiotypic antibody that binds to glucocorticoid receptor, J. Biol. Chem. 261:5094 (1986).

10. J. I. Choca, M. M. Kwatra, M. M. Hosey, and R. D. Green, Specific photo-affinity labeling of inhibitory adenosine receptors, Biochem. Biophys. Res. Comm. 131:115 (1985).

11. W. L. Cleveland, N. H. Wasserman, R. Sarangarajan, A. S. Penn, and B. F. Erlanger, Monoclonal antibodies to the acetylcholine receptor by a normally functioning auto-anti-idiotypic mechanism, Nature 305:56 (1983).

12. J. W. Daly, R. F. Bruns, and S. H. Snyder, Adenosine receptors in the central nervous system - relationship to the central actions of methylxanthines, Life Sci. 28:2083 (1981).

13. D. R. Davies and H. Metzger, Structural basis of antibody function, Ann. Rev. Immunol. 1:87 (1983).

14. M. O. Dayhoff, R. M. Schwartz, and B. C. Orcutt, Atlas of protein sequence and structure, Natl. Biomed. Res. Fnd. 5(Suppl. 3):345 (1979).

15. M. J. Dowdall, A. F. Boyne, and V. P. Whittaker, Adenosine triphosphate constituent of cholinergic synaptic vesicles, Biochem. J. 140:1 (1974).

16. K. Eichmann, Expression and function of idiotypes on lymphocytes, Adv. Immunol. 26:195 (1978).

17. B. F. Erlanger, Anti-idiotypic antibodies. What do they recognize. Immunol. Today 6:10 (1985).

18. B. F. Erlanger, F. Borek, S. M. Beiser, and S. Lieberman, Steroid protein conjugates. I. Preparation and characterization of conjugates of bovine serum albumin with testosterone and with cortisone, J. Biol. Chem. 228:713 (1957).

19. B. F. Erlanger, W. L. Cleveland, N. H. Wasserman, B. L. Hill, A. S. Penn, H. H. Ku, and R. Sarangarajan, in: "Molecular Basis of Nerve Activity," W. de Gruyter and Company, Berlin and New York (1985).

20. B. F. Erlanger, N. H. Wasserman, W. L. Cleveland, A. S. Penn, B. L. Hill, and R. Sarangarajan, in: "Monoclonal Antibodies: Probes for Receptor Structure and Functions," A. R. Liss, Inc., New York (1984).

21. I. H. Fox and W. N. Keeley, Role of adenosine and 2'-deoxyadenosine in mammalian cells, Ann. Rev. Biochem. 47:655 (1978).

22. B. W. Fulpius, A. K. Lefvert, S. Cueonoud, and A. Mourey, Properties and serum levels of specific populations of anti-acetylcholine receptor antibodies - myasthenia gravis, Ann. N.Y. Acad. Sci. 377:307 (1981).

23. S. Green, P. Walter, V. Kumar, A. Krust, J. M. Bornert, P. Argos, and P. Chambon, Human oestrogen receptor cDNA: sequence, expression and homology to v-erb-A, Nature 320:134 (1986).

24. G. L. Greene, P. Gilna, M. Waterfield, A. Baker, Y. Hort, and J. Shine, Science 231:1150 (1986).

25. R. Gillemin, Endorphins, brain peptides that act opiates, N. Eng. J. Med. 296:226 (1977).

26. T. Heidmann, and J.-P. Changeux, Structural and functional properties of acetylcholine receptor protein in its purified and membrane-bound states, Ann. Rev. Biochem. 47:317 (1978).

27. S. M. Hollenberg, C. Weinberger, E. S. Ong, G. Cerelli, A. Oro, R. Lebo, E. P. Thompson, M. G. Rosenfeld, and R. M. Evans, Primary structure and expression of a functional human glucocorticoid receptor cDNA, Nature 318:635 (1985).

28. C. J. Homcy, S. G. Rockson, and E. Haber, An anti-idiotypic antibody

that recognizes the beta-adrenergic receptor, J. Clin. Invest. 69:1147 (1982).

29. N. K. Jerne, Towards a network of the immune system, Ann. Immunol. (Inst. Pasteur) 125C:373 (1974).

30. T. L. Lentz, T. G. Burrage, A. L. Smith, J. Crick, and G. H. Tignor, Is the acetylcholine receptor a rabies virus receptor Science 215:182 (1982).

31. J. Lindenmann, Ann. Immunol. (Inst. Pasteur) 130C:311 (1979).

32. J. Lindstrom, S. Tzartos, and W. Gullick, Structure and function of the acetylcholine receptor molecule studied using monoclonal antibodies, Ann. N.Y. Acad. Sci. 377:1 (1981).

33. R. Miesfeld, S. Okret, A.-C. Wilkstrom, O. Wrange, J.-A. Gustafsson, and K. R. Yamamoto, Characterization of a steroid hormone receptor gene and messenger RNA in wild type and mutant cells, Nature 312:779 (1984).

34. C. R. Merrill, D. Goldman, S. A. Sedman, and M. H. Ebert, Ultrasensitive stain for proteins in polyacrylamide gels shows regional variation in cerebrospinal fluid proteins, Science 211:1437 (1981).

35. J. I. Nagy and L. A. LaBella, Immunohistochemistry of adenosine deaminease: implications for adenosine neurotransmission, Science 224:166 (1984).

36. S. B. Needleman and C. D. Wunsch, A general method applicable to search for similarities - amino acid sequence of two proteins, J. Mol. Biol. 48:443 (1970).

37. J. T. Nepom and M. Tardieu, Surv. Immunol. Res. 1:255 (1982).

38. A. Nisonoff and E. Lamoi, Implications of the presence of an internal image of the antigen in anti-idiotypic antibodies - possible application to vaccine production, Clin. Immunol. Immunopathol. 21:397 (1981).

39. Y. Oudin and M. Michael, Immunochimie - une nouvelle forme d'allotypie des globulines gamma du serum de lapian, apparemment liee a la fonction et a la specificite anticorps, C.R. Acad. Sci. (Paris) 257:805 (1963).

40. J. Patrick and J. Lindstrom, Autoimmune response to acetylcholine receptor, Science 180:871 (1973).

41. L. S. Rodkey, Autoregulation of immune responses via idiotype network interactions, Microbiol. Rev. 44:631 (1980).

42. I. M. Roitt, Y. M. Thanavala, D. K. Male, and F. C. Hay, Anti-idiotypes as surrogate antigens - structural considerations, Immunol. Today 6:265 (1985).

43. K. Sege and P. A. Peterson, Use of anti-idiotypic antibodies as cell surface receptor probes, Proc. Natl. Acad. Sci. U.S.A. 75:2443 (1978).

44. A. B. Schreiber, P. O. Couraud, C. Andre, B. Vray, and A. D. Strosberg, Anti-prenolol anti-idiotypic antibodies bind to beta-adrenergic receptors and modulate catecholamine-sensitive adenylate cyclase, Proc. Natl. Acad. Sci. U.S.A. 77:7385 (1980).

45. J. A. Schroer, T. Bender, R. J. Feldmann, and K. J. Kim, Mapping epitopes of the insulin molecule using monoclonal antibodies, Eur. J. Immunol. 13:693 (1983).

46. R. M. Schwartz and M. O. Dayhoff, Atlas of protein sequence and structure, Natl. Biomed. Res. Fnd. 5(Suppl. 3):345 (1979).

47. S. J. Snyder, R. F. Bruns, J. N. Daly, and R. B. Innis, Multiple neurotransmitter receptors in the brain: amines, adenosine, and cholecystokinin, Fed. Proc. 40:142 (1981).

48. G. L. Stiles, D. R. Daly, and R. M. Olsson, The Al adenosine receptor identification of the binding subunit by photoaffinity cross linking, J. Biol. Chem. 260:10806 (1985).

49. B. A. Suarez-Isla, K. K. Wan, J. Lindstrom, and M. Montal, Single channel recordings from purified acetylcholine receptors reconstituted in bilayers formed at the tip of patch pipets, Biochemistry 22:2319 (1983).

50. D. Van Calker, M. Muller, and B. Hamprecht, Adenosine regulates via two different types of receptors, the accumulation of cyclic AMP in cultured brain cells, J. Neurochem. 33:999 (1979).

51. N. H. Wasserman, E. Bartels, and B. F. Erlanger, Conformational properties of the acetylcholine receptor as revealed by studies with constrained depolarizing ligands, Proc. Natl. Acad. Sci. U.S.A. 76:256 (1979).

52. N. H. Wasserman, A. S. Penn, P. I. Freimuth, N. Treptow, S. Wentzel, W. L. Cleveland, and B. F. Erlanger, Anti-idiotypic route to anti-acetylcholine receptor antibodies and experimental myasthenia gravis, Proc. Natl. Acad. Sci. U.S.A. 79:4810 (1982).

53. C. Weinberger, S. M. Hollenberg, M. G. Rosenfeld, and R. M. Evans, Domain structure of human glucocorticoid receptor and its relationship to the v-erb-A oncogene product, Nature 318:670 (1986).

54. W. J. Wojcik, and N. H. Neff, Location of adenosine release and adenosine Al receptors to rat striatal neurons, Life Sci. 33:755 (1983).

55. J. Wolf, C. Londos, and D.M.F. Cooper, Adv. Cyc. Nucl. Res. 14:199 (1981).

56. J. Zemlicka and F. Sorm, Nucleic acids components and their analogues. 60. Reaction of dimethylcholoromethyleneammonium chloride with 2',3'5'-tri-O-acetylinosine. A new synthesis of 6-chloro-9-(beta-D-ribofuranosyl) purine, Coll. Czech. Comm. 30:1880 (1965).

57. H. Zimmer and C. R. Denston, Adenosine triphosphate - cholinergic vesicles isolated from the electric organ of Electrophorus electricus, Brain Res. 111:365 (1976).

58. H. Zimmerman and E.J.M. Grondal in: "Molecular Basis of Nerve Activity," J.-P. Changeux, F. Hucho, A. Maelicke, and E. Neumann, eds., W. de Gruyter and Company, Berlin and New York (1985).

IDIOTYPIC INTERACTIONS IN THE TREATMENT OF HUMAN DISEASES

Raif S. Geha

Division of Allergy
The Children's Hospital
Boston, Massachusetts

INTRODUCTION

The importance of the idiotypic network in the regulation of the immune response of experimental animals has been amply established. The role of the idiotypic anti-idiotypic interactions in the regulation of the human immune response to antigen has been less extensively studied. In this review we will discuss data obtained from our laboratory on the role the idiotypic network plays in the regulation of human immunity in health and in disease states.

Anti-Id Antibodies to Human Anti-Tetanus Toxoid Antibodies

The immune response to tetanus toxoid (TT) has been extensively studied because almost all adult donors exhibit in response to TT delayed skin hypersensitivity, T cell proliferation in vitro, and possess substantial serum antibody titers to TT and their peripheral blood lymphocytes, under appropriate conditions, can be shown to synthesize anti-TT antibodies in vitro.

Rabbit anti-Id antibodies have been raised against $F(ab')_2$ fragments of IgG anti-TT and rendered idiotype-specific following appropriate absorptions with autologous TT non-reactive IgG $F(ab')_2$ and with pooled IgG (15,16). These antisera precipitated from 30 to 50% of rabiolabeled immunogen, i.e., ^{125}I $F(ab')_2$ anti-TT (Figure 1). This was not surprising because the human IgG anti-TT response is a heterogeneous one. Thus, idiotypic determinants which are expressed on antibody molecules which are present in very small amounts may not be able to elicit an antibody response. The anti-Id antisera obtained always exhibited vigorous reactivity with sites related to antigen binding because a) TT antigen vigorously inhibited the binding of ^{125}I idiotype to anti-Id (Figure 2); and b) anti-Id inhibited the binding of TT antigen to IgG. The anti-Id antibodies obtained showed poor or little cross reactivity with IgG anti-TT from unrelated donors. Because in initial studies we have absorbed the anti-Id antisera with pooled IgG which contained anti-TT, we may have removed antibodies which recognized cross reactive idiotypes (CRI). We have recently reexamined the presence of CRI using as probes anti-Id antisera which were carefully absorbed with pooled human IgG which was depleted of reactivity to TT antigen. The resulting antisera exhibited variable and weak cross reactivity with IgG anti-TT idiotypes from donors unrelated to the source of the immunizing idiotype. Cross reactivity ranged from 0

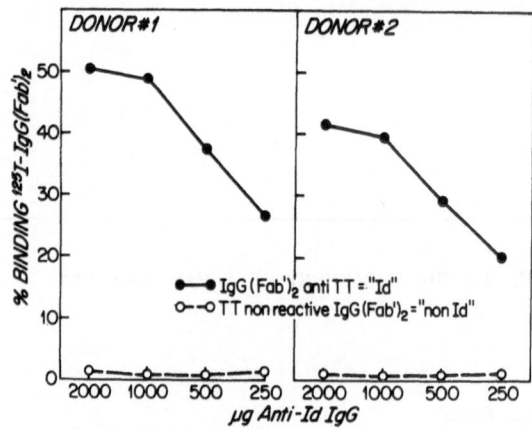

Figure 1. Idiotype binding by rabbit anti-idiotypic IgG. Approximately 50 ng of ^{125}I labeled IgG F(ab')$_2$ anti-TT "idiotype" and of TT nonreactive IgG F(ab')$_2$ "nonidiotype" were added to various amounts of rabbit anti-IgG raised against the "idiotype" of the individual subject. The percent bound was calculated as the ratio of the counts per minute (cpm) precipitated by the anti-Id to the cpm precipitated by rabbit antihuman Fab x 100.

to 20% reactivity of individual antisera of control and averaged from 5 to 10% of control reactivity with various antisera as determined by a) direct binding of anti-I to radiolabeled idiotype of unrelated donors; and b) inhibition by anti-Id of TT binding to IgG anti-TT from unrelated donors.

The relatively small degree of idiotypic cross reactivity of IgG anti-TT idiotypes among unrelated subjects in the IgG anti-TT system is in agreement with the observations of other investigators who studied cross reactive idiotypes on antibodies to foreign proteins from healthy subjects. Altevogt and Wigzell (1) used rabbit anti-Id serum raised against IgG F(ab')$_2$ anti-TT from a single donor and found that only one out of four unrelated donors tested showed cross reactivity. Pasquali et al. (40) analyzed idiotypic

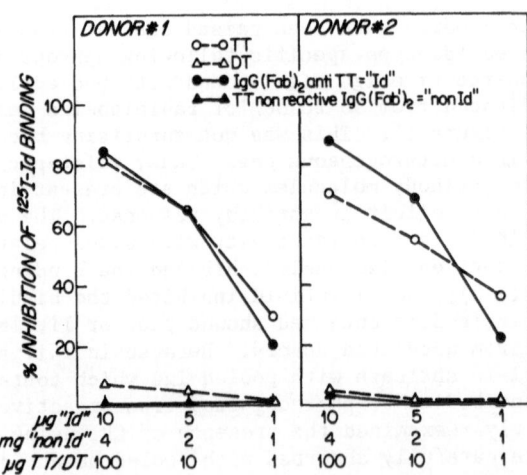

Figure 2. Inhibition of ^{125}I-"idiotype" binding to anti-Id IgG (500 μg) by "idiotype," "nonidiotype," and DT.

136

cross reactivity on IgM rheumatoid factor (RF). Rabbit anti-Id to IgM-RF from a patient with rheumatoid arthritis reacted with the patient's RF but not with ten of 11 polyclonal and monoclonal RF from unrelated individuals. In their study of anti-Rh antibodies, Natvig et al. (37) could detect CRI in only two out of 22 subjects. The results of these studies contrast with those of Cheung et al. (9) who demonstrated CRI on anti-casein antibodies of 12 out of 16 IgA deficient patients detected by a rabbit anti-Id to anti-casein IgG from an index patient. The reason for the high prevalence of CRI in these patients is not clear. It is possibly related to the nature of the antigen studied. In contrast to TT, a high molecular weight bacterial protein, casein is the family of proteins also present in humans which are of varying molecular weights (12,000-24,000) and therefore may present a limited number of immunogenic sites resulting in restricted antibody heterogeneity. This factor may be one reason why autoantibodies tend to share cross reactive determinants. It is also possible that certain V restrictions are linked to IgA deficiency rendering IgA deficient patients more likely to share certain variable region genes, e.g., those used in anti-casein antibodies, than normal subjects. Finally, repeated immunization of IgA deficient patients with casein via their gastrointestinal tracts may have resulted in the selective predominance of anti-casein antibodies with CRI. Predominance of CRI is known to occur after repeated immunization in mice (11). In this regard Bose et al. (3) have presented evidence for CRI in patients repeatedly immunized with ragweed antigen in the course of allergic immunotherapy and Saxon et al. (42) has presented evidence for CRI at the T cell level in subjects repeatedly and vigorously hyperimmunized with TT antigen. It should be noted that in the latter two studies as well as in the anti-casein study the contribution of anti-Id antibodies bearing the "internal image" of antigen has not been assessed.

Studies on cross reactive idiotypes of anti-TT antibodies in two families showed that idiotypic cross reactivity among members was significantly higher than among unrelated subjects. The exact interpretation of CRI among family members is difficult in the absence of primary sequence data. Idiotypic antigens are serologic markers which indirectly identify portions of the variable regions of immunoglobulin light and heavy chains. A central question is whether the idiotypic cross-reactivity observed by serologic methods will be found to be due to similar amino acid V region sequences. In most mouse systems, this has been found to be true. In some instances, a substitution of one amino acid has resulted in major changes in the profile of idiotypic reactivity (41). For human proteins, the V regions of rheumatoid factors of the PO (for Pompa protein) or La (for Lay) proteins are homologous and IgM anti-DNA molecules isolated from sera of different patients with systemic lupus erythematosus also have similar sequences (31). There are, however, exceptions in which idiotypic cross-reactivity of murine antibodies has been found to be due to very small regions, or single amino acids, carbohydrate groups or no sequence homology at all. It seems unlikely, however, that similar variable regions as detected by our anti-Id antisera could be generated in family members exclusively by somatic diversification. The results, rather, suggest the inheritance of antibody genes related to the idiotypic determinants in humans.

Binding of Anti-Id to Human B and T Cells

Rabbit anti-Id IgG was found to bind to 4-10/1,000 human B cells (17). The binding was completely inhibited by cold "idiotype" and partially but specifically inhibited by TT antigen (Table 1). This latter observation suggests that the anti-Id recognized determinants that were related as well as determinants that were unrelated to the antigen binding site. The idiotypic determinants detected on the B cell surface were shown to be synthesized by the B cells because pulsing the B cells with radiolabeled amino acids followed by immunoprecipitation of cell surface proteins with anti-Id resulted

Table 1. Binding of Anti-Idiotypic Antiserum to B Cells

| Donor # | % of cells showing fluorescence with GAHIG-F* after treatment with | | | |
| | Preimmune Rabbit IgG | Post Immune Rabbit IgG | | |
			+TT	F(ab')$_2$ Anti TT
1	0.1	4.8	2.1	0.5
2	0.5	8.1	3.0	0.8
3	0.4	6.6	2.6	1.3
4	0.2	4.3	1.8	0.3
5	0.6	10.5	5.1	1.2

*In each experiment 10,000 cells were counted. Each donor was studied on three separate occasions. F(ab')$_2$ rabbit IgG and F(ab')$_2$ GAHIG were used.

in the precipitation of material which comigrated on SDS gels with immunoglobulin. Preclearing the cell lysate with anti-Ig resulted in the loss of the ability of the anti-Id to precipitate radiolabeled material from the B cells.

Rabbit anti-Id was also capable of binding to human T cells. The frequency of Id + T cells was very low. It ranged from 2-4/1,000 T cells (16). The rabbit anti-idiotypic antibody bound to T cells, and not to B cells that contaminated the T cell preparations. These lines of evidence argued in favor of binding to T cells. First, the frequency of B cells that bind the rabbit anti-Id (anti-TT) was less than 1%. Because the T cell preparations contained less than 1% B cells, idiotype-positive B cells in these preparations would occur at a frequency of less than one per 10,000 cells. This is much lower than the observed frequency of idiotype-positive cells (24 to 38 per 10,000) in the T cell-rich preparations. Second, capping of cell surface immunoglobulins on 70% of B cells by preincubation with GAHIG, a polyclonal goat antihuman immunoglobulin, resulted in a negligible diminution (< 15%) in the frequency of idiotype-positive cells detected in the T cell preparations. Third, double immunofluorescence staining revealed that less than 10% of the Id+ cells had surface Ig.

The binding of rabbit anti-Id to T cells was idiotype specific. It was inhibited by the IgG anti-TT used for immunization and by TT antigen, but not by TT non-reactive IgG nor by DT antigen. TT was less efficient than IgG F(ab')$_2$ anti-TT in inhibiting anti-Id binding to the T cells. This phenomenon was previously seen with B cells and may reflect the presence of shared idiotypes on receptor molecules that differ in their specificity for antigen (13,23,39).

The partial, rather than complete, inhibition of anti-Id binding to T cells by IgG anti-TT contrasts with the complete inhibition seen in the case of the B cells. It is possible that after its injection into the rabbit, IgG F(ab')$_2$ anti-TT dissociated into H and L chains that then induced anti-V_H and anti-V_L antibodies. Either of these classes of antibodies could potentially react with T cells, and not with B cells. Such a reaction would not be inhibited by undissociated IgG F(ab')$_2$ anti-TT. In this regard, expression of V_H-related idiotypes, rather than $V_H \neq V_L$ idiotypes by T cells has been reported (8,29).

The reactivity of anti-Id antisera with T cells suggested that the idiotypic determinants expressed by T cells were shared with those expressed by

B cells and by serum antibody. It is possible, however, that circulating T cell-derived antigen-specific material co-purified with the IgG anti-TT used to raise the anti-Id as suggested by the work of Iverson et al. (10) and Cone et al. (25). If that was the case, then the rabbit antiserum could have contained both anti-T cell Id reactivity and anti-B cell Id reactivity, and these two reactivities could be directed against unrelated determinants. Two lines of evidence argue against the presence of antibodies directed against T cell-derived antigen-specific material in the rabbit antiserum. First, the IgG F(ab')$_2$ anti-TT used for immunization of the rabbits resolved in only one band on PAGE. Second, absorption with EBV transformed B cells derived from the IgG F(ab')$_2$ anti-TT donors, but not with B cells from an unrelated donor, removed the reactivity of the anti-Id antiserum with T cells (Figure 3).

In experimental animals there is strong evidence to suggest that B and T cells share idiotypic determinants because polyclonal as well as some mono-clonal antibodies to highly purified myeloma proteins with known antigenic specificity bind to suppressor T cells and to suppressor T cell hybridomas and their soluble factors (7,36). Sharing of idiotypic determinants between T and B cells, however, does not imply structural similarity of their antigen receptor at the primary amino acid sequence level but simply implies similarity in the three dimensional structure of their antigen receptors. Indeed, it is now abundantly clear that Id+ T cells do not express V_H gene products (28,30,36). Precedents for cross reactivity of antibody with molecules that have different primary amino acid structures are well known: a case in point is the cross reactivity of anti-idiotypic antibodies to anti-retrovirus 3 hemagglutinin with the receptor for the hemagglutinin expressed on somatic cells (38).

Idiotypic determinants were expressed on T8+ cells but not on T4+ cells (Table 2). T8+ cells have been reported to bind directly to antigen (33)

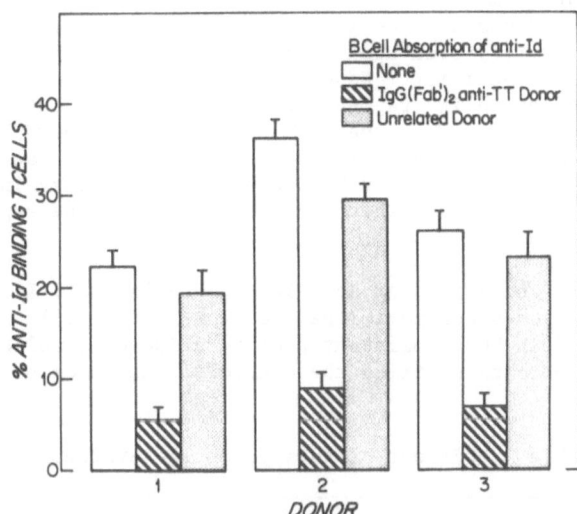

Figure 3. Effect of adsorption of anti-Id antisera on their reactivity with T cells. The antisera were absorbed with no cells, EBV-B cells derived from the IgG F(ab')$_2$ anti-TT donor, or EBV-B cells derived from an unrelated donor. The antisera were then tested by indirect immunofluorescence for their capacity to specifically bind to T cells from the IgG F(ab')$_2$ anti-TT donor. The number of fluorescent T cells is shown on the ordinate; the donor tested is shown on the abscissa (from 16).

Table 2. Distribution of T Cells Specifically Binding Rabbit Anti-Id[a]

T Cells	Subject 1	Subject 2	Subject 3
Unfractionated	28[b]	37	30
T4+	3	3	4
T8+	61	90	87

[a]The frequency of positive cells represents the difference between the frequency of cells binding FITC-GAHIG after preincubation with rabbit anti-Id IgG F(ab')$_2$ minus the frequency of cells binding FITC-GAHIG after reincubation with rabbit preimmune IgG F(ab')$_2$. The latter never exceeded 1 per 10,000.
[b]Immunofluorescent cells per ten thousand cells.

and anti-V$_H$ antibodies and to inhibit antigen binding to human T cells (32). T8+ cells contain predominantly suppressor and cytotoxic cells. Both types of cells have been shown in experimental animals to express idiotypic determinants (7,38,49).

Effect of Heterologous Anti-Id on the Human Immune Response

Rabbit anti-Id antibodies to human IgG anti-TT have demonstrable effect on the TT-specific immune response by B and T cells in vitro. Anti-Id IgG was found to inhibit the pokeweed mitogen driven (PWM) production of IgG anti-TT antibodies by peripheral blood mononuclear cells (Table 3). Anti-Id also inhibited IgG anti-TT antibody production in B cells stimulated with supernatants of PWM stimulated T cells demonstrating that anti-Id can exert direct inhibitory effects on B cells. Anti-Id IgG by itself induced no Ig synthesis in B cells (17) even upon addition of T cell supernatants known to certain BCGF and BCDF activity. However, when anti-Id antibodies were digested with pepsin and their fragments were used to stimulate B cells, there was induction of IgG anti-TT synthesis upon addition of BCGF/BCDF containing supernatants (Brozek et al. unpublished observations). These results demonstrate that anti-Id antibodies can have opposite modulatory influences on human B cells and suggest that they can play a role in the regulation of the human immune response.

In addition to the effect of anti-Id on B cells, anti-Id had demonstrated effects on the antigen-specific immune T cell response (16). Anti-Id by itself caused a modest but consistent proliferation of T cells with stimulation indices of two to three times the control. The major effect of anti-Id

Table 3. Effect of Anti-Id on IgG Synthesis

Stimulus	Total IgG	Immunoglobulin Synthesis	
		IgG anti-TT	IgG anti-DT
Medium	210	< 10	< 10
Anti-Id IgG	180	< 10	< 10
PWM	13,500	187	86
PWM + anti-Id IgG	12,800	82	80

Table 4. Induction of Suppressor T Cells by Anti-Idiotypic Antibody[a]

Subject #	Preincubation of T Cells Added to the Culture	Proliferation of Culture Stimulated with:		
		--	TT	DT
1	Medium	187±63[b]	14,556±1,280	13,782±583
	Rabbit Preimmune IgG	196±28	13,533± 622	13,805±497
	Rabbit Anti-Id IgG	265±41	8,677± 447	13,725±721
2	Medium	585±36	17,503±1,105	8,615±263
	Rabbit Preimmune IgG	643±28	16,825± 648	9,376±408
	Rabbit Anti-Id IgG	609±64	9,672± 579	8,861±225
3	Medium	428±45	12,392± 272	10,706±320
	Rabbit Preimmune IgG	531±43	12,014± 380	9,814±286
	Rabbit Anti-Id IgG	516±29	7,631± 549	9,356±351

[a]T cells were preincubated for 2 days with rabbit IgG (250 µg/ml) were washed and were added at a 1:1 ratio to untreated, autologous T cells in the presence of 20% autologous monocytes. Results represent mean ± S.E. of triplicate cultures. Values underlined were significantly different ($p < 0.05$) from controls.
[b]Counts per minute of (^{3}H) thymidine incorporated per culture.

Table 5. Induction of Suppressor T Cells by Anti-Idiotypic Activity[a]

Donor #	Preincubation of T Cells Added to the Culture	IgG Anti-TT (ng/ml) in TT-stimulated Cultures	IgG Anti-DT(ng/ml) in DT-stimulated Cultures
1	Medium	126 ± 9	84 ± 7
	Rabbit Preimmune IgG	115 ± 12	81 ± 11
	Rabbit Anti-Id IgG	78 ± 6	80 ± 8
2	Medium	89 ± 8	67 ± 14
	Rabbit Preimmune IgG	93 ± 10	65 ± 8
	Rabbit Anti-Id IgG	56 ± 4	62 ± 9
3	Medium	95 ± 11	77 ± 5
	Rabbit Preimmune IgG	88 ± 6	81 ± 12
	Rabbit Anti-Id IgG	53 ± 7	75 ± 8

[a]Results represent mean ± S.E. of triplicate cultures. T cells were preincubated for 2 days with rabbit IgG (250 µg/ml), were washed and added to autologous T and B cells at a ratio of 2:2:1 and the cultures were stimulated 4 days with antigen (TT and DT, 20 ml), were washed and recultured for 8 days. Supernatants were then collected and assayed for IgG anti-TT and IgG anti-DT. Cultures not stimulated with antigen made neither IgG anti-TT nor IgG anti-DT. IgG anti-TT was present only in TT primed cultures and IgG anti-DT was present only in DT primed cultures.

on T cells was that it induced substantial antigen-specific suppressor cell activity. The targets of this suppression were antigen-induced T cell proliferation (Table 4) and antigen-driven helper T cell-dependent antibody synthesis by B cells (Table 5). In the case of proliferation the target of suppression would be a T cell, although a role for the monocytes in the delivery of the suppressor signals cannot be excluded. In the case of antidriven antibody synthesis, T and B cells could have been the targets of suppression.

It was also demonstrated that Id+ T cells can exert suppressor activity in the presence of antigen alone. Removal of Id+ cells on anti-Id coated plates resulted in the enhancement of T cell proliferation and helper function. Suppression of immune response by antigen-binding Lyt-2+ T cells has been described in experimental animals (44).

The Auto Anti-Id Antibodies in the Normal Human Immune Response

Auto anti-Id to anti-TT antibodies were demonstrated in the circulation of normal adults following booster immunization with TT. IgG (18) capable of binding autologous IgG F(ab')$_2$ anti-TT, derived from serum obtained seven and ten days after immunization, was detectable in the serum by the end of the second week post-immunization (Figure 4). This binding was shown to be idiotype-specific and not to result from rheumatoid factor-like activity. Auto anti-Id antibodies detected at different intervals post-immunization recognized overlapping but also different idiotypes on IgG F(ab')$_2$ anti-TT obtained shortly post-immunization (day 7-10).

Auto anti-Id IgG was shown to recognize idiotypic determinants involved in TT binding because IgG taken eight weeks and more after immunization and

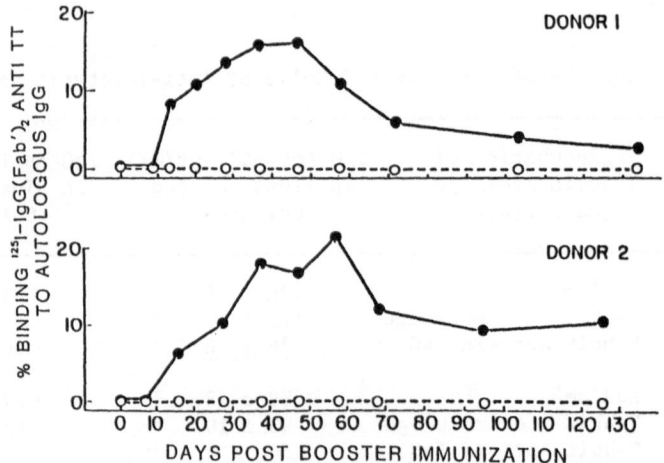

Figure 4. Binding of ^{125}I IgG F(ab')$_2$ anti-TT to autologous IgG determined by precipitation with S. aureus. Numbers on the abscissa represent the days post-booster immunization with TT. The numbers on the ordinate represent percent binding of 20 ng (50,000 cpm) of ^{125}I IgG F(ab')$_2$ anti-TT (0—0) and of 20 ng of ^{125}I TT nonreactive IgG F(ab')$_2$ (●—●) to 250 µg of autologous IgG. Percent binding was calculated by using as total binding the amount of IgG F(ab')$_2$ bound by rabbit anti-human Fab. In the case of IgG F(ab')$_2$ anti-TT, the amount bound to Sepharose 4B TT was almost (>90%) equivalent to the total binding. The cpm of ^{125}I IgG F(ab')$_2$ anti-TT bound to S. aureus alone was 190 cpm in donor 1 and 85 cpm in donor 2. All tests were done in triplicate and repeated twice (from 15).

depleted of anti-TT reactivity specifically inhibited the binding of ^{125}I TT to autologous IgG collected at days 7 and 10 post-immunization. Significant auto anti-Id activity was still detectable in both assays (idiotype binding and inhibition of TT antigen binding) at the end of the study period four months post-immunization. In experimental animals the duration of the auto anti-Id response has been reported to vary in length from two weeks to a few months (eight to 15). This variability probably results from difference in antigens used for immunization, modes of immunization, and sensitivity of the assays used to detect auto anti-Id antibody. Our findings of a prolonged auto anti-Id response after booster immunization with TT may be due to a long life of anti-Id antibody-secreting B cells and/or to continuous stimulation of anti-Id synthesis by free antibody and/or by idiotype-bearing cells.

To study the modulation of the expression of idiotypes by circulating IgG after immunization with TT, a rabbit anti-Id antibody was used as a probe. This rabbit anti-Id was raised against IgG F(ab')$_2$ anti-TT present at days seven and ten post-immunization, i.e., against "early" anti-TT idiotypes. The antiserum precipitated only 35 to 40% of the immunizing IgG F(ab')$_2$ anti-TT. The reactivity of this anti-Id with IgG diminished starting two weeks post-immunization and bottomed at about two months post-immunization at a time of peak auto anti-Id activity (Figure 5) indicating a decrease in the level of "early" anti-TT idiotypes. The decrease in the expression of "early" anti-TT idiotypes was long-lasting, for it remained evident for four months after booster immunization, a time by which the levels of auto anti-Id were greatly reduced. Although the mechanisms responsible for this long-lasting modulation of idiotype expression remain unknown, it is clear that the decrease in the expression of "early" anti-TT idiotypes took place concomitantly with the appearance of auto anti-Id antibody. These results and those of Schrater and co-workers (43) in the mouse suggest that the auto anti-Id response may have contributed to the modulation of idiotype expression observed after booster immunization with TT.

The modulation of idiotype expression after immunization with TT must not have been limited to a decrease in the levels of some of the "early"

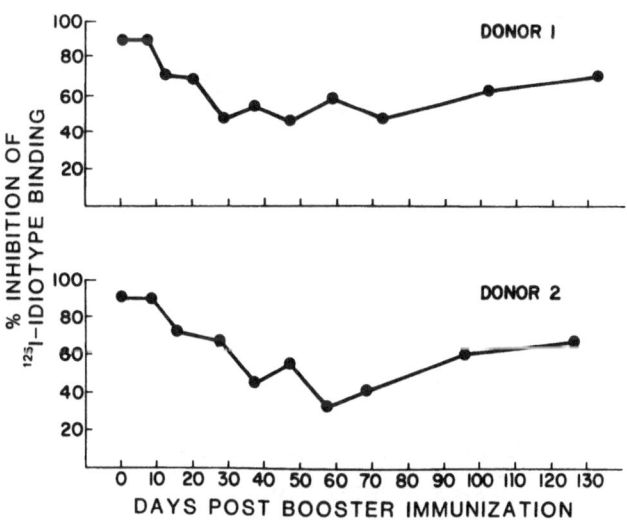

Figure 5.   Inhibition of the binding of ^{125}I "idiotype" [IgG F(ab')$_2$ anti-TT] to rabbit anti-idiotypic IgG derived from the idiotype donor. In these experiments 500 µg of rabbit anti-Id-IgG and 20 ng (3000 to 5000 cpm/ng) of ^{125}I idiotype were used. IgG from the idiotype donor was used in the amount of 250 µg (from 15).

anti-TT idiotypes, because this decrease occurred in the face of a rise in hemagglutinating IgG antibody titers. Thus, it is quite probable that there was a concomitant increase in the levels of other anti-TT idiotypes. Similar conclusions were reached previously by MacDonald and Nisonoff (34) in their longitudinal study of idiotype expression in rabbits separately immunized with the p-azo benzoate hapten.

The presence of circulating auto anti-Id was associated with the presence of circulating Id binding cells. Indeed, circulating cells capable of binding autologous IgG F(ab')$_2$ anti-TT appeared by the third week after boosting and remained detectable throughout the three to four-month study period (Figure 6). The frequency of idiotype binding cells paralleled more or less the magnitude of the serum auto anti-Id antibody response, which suggests that auto anti-Id bearing cells can remain activated for prolonged periods of time after immunization.

Because of the presence of auto anti-Id antibody in the serum, great care was taken to ascertain that the binding of autologous IgG F(ab')$_2$ anti-TT to peripheral blood lymphocytes (PBL) was not due to passively absorbed auto anti-Id. Since idiotype binding cells could be detected after treatment of the PBL with trypsin and after overnight incubation to allow for the shedding of passively absorbed immunoglobulins, it is safe to conclude that passively absorbed auto anti-Id did not play a significant role in the experiments. This was further confirmed by the demonstration that pokeweed mitogen (PWM) could induce the synthesis of auto anti-Id in vitro.

The idiotype binding cells detected were predominantly B cells. Very few idiotype binding T cells were detected. This, however, should not be interpreted to indicate absence of auto anti-Id bearing T cells. In experimental animals several investigators have presented evidence for auto anti-Id bearing T cells. Tasiaux and associates (45) have detected by immunofluorescent techniques auto anti-Id bearing cells in rabbits immunized repeatedly with tobacco mosaic virus. Janeway and co-workers (26) and Woodland and

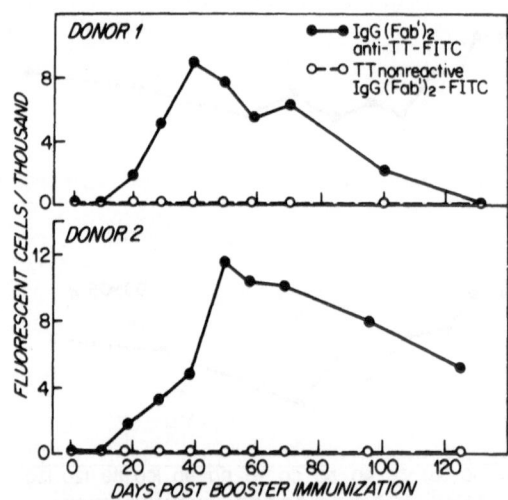

Figure 6. Binding of nonadherent peripheral blood lymphocytes to fluorescein-conjugated autologous IgG F(ab')$_2$. Numbers on the abscissa represent days after booster immunization with TT. Numbers on the ordinate represent the frequency of cells staining with autologous IgG F(ab')$_2$ anti-TT (O—O) and autologus TT-non-reactive IgG F(ab')$_2$ (●--●) (from 18).

Cantor (50) have presented functional evidence for a T helper cell that recognizes idiotypes expressed on B cells and Ju and associates (27) and Weinberger and co-workers (48) have presented evidence for anti-idiotype bearing suppressor effector T cells.

A direct effect of auto anti-Id on TT antigen-specific antibody synthesis could be demonstrated. Auto anti-Id (day 38 IgG, Figure 4) partially but significantly inhibited the PWM-induced and the spontaneous synthesis of anti-TT antibody by PBL taken shortly (ten days) after immunization (Figure 7). The inhibition of anti-TT synthesis by auto anti-Id was antigen-specific and idiotype-specific. Since auto anti-Id antibody recognizes only a fraction of the idiotypes expressed IgG anti-TT and presumably only a fraction of the anti-TT idiotypes expressed by PBL taken shortly after immunization, its effect on total IgG anti-TT synthesis was only a partial effect, albeit a significant one. It was directly demonstrated that the synthesis of those idiotypes that were recognized by the auto anti-Id antibody was the one predominantly affected. Anti-TT synthesis by PBL present in the circulation at the same time as the auto anti-Id antibody was not affected by that antibody (Figure 7), which suggests that some anti-TT idiotypes expressed by PBL early after immunization are no longer expressed later in the course of the immune response.

In contrast to TT antigen, which stimulates anti-TT synthesis at low doses (47), auto anti-Id failed to stimulate anti-TT synthesis when added at low concentrations to cultures of PBL taken at day 0 or day 10 post-immunization. This may have resulted from the failure of auto anti-Id antibody to activate TT-specific helper T cells and/or because of selective activation of suppressor T cells. In this regard there is evidence that the TT determinants recognized by helper T cells differ from those recognized by serum

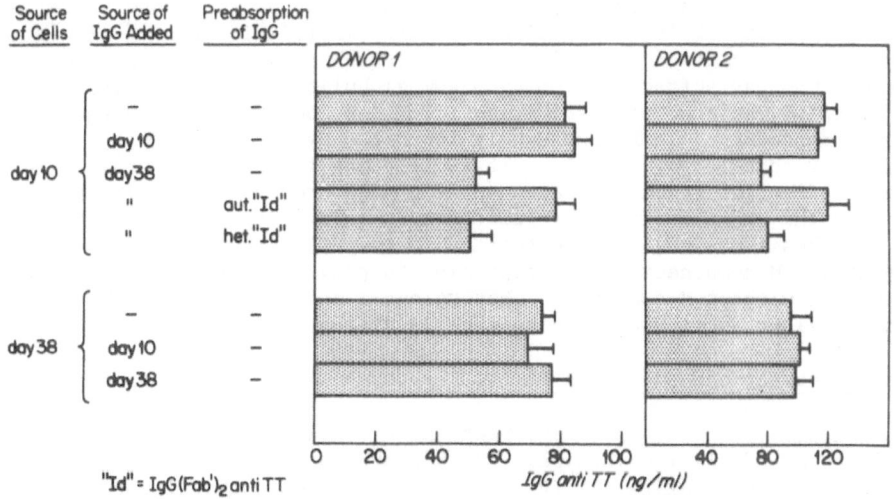

"Id" = IgG (Fab')₂ anti TT

IgG anti TT (ng/ml)

Figure 7. Effect of IgG taken post-immunization on IgG anti-TT synthesis by PWM-stimulated autologous PBL. Taken 10 days after and 38 days after booster immunization with TT in the two subjects studied. Number of days represent days elapsed after booster immunization. Values represent mean ± SD of triplicate cultures. IgG samples tested for the capacity to inhibit IgG anti-TT synthesis were preabsorbed extensively with Sepharose 4B-TT. Absorptions with "Id", i.e., IgG F(ab')₂ anti-TT, were performed by absorbing 2.5 mg of IgG in 1 ml of PBS with 0.25 mg of IgG F(ab')₂ anti-TT cross linked to 0.25 ml of Sepharose 4B (from 18).

Table 6. In Vitro Synthesis of IgG and M Component
by PBL of Patient with M Component

Culture Period	Stimulus	Inhibitor	^{3}H Counts per Minute precipitated by*	
			Anti-IgG	Anti-Id**
0-19 h	none	---	1,755 ± 474	1,419 ± 426
120-168 h	none	---	2,619 ± 448	2,360 ± 584
		Anti-idiotypic IgG	624 ± 190 (p < 0.05)	422 ± 206 (p < 0.05)
		Anti-idiotypic IgG F(ab')$_2$	2,167 ± 668	1,857 ± 343

*Counts per minute of specific radioactivity precipitated from 1/10 of 1 ml
of PBL culture fluid supernates (4 x 10^6 PBL/ml). Values represent mean ±
SD of two replicate cultures; the supernate of each was tested in duplicate.
**Id = anti-M component idiotype.

antibody to TT (4). Although anti-Id antibody cross reacts with TT determinants recognized by antibody, it is likely that it does not cross react with
those determinants recognized by the helper T cells and hence fails to activate these T cells.

Auto Anti-Id Antibody in Abnormal Human Immune Responses

The relatively frequent presence of serum immunoglobulin M components
in patients with immunodeficiency raises the question as to whether a deficient idiotype network in such patients results in failure to self-regulate
immunoglobulin production by anti-Id. In one such patient who was extensively
studied and who was suffering from hypogammaglobulinemia the majority of
circulating IgG was accounted for by an IgG$_1$K component. In vitro synthesis
of this M component could be profoundly inhibited by anti-idiotypic IgG
raised in a rabbit (35) (Table 6). It is tempting to speculate that failure
to make an effective regulatory auto anti-Id response in this immunodeficient
patient set the stage for the unregulated synthesis of the M component.
Such a hypothesis may not only be applicable to patients with general immunodeficiency and M component but perhaps also to patients with B cell proliferation with or without M component. Heterologous anti-Id has been shown to
inhibit B cell production of M components in vitro in some of these patients.

Idiotypic Interactions and the Allergic Response

In animals IgE antibodies have been shown to share idiotypic determinants
with antibodies of the IgG isotype. Furthermore, anti-Id antibodies have
been shown to down-regulate the IgE antibody response in experimental animals
(2,12).

Sharing of idiotypic determinants between IgE antibodies and IgG antibodies has also been shown in humans (19). Indeed, rabbit anti-Id antibodies
to human IgG anti-TT elicited a Prausnitz-Kustner reaction in sites of the
forearms of normal subjects sensitized with IgG anti-TT antibodies derived
from the same donor of the IgG anti-TT antibodies used for immunization (Table
7). It was very important in these studies to ascertain that the material
used to raise the anti-Id consisted solely of IgG anti-TT and was not contaminated with IgE anti-TT. This was done by absorbing the immunosorbent
purified IgG F(ab')$_2$ anti-TT with Sepharose anti-IgE prior to its injection

Table 7. Elicitation of P-K Reactions by Antigen and by Anti-Id Antibody

Sensitizing Fraction	IgG mg/ml	IgE ng/ml	Maximal Dilution of Sensitizing Fraction Resulting in Positive P-K Reaction Following Challenge:		
			TT	Anti-Id IgG	Grass
Normal saline	--	--	<1:10	<1:10	<1:10
Serum	10.8	1,920	1:500	1:100	1:1000
Serum, heat-treated (56°, 1 h)	ND	ND	<1:10	<1:10	<1:10
Ig-rich fraction (50% ammonium sulfate cut)	9.2	1,430	1:500	1:100	1:1000
Ig-rich fraction not bound to the anti-IgE column	9.0	12	<1:10	<1:10	<1:10
IgE-rich fraction eluted from the anti-IgE column (IgE-rich fraction)	7×10^{-2}	1,280	1:500	1:100	1:1000

All serum fractions were prepared from the serum of the donor against whose $F(ab')_2$ anti-TT the anti-Id was raised. Each P-K test was performed on at least two separate occasions at a 10 day interval using the same recipient with exactly the same results. All readings were done blinded. ND = not detectable.

Table 8. Effect of Anti-Id IgG on IgE Synthesis

Source of PBL	Addition to the Culture	Total pg/ml	IgE Synthesis Anti-TT U/ml	Anti-AgE U/ml
Donor 1	Preimmune IgG	1,870 ± 80	232 ± 17	357 ± 20
	Anti-Id IgG	1,607 ± 115	163 ± 8 ($p < 0.02$)	326 ± 18
Donor 2	Preimmune IgG	2,446 ± 85	228 ± 16	273 ± 21
	Anti-Id IgG	2,377 ± 101	121 ± 13 ($p < 0.02$)	284 ± 14
Donor 3	Preimmune IgG	318 ± 37	120 ± 10	---
	Anti-Id IgG	258 ± 25	77 ± 8 ($p < 0.05$)	

Values represent mean ± SD of triplicate cultures. Rabbit IgG was added at a concentration of 1 mg/ml for the first 48 h of culture, then the cells were washed and recultured at a concentration of 2×10^6 viable cells/ml for additional days. Anti-Id was directed against IgG anti-TT. All three donors had serum IgE anti-TT.

into the rabbit. The resultant injected material contained no detectable IgE. Thus the elicitation of a wheal and flare reaction by the anti-Id in skin sites sensitized with serum from the "idiotype" donor was indeed due to shared Id determinants between IgG and IgE.

Like in the case of IgG, anti-Id antibodies were demonstrated to inhibit the antigen-specific IgE antibody response in vitro (20). Lymphocytes from donors whose serum contained IgE antibodies to TT synthesized IgE anti-TT in vitro spontaneously following immunization. This synthesis was inhibited upon addition of anti-Id antibodies (Table 8). The target of anti-Id suppression appeared to be B cells as well as radio-sensitive T cells. Indeed, anti-Id inhibited IgE anti-TT synthesis by cultures of purified B cells. Furthermore, T cells preincubated with anti-Id, then washed, inhibited IgE anti-TT synthesis by B cell cultures.

Repeated immunization with antigen appears to be conducive to the production of auto anti-Id as previously discussed. Perhaps this is because complexes of antigen and Id are particularly immunogenic. Allergic diseases involve repeated stimulation by antigen either naturally or in the course of immunotherapy. Thus, the presence of auto anti-Id antibodies to allergen-specific antibodies in humans would be expected. Auto anti-Id has been described in isolated allergic patients receiving immunotherapy (3). In a rather large series Castracane and associates (6) have reported the presence of auto anti-Id to ragweed antibodies in normal subjects (n=12) and, to a lesser extent, in untreated allergic subjects (n=13). In allergic subjects treated with immunotherapy (n=7) the level of auto anti-Id appeared to go up to the normal range. These results suggested that decreased production of auto anti-Id in allergic subjects allows the escape of IgE antibody synthesis from immunoregulatory influences.

Allergen-specific antibodies have been, in general, found to share cross reactive idiotype CRI (3,6). These CRI may be the result of a limited number of V genes committed to the antibody response to allergens which are proteins of rather low molecular weight. CRI may be further heightened by repeated antigenic stimulation which, in animals, leads to the emergence of dominant idiotypes (11). It must be noted, however, that the presence of anti-Id antibodies bearing internal image of antigen in anti-Id reagents and/or poor absorption of antibodies directed against a non-hypervariable region of the V domain represented in a small proportion of human immunoglobulins (31) may have contributed to the high degree of idiotypic cross reactivity observed in some studies.

Taken together, the data discussed strongly suggest a role for auto anti-Id antibody in the regulation of the allergic response. Longitudinal

Table 9. Reactivity of Serum IgG with Autologous B Cells from a Patient with Acquired C1 Esterase Deficiency and Chronic Lymphocytic Leukemia and from a Normal Subject

Source of B Cells	Trypsin Treatment	Surface Isotype % Positive Cells with		Anti-Idiotype Reactivity % Positive Cells with			
				Patient IgG		Normal IgG	
		anti μ	anti γ	total	Δ	total	Δ
Patient	–	73	16	53	37	18	2
	+	25	12	70	58	14	2
Normal Subject	–	70	7	12	5	7	0

studies that examine the level of auto anti-Id, the modulation of idiotypes on allergen-specific IgE and the effect of auto anti-Id on IgE synthesis still need to be performed.

Auto Anti-Id Antibody in Acquired Cl Esterase Inhibitor Deficiency

A potential complication of B cell tumor therapy with anti-idiotypic antibody could be the development of the syndrome of acquired Cl esterase inhibitor deficiency and angioneurotic edema. This syndrome has been described in adult patients suffering from a variety of B cell malignancies (5,22). It is characterized by decreased levels of Cl esterase inhibitor Cl, C2, and C4 but with normal levels of C3. Anti-idiotypic antibodies directed against circulating monoclonal immunoglobulins present on the surface of the B cell tumors (Table 9) and in circulation (Figure 8) have been demonstrated in this syndrome (21). The interaction of anti-Id with idiotype leads to deposition of Clq on the surface of the B cells (Figure 9).

Cl inhibitor binds covalently to Clr and Cls and dissociates them from Clq. This disassembly of macromolecular Cl results in the formation of Clr-Cls-Cl-inhibitor complexes, which have been detected in the serum of some patients, including patients with acquired Cl-inhibitor deficiency. The rate of Cl-inhibitor consumption in these patients is almost twice the rate in normal controls or in patients with hereditary angioedema.

The activation of C4 and C2 in patients with acquired angioedema and Cl-inhibitor deficiency does not result in the formation of an effective classical-pathway C3 convertase (C4b2a), and consequently C3 and all the later-acting components are present in normal amounts in the serum of these patients. This aberrant fixation of complement by the idiotype-anti-idiotype complex may be due to one or more of several factors. It is apparent that, in some cases, the ratio of idiotype to anti-idiotype is very high and the reaction is well into the zone of antigen excess. Under such circumstances it might be expected from studies with IgG oligomers that the kinetics of Cl fixation would be relatively slow (14,46). Since the rate of Cl-Cl inhibitor interaction is very rapid, Cl-inhibitor may be preferentially consumed (51).

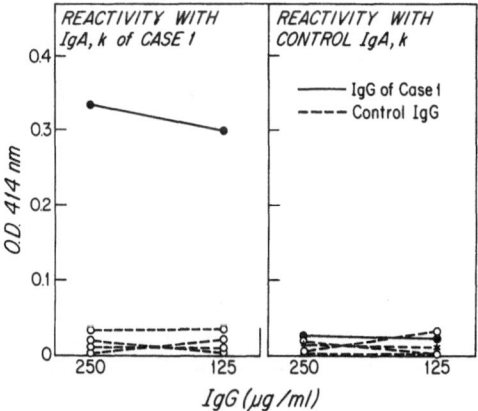

Figure 8. Reactivity of serum IgG from patient 1 and from four control patients, who had IgA multiple myeloma and normal levels of Cl inhibitor, with IgA M components isolated from patient 1 (panel A) and from one of the control patients (panel B). The asterisks at the bottom of panel B identify the control patient whose IgA was used. Results similar to those shown in panel B were obtained when IgA M components from the other three control patients were studied (from 21).

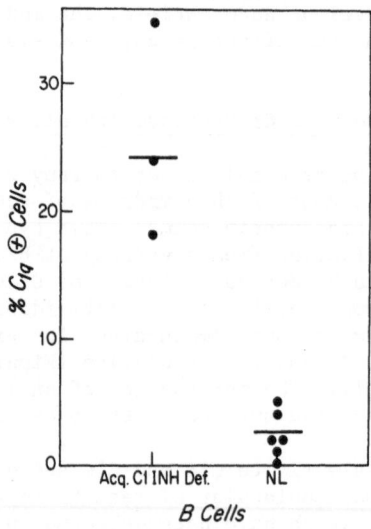

Figure 9. Percentage of circulating E-rosette-negative (B) cells bearing
C1q, and determined by indirect immunofluorescence with mouse
monoclonal antibody to C1q and goat antimouse IgG-FITC (fluores-
cein isothiocyanate). Background staining of B cells with mouse
ascites and goat anti-mouse IgG-FITC was always less than 5% and
was subtracted from the experimental value (from 21).

However, since these patients have very low levels of C4, such slow C1
activation does not appear to be a sufficient explanation for the findings
observed. It is possible that the stereochemistry of Fab-Fab interactions
as in an idiotype-anti-idiotype complex, could impede the formation of C4b2a
complexes or render them exquisitely susceptible to attack by the control
proteins, C4b-binding protein and C3b/C4b inactivator (factor I), so that
rapid decay of the classical pathway C3 convertase C4b2a is induced. It is
also possible that regulatory elements integral to the B cell membrane,
where idiotype-anti-idiotype interactions take place, impede the formation
of C3 convertase (24). The outcome of these events is the failure of C3
activation.

CONCLUSION

It is clear that idiotypic-anti-idiotypic interactions play an important
role in the regulation of the human humoral and cell mediated immune response.
Like all regulatory mechanisms, idiotype-anti-idiotypic interactions may be
protective to the individual, e.g., dampening the magnitude of undesirable
responses such as the IgE allergic response, coating monoclonal malignant
cells with antibody rendering them better targets for destruction. In other
situations, these interactions may be harmful, e.g., formation of idiotypic-
anti-idiotypic complexes in circulation, as in systemic lupus erythematosus
and their potential deposition in vital tissues such as kidney and the potential for anti-idiotypic antibodies to antitransmitter or antihormone antibodies to act on antireceptor antibodies and, therefore, to function as agonists or antagonists. An understanding of idiotypic-anti-idiotypic interactions is important in the devising of therapeutic strategies as discussed
elsewhere in this book for the treatment of tumors, for vaccination and in
the treatment of autoimmune disease.

REFERENCES

1. P. Altevogt and H. Wigzell, V_H-associated idiotype in human anti-tetanus antibodies, Scand. J. Immunol. 17:183 (1983).
2. K. Blaser, T. Nakagawa, and A. L. DeWeck, Suppression of the benzyl-penicilloyl (BPO) specific IgE formation with isologous anti-idiotypic antibodies in BALB/c mice, J. Immunol. 125:24 (1980).
3. R. Bose, D. G. Marsh, J. Duchateau, A. H. Sehon, and G. Delespesse, Demonstration of auto anti-idiotypic antibody cross reacting with public idiotypic determinants in the serum of rye-sensitive allergic patients, J. Immunol. 135:2474 (1984).
4. M. D. Broff, M. E. Jonsen, and R. S. Geha, Nature of the immunogenic moiety recognized by the human T cell proliferating in response to tetanus toxoid antigen, Eur. J. Med. 11:365 (1981).
5. J. R. Caldwell, S. Ruddy, P. H. Schur, and K. F. Austen, Acquired C1 deficiency in lymphosarcoma, Clin. Immunol. Immunopathol. 1:39 (1972).
6. J. M. Castracane, T. J. Hall, and J. E. Rocklin, Generation of anti-idiotypic (aId) antibodies in ragweed sensitive patients under-going specific immunotherapy, Clin. Res. 608A (1985).
7. J. Cerny, C. Heusser, R. Wallich, G. J. Hammerling, and D. D. Eardley, Immunoglobulin idiotypes expressed by T cells. I. Expression of dis-tinct idiotypes detected by monoclonal antibodies on antigen-specific suppressor T cells, J. Exp. Med. 156:719 (1982).
8. T. C. Chanh and M. D. Cooper, T cell hybrids that express a V_H idiotype-related determinant on a glycoprotein distinct from H-2, Thy-1, and Lyt-1 molecules, J. Exp. Med. 158:452 (1983).
9. M.K.L. Cheung and C. Cunningham-Rundles, Cross reactive idiotypes in immunoglobulin A-deficient sera, J. Clin. Invest. 75:1722 (1985).
10. R. E. Cone, R. W. Rosenstein, J. H. Murray, G. M. Iverson, W. Ptaz, and R. K. Gershon, Characterization of T cell surface proteins bound by heterologous antisera to antigen-specific T cell products, Proc. Natl. Acad. Sci. U.S.A. 78:6411 (1981).
11. J. D. Conger, G. K. Lewis, and J. W. Goodman, Idiotype profile of an immune response. I. Contrasts in idiotypic dominance between primary and secondary responses and between IgM and IgG plaque-forming cells, J. Exp. Med. 17:173 (1981).
12. A. Dessein, S. Ju, M. D. Dorf, B. Benacerraf, and R. N. Germain, IgG response to synthetic polypeptide antigens. II. Idiotypic analysis of the IgE response to L-glutamic acid-L-alanine-L-tyrosine (GAT), J. Immunol. 124:71 (1980).
13. K. Eichmann, A. Coutinho, and F. Melcher, Absolute frequencies of lipopolysaccharide-reactive B cells producing A5A idiotype in unprimed, streptococcal A carbohydrate-primed, anti-A5A idiotype-sensitive and anti-A5A idiotype-suppressed A/J mice, J. Exp. Med. 146:1436 (1977).
14. G. Füst, G. A. Medgyesi, E. Rajnavölgyi, M. Csésci-Nagy, K. Czikora, and J. Gergely, Possible mechanisms of the first step of the classical complement activation pathway: binding and activation of C1, Immunology 35:873 (1978).
15. R. S. Geha, Detection of auto anti-idiotypic antibody during the normal human immune response to tetanus toxoid antigen, J. Immunol. 129(1):139 (1982).
16. R. S. Geha, Idiotypic determinants on human T cells and modulation of human T cell responses by anti-idiotypic antibodies, J. Immunol. 133:1846 (1984).
17. R. S. Geha, Expression of idiotypic determinants on human B cells and modulation of human B cell activation by anti-idiotypic antibodies, in: "Human B Lymphocyte Function. Activation and Regulation," A. S. Fauci and R. E. Ballieux, eds., Raven Press, New York (1982).
18. R. S. Geha, Presence of circulating anti-idiotype bearing cells after booster immunization with tetanus toxoid (TT) and inhibition of anti-TT antibody synthesis by auto-anti-idiotypic antibody, J. Immunol. 130:1634 (1983).

19. R. S. Geha, Elicitation of the Prausnitz-Kustner reaction by anti-idiotypic antibodies, J. Clin. Invest. 69:735 (1982).

20. R. S. Geha and M. Comunale, Regulation of immunoglobulin E antibody synthesis in man by anti-idiotypic antibodies, J. Clin. Invest. 71:46 (1983).

21. R. S. Geha, I. Quinti, K. F. Austen, M. Cicardi, A. Sheffer, and F. S. Rosen, Acquired C1-inhibitor deficiency associated with anti-idiotypic antibody to monoclonal immunoglobulins, N. Eng. J. Med. 312:534 (1985).

22. J. A. Gelfand, G. R. Boss, C. L. Conley, R. Reinhart, and M. M. Frank, Acquired C1 esterase inhibitor deficiency and angioedema: a review, Medicine 58:321 (1979).

23. B. Goldberg, W. E. Paul, and C. A. Bona, Idiotype-anti-idiotype regulation. IV. Expression of common regulation idiotypes on fructosan-binding and non-fructosan-binding monoclonal immunoglobulin, J. Exp. Med. 158:515 (1983).

24. K. Iida and V. Nussenzweig, Functional properties of membrane-associated complement receptor CR1, J. Immunol. 130:1876 (1983).

25. G. M. Iverson, D. D. Eardley, C. A. Janeway, and R. K. Gershon, Use of anti-idiotype immunosorbents to isolate circulating antigen-specific T cell-derived molecules from hyperimmune sera, Proc. Natl. Acad. Sci. U.S.A. 80:1435 (1983).

26. C. A. Janeway, Jr., D. L. Bert, and F. W. Shen, Cell cooperation during in vivo anti-hapten antibody responses. V. Two synergistic Ly-1+23-helper T cells with distinctive specificities, Eur. J. Immunol. 10:231 (1980).

27. S. T. Ju, F. L. Owen, and A. Nisonoff, Structure of immunosuppression of a cross-reactive idiotype associated with anti-p-azophenylarsonate antibodies to strain A mice, Cold Spring Harbor Symp. Quant. Biol. 41:699 (1976).

28. E. Kraig, M. Kronenberg, J. A. Kapp, C. W. Pierce, A. F. Abruzzini, C. M. Sorensen, L. E. Samelson, R. H. Schwartz, and L. E. Hood, T and B cells that recognize the same antigen do not transcribe similar heavy chain variable region gene segments, J. Exp. Med. 158:192 (1983).

29. U. Krawinkel, M. Cramer, T. Imanishi-Kari, R. S. Jack, K. Kajewsky, and O. Makela, Isolated hapten-binding receptors of sensitized lymphocytes. I. Receptors from nylon wool-enriched mouse T lymphocytes lack serological markers of immunoglobulin constant domain but express heavy chain variable portions, Eur. J. Immunol. 8:566 (1977).

30. M. E. Kronenberg, E. Kraig, G. Siu, J. A. Kapp, J. Kappler, P. Marrack, C. W. Pierce, and L. Hood, Three T cells hybridomas do not contain detectable heavy chain variable gene transcripts, J. Exp. Med. 158:210 (1983).

31. H. G Kunkel, Cross-reacting idiotypes in the human system, in: "Biology of Idiotypes," M. Green and A. Nisonoff, eds., Plenum Publishing Corporation, New York (1984).

32. T. Lea and T. E. Michaelsen, Anti-V$_H$ antibodies interfere with antigen binding by human T lymphocyates, Clin. Exp. Immunol. 49:657 (1982).

33. T. Lehner, Antigen-binding human T suppressor cells and their association with HLA-DR locus, Eur. J. Immunol. 13:370 (1983).

34. A. B. MacDonald and A. Nisonoff, Quantitative investigations of idiotype antibodies. III. Persistence and variations in idiotypic specificities during the course of immunization, J. Exp. Med. 131:583 (1970).

35. F. Mudawwar, Z. Awdeh, K. Ault, and R. S. Geha, Regulation of monoclonal immunoglobulin G synthesis by anti-idiotypic antibody in a patient with hypogammaglobulinemia, J. Clin. Invest. 65:1201 (1980).

36. K. Nakanishi, K. Sugimura, Y. Yaoita, K. Maeda, S. Kashiwamura, T. Honjo, and T. Kishimoto, A T15-idiotype-positive T suppressor hybridoma does not use the T15 V$_H$ gene segment, Proc. Natl. Acad. Sci. U.S.A. 79:6984 (1982).

37. J. B. Natvig, H. G. Kunkel, R. E. Rosenfield, J. F. Dalton, and S.

Kochwa, Idiotypic specificities of anti-Rh antibodies, *J*. *Immunol*. 116:1536 (1976).

38. J. T. Nepom, H. L. Weiner, M. A. Dichter, M. Tardieu, D. R. Spriggs, C. F. Gramm, M. L. Powers, B. N. Fields, and M. I. Greene, Identification of a hemmaglutinin specific idiotype associated with reovirus recognition shared by lymphoids and neural cells, J. Exp. Med. 155:155 (1982).

39. J. Oudin and P. A. Cazenave, Similar idiotypic specificities in immunoglobulin fractions with different antibody function or even without detectable antibody function, Proc. Natl. Acad. Sci. U.S.A. 68:2616 (1971).

40. J.-L. Pasquali, S. Fong, C. Tsoukas, J. H. Vaughn, and D. A. Carson, Inheritance of immunoglobulin M rheumatoid-factor idiotypes, J. Clin. Invest. 66:863 (1980).

41. A. Radbruch, S. Zaiss, C. Kappen, M. Bruggemann, K. Beyreuther, and K. Rajewski, Drastic change in idiotype but not antigen binding specificity of autoantibodies by a single amino acid substitution, Nature 315:506 (1985).

42. A. Saxon and E. Barnett, Human auto-anti-idiotype regulating T cell-mediated reactivity to tetanus toxoid, J. Clin. Invest. 73:343 (1984).

43. A. F. Schrater, E. A. Goidl, G. J. Thorbecke, and G. W. Siskind, Production of auto-anti-idiotypic antibody during the normal immune response to TNP-Ficoll. I. Occurrence in AKR/J and BALB/c mice of hapten-augmentable, anti-TNP plaque-forming cells and their accelerated appearance in recipients of immune spleen cells, J. Exp. Med. 150:138 (1979).

44. M. Taniguchi and J.F.A.P. Miller, Enrichment of specific suppressor T cells and characterization of their surface markers, J. Exp. Med. 146:1450 (1977).

45. N. Tasiaux, R. Leuwenkroon, C. Bryuns, and J. Urbain, Possible occurrence and meaning of lymphocytes bearing auto-anti-idiotypic receptors during the immune response, Eur. J. Immunol. 8:464 (1978).

46. J. Tschopp, Kinetics of activation of the first component of complement (c1) by IgG oligomers, Mol. Immunol. 19:651 (1982).

47. D. J. Volkman, H. C. Lane, and A. S. Fauci, Antigen induced in vitro antibody production by humans: a model for B cell activation and immunoregulation, Proc. Natl. Acad. Sci. U.S.A. 78:2528 (1981).

48. J. Z. Weinberger, R. N. Germain, B. Benacerraf, and M. E. Dorf, Hapten-specific T cell responses to 4-hydroxy-3-nitrophenyl acetyl. V. Role of idiotypes in the suppressor pathway, J. Exp. Med. 152:161 (1980).

49. J. Z. Weinberger, R. N. Germain, S. I. Ju, M. I. Green, B. Benacerraf, and M. E. Dorf, Hapten-specific T cell responses to 4-hydrozy-3-nitro-phenyl acetyl. II. Demonstration of idiotypic determinants on suppressor T cells, J. Exp. Med. 150:761 (1979).

50. R. Woodland and H. Cantor, Idiotype-specific T helper cells are required to induce idiotype-positive B memory cells to secrete antibody, Eur. J. Immunol. 8:600 (1978).

51. R. J. Ziccardi, A new role for C-1 inhibitor in homeostasis: control of activation of the first component of human complement, J. Immunol. 128:2505 (1982).

REGULATION OF AUTOIMMUNE DISEASES

Norman Talal

Department of Medicine
The University of Texas Health Science Center and
The Veterans Administration Hospital
San Antonio, TX 78284

The field of autoimmunity, like immunology itself, is undergoing rapid change due to progress in molecular biology and technology. Autoimmunity is traditionally defined as the body's immune system turning against itself to produce lymphocytes reactive with self-components. These lymphocytes may be B cells secreting autoantibodies like those responsible for hemolytic anemia, T cells attacking and destroying target organs such as the thyroid, or most often, a combination of both.

The old concept that individuals are tolerant to self because of the elimination of "forbidden" clones during fetal development was abandoned almost a decade ago. Normal healthy individuals have B lymphocytes capable of reacting with self-antigens through Ig receptors. Such cells can be triggered to proliferate and secrete autoantibodies of a wide range of specificities. This potential for autoimmunity exists in everyone and becomes manifest rather frequently. Examples are drug-induced autoimmunity, autoimmunity associated with aging, and the autoimmunity that occurs in chronic infectious diseases. Why autoimmunity doesn't occur still more often is generally explained by the actions of an appropriately balanced immunoregulatory system that normally functions to mount brisk immune responses to foreign antigens and to prevent reactions to self. But exactly how immunoregulation works in all its intricacies and mechanisms has become a very complicated problem.

Ten years ago we simply attributed regulation to an equilibrium established between helper (OKT4) and suppressor (OKT8) T cells. Autoimmune patients and autoimmune mice were found to be deficient in suppressor function and to manifest polyclonal B cell activation. However, we now appreciate that this is an oversimplification and that there is not always a correlation between the number and function of suppressor T cells and autoimmune disease activity.

Autoimmune diseases are multifactorial (5). At least four major components play a crucial role in pathogenesis (Figure 1). In a given patient, one, two, three or all four factors may be required for the disease to become clinically manifest. The actual contribution from each factor may vary in different patients. For example, a teenage girl with a strong family history of SLE may be clinically asymptomatic but have a false-positive VDRL or serum antinuclear factor as the first indication of a lupus diathesis. An autoimmune disease may appear for the first time in another patient following a

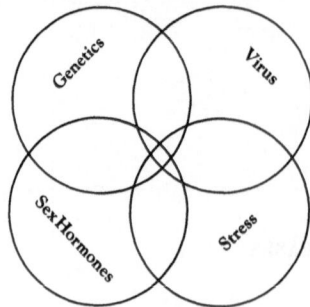

Figure 1. Four major factors (genetic viral, hormonal, and psycho-
          neurologic) interact in varying proportions to contribute
          to the etiology of autoimmune disease.

particularly stressful life cycle event such as the loss of a loved one.
Furthermore, although unproven to date, there may be a viral or other etio-
logic agent for autoimmunity that, once discovered, will make these other
factors seem less important.

GENETIC FACTORS (3,4)

    T cell activation requires appropriate presentation of antigen on the
surface of an antigen presenting cell (APC), usually a macrophage strongly
expressive of class II histocompatibility cell surface antigens (Figure 2).
These cell surface molecules, collectively called Ia (or DR in man), are now
known to be the products of several IR gene loci in the Major Histocompatibility Complex (MHC) (I-A and I-E in the mouse; DP, DQ, and DR in man).
Each molecule is composed of an α and β chain. There are at least five α
chain gene loci and seven β chain gene loci. The Ia molecules are capable
of functionally, perhaps physically, interacting with foreign antigens to
activate T cells in conjunction with the secretion of the macrophage product
interleukin-1 (IL-1).

    Studies at both the gene level and at the cell surface molecular level
(Ia molecules) indicate a vast polymorphism in the population, particularly
with regard to the DR and DQ β chains. Studies with monoclonal antibodies
to murine Ia molecules employing cross-backing techniques demonstrate that
each molecule encodes multiple epitopes which are spatially distinct. Even
more interesting, it seems that common epitopes can be expressed on structurally distinct Ia molecules. This complex polymorphism, thought to arise
from gene conversion events, may explain the correlation of particular HLA
types with an increased susceptibility for certain autoimmune diseases. The
polymorphism in Ia structure may be the molecular basis for the well-recog-
nized association of certain HLA types with specific diseases, the best
example being B8 DR 3 with coeliac disease, dermatitis herpetiformis, myasthenia gravis, Grave's disease, chronic active hepatitis, idiopathic Addison's
disease, and insulin-dependent diabetes mellitus.

    As our analytic abilities have progressed technically due to studies of
restriction fragment length polymorphism, we now appreciate that the DR designations represent broad public specificities with the strongest disease
correlations perhaps occurring with smaller areas or epitopes on the class
II molecule. Our conventional typing reagents are not capable of discrimina-
ting the finer specificities of these epitopes. This may explain why HLP

associations fall short of 100% (for example, 70% of rheumatoid arthritis patients are DR4 positive, 59% of multiple sclerosis patients are DR2 positive). The importance of relatively small differences in Ia structures is also illustrated by the immune alterations found in the bml2 mutant mouse. A difference of only three amino acids in the I-A$^\beta$ chain converts the C57B1/6 mouse into the bml2 mutant with the resultant effect of changing a strain highly susceptible to experimental autoimmune myasthenia gravis into one that is resistant.

We are also becoming more aware of the importance of class III genes in the MHC and their potential role in autoimmunity. The class III region includes genes that code for the second and fourth components of complement, for factor B, and for the enzyme 21-hydroxylase. C4 null genes and genetic deficiencies of complement are associated with autoimmune disease, particularly with systemic lupus erythematosus. The MHC region in the mouse also regulates numerous sex-related functions, one being a sex-limited protein that maps to the class III region. The possible relationship between sex factors and autoimmunity is discussed later.

INTERLEUKINS AND INTERFERON

The helper/inducer T cell (OKT4) responds to IL-1 and to antigen on APCs (Figure 2) to produce interleukin-2 (IL-2), a critical immune hormone that interacts with specific receptors on T cells and natural killer (NK) cells to mediate lymphocyte proliferation, γ interferon production and the production of other lymphokines that regulate B cells (e.g., B cell growth and differentiation factors). The polyclonal B cell activation that occurs in autoimmunity probably arises from multiple mechanisms, some dependent and some independent of T cells and IL-2. Indeed, IL-2 production and response is deficient in many autoimmune conditions.

Recent studies have shown that the T cell antigen receptor is also composed of two chains (α and β) and is structurally homologous to both immunoglobulin and HLA. All three families of molecules are thought to derive from a single primordial gene product through an evolutionary process of

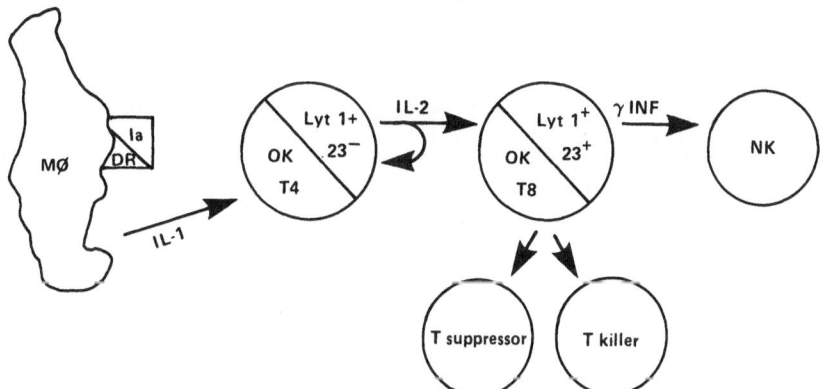

Figure 2. An immunoregulatory circuit indicating the relationship of antigen presenting cells (APCs), IL1, IL2, T cell subsets, γ interferon and NK cells. The activation of OKT4 helper/inducer cells by APCs leads to an entire cascade of events controlled by IL2 interactions with specific receptors. These immunoregulatory events are perturbed in autoimmune diseases.

gene duplication and mutation. The T cell receptor expresses idiotype and binds both Ia and antigen. The outcome of this binding is extremely important for normal immunoregulation or for autoimmunity. For example, normal individuals who are HLA-B8-DR3 have evidence of immunologic hyperresponsiveness as evidenced by studies of humoral and cellular immunity. Whether this IR gene effect is exerted at the level of the antigen presenting cell or at the level of the responding T cell is not yet known.

Gamma interferon induces the expression of class II molecules on APCs and has been postulated as the cause of aberrant Ia expression on thyroid cells in thyroiditis. Such expression could convert parenchymal cells into APCs which might then lead to aberrant immune reactions locally and target organ specific autoimmunity. A local virus infection has been proposed as the stimulus for this interferon production.

AUTOANTIBODIES

Autoantibodies, like myeloma proteins, were once considered highly abnormal B cell products. We now appreciate that both autoantibodies and myeloma proteins are rather conventional Igs that can teach us much about normal immune mechanisms.

Antibodies to DNA occur in the majority of lupus patients but are difficult to induce in experimental animals. Several monoclonal macroglobulins which react with Klebsiella polysaccharides also share idiotypic determinants with monoclonal lupus anti-DNA autoantibodies and have similar polynucleotide-binding properties. The reaction with the polynucleotides is specifically inhibited by Klebsiella polysaccharides which also inhibit binding to the anti-idiotype. This idiotype is thought to derive from a single germ line gene whose original specificity is probably not anti-DNA but anti-bacterial.

In another instance, a single amino acid substitution arising as a mutation in a monoclonal antibody to polyphorylcholine (a constituent of pneumococcus) resulted in a loss of the original specificity and acquisition of reactivity with DNA and cardiolipin, features characteristic of anti-DNA antibodies in lupus.

These studies, taken together, suggest that autoantibodies such as anti-DNA may arise through a process of somatic mutation from an original antibody whose specificity might be anti-bacterial or anti-viral.

A dominant cross-reactive idiotype has recently been reported in lupus patients but also in a majority of healthy family members of these patients who did not bind DNA. Thus, the idiotype and the DNA-binding site represent different epitopes on the Ig molecule in these individuals. Again, somatic mutation might be responsible for the acquisition of anti-DNA specificity in the lupus patients.

IDIOTYPE NETWORK

Viruses may lead to autoimmune disease by interfering with idiotypic network regulation in addition to direct target organ attack or molecular mimicry. Idiotypes are recognized in vivo leading to physiologic anti-idiotypic responses that may be important for autoimmunity in several ways: 1) prevention of autoimmunity by limiting the expansion of autoreactive B or T cell clones or helpers for such clones; 2) generation of autoimmunity through cross-reactions between foreign and host epitopes (e.g., helper cells for an anti-pathogen response might also help an autoantibody response); 3) generation of autoimmunity because auto-anti-idiotypic antibodies to viral antibodies could theoretically react with cell surface receptors for that virus. This would be analogous to the demonstrated ability of anti-idiotypes to anti-insulin antibodies to bind to insulin receptors, imitating the action of insulin and even causing diabetes mellitus.

Anti-idiotypic antibodies may also have therapeutic potential since an anti-idiotype to anti-DNA can transiently suppress glomerulonephritis in autoimmune mice.

SEX HORMONES

Autoimmune diseases are much more common in women than in men (1). Normal females are more immunologically reactive than normal males and are thought, therefore, to be more susceptible to autoimmune disorders. These observations are explained by the ability of sex steroid hormones to modulate immune reactivity with androgens suppressing and estrogens augmenting. This field began with studies performed in the classic B/W mouse model for lupus in which female mice develop autoantibodies, immune complex glomerulonephritis, and die from renal failure several months earlier than males. An accelerated disease indistinguishable from females develops in male B/W mice castrated prior to puberty. Although gonadectomy does not benefit female B/W mice, the administration of male hormone suppresses their disease and allows them to live a normal life span. Most importantly, this beneficial effect of androgen can be demonstrated as late as six months of age, a time when SLE is already well established in female B/W mice.

These studies have their clinical counterpart in SLE where there is a deviation in the normal metabolism of estradiol resulting in an elevation of estrogenic metabolites and the creation of a hyperestrogenic state. There is also evidence for decreased total androgens in SLE, so that sex hormone factors are now considered important in the pathogenesis of autoimmune disease.

Both SLE patients and mice demonstrate a delayed clearance of particulate immune complexes. Female B/W mice develop this abnormality earlier than males. Furthermore, this defect can be suppressed in female B/W mice by exposing them to sustained androgen. By contrast, defective clearance develops earlier in male B/W mice given sustained estrogen. These results suggest an important influence of sex steroid hormones on the clearance of immune complexes, and offers an explanation for the clinical benefit achieved in mice by androgen administration.

There is evidence for sex steroid hormone receptors in the lymphoid organs of both humans and mice. Moreover, sex hormones act to influence lymphocyte number and function. The OKT8 suppressor cells in man and the Lyt-2$^+$ suppressor cells in mice are important target sites for sex hormone modulation. Estrogen depleted Lyt-2$^+$ cells, whereas testosterone increased or maintained this subpopulation of cells in spleen and lymph nodes. Similarly, the suppressor cell activity and IL-2 production on a per cell basis in estrogen-treated animals was diminished, whereas testosterone-treated animals had normal or enhanced activity.

The therapeutic effect of androgen on spontaneous autoimmunity can also be demonstrated in another lupus model, the MRL/lpr mouse. Autoantibody levels, renal function and survival are all improved even in this very aggressive disease.

In patients, myasthenia gravis (MG) occurs three times more commonly in women than in men. In experimental MG, AChR specific lymphocyte proliferative and autoantibody responses were suppressed by ovariectomy and enhanced by orchidectomy. Moreover, testosterone-implanted animals demonstrated lower lymphocyte and autoantibody response to AChR as compared to sham-implanted animals.

Chronic thyroiditis occurs four times more frequently in women, but only after puberty. Experimental autoimmune thyroiditis can be induced in mice by administration of mouse thyroglobulin emulsified in complete Freund's adjuvant followed by injection of lipopolysaccharide. Evidence for the suppressive effect of androgen on autoimmunity was also obtained using this experimental thyroiditis model. Similar results have been obtained studying spontaneous autoimmune thyroiditis in rats. Castration of male rats increased both autoantibodies and thyroiditis lesions so that their disease was equivalent to females.

The female/male ratio in rheumatoid arthritis (RA) is 4:1. Cell wall peptidoglycan-polysaccharide fragments derived from bacteria such as group A streptococci induce chronic polyarthritis in rats which resembles RA clinically, histologically and radiologically. An interesting sex difference is demonstrated when group A streptococcal cell wall fragments are injected into LEW/N rats. LEW/N female rats are highly susceptible to arthritis whereas LEW/N males are resistant. Castrated LEW/N males, or β-estradiol-treated males whether or not castrated, developed an arthritis as severe as that seen in LEW/N females.

Thus, the influence of sex hormones has been demonstrated in several animal models of autoimmunity as well as in patients.

PSYCHONEUROIMMUNOLOGY

The immune and nervous systems are two nonclassic target sites for sex hormone action. Sex hormone receptors in the brain promote evolution and species survival by regulating patterns of behavior related to reproduction and territorial defense. The immunological enhancement brought about by estrogen may also have contributed to species survival throughout evolution by protecting women from infections and generating humoral immune mechanisms that protect the fetus from rejection.

In considering the effect of sex hormones on the central nervous system, one must also reflect upon the influence of stress and psychoneurologic factors not only as important consequences of autoimmune disease but also as possible causative factors. The existence of important physiologic connections between the neuroendocrine, classical endocrine and immune system is now well established.

All three systems are under the influence of higher centers in the brain; stress, mood, and emotions can directly or indirectly act on all three systems. A stressful event might through immune or other mechanisms be enough to trigger the onset of autoimmunity. Often this event is the real or threatened loss of an important interpersonal relationship. Psychosocial factors such as bereavement can alter immune function either by direct neural mechanisms or by indirect mechanisms involving pituitary hormones or neuropeptides. The presence of endorphin and ACTH receptors on lymphocytes offers a clue as to one possible mechanism whereby the brain may influence lymphocyte behavior.

LESSONS FROM AIDS

The Acquired Immunodeficiency Syndrome (AIDS) has many lessons for autoimmunity. It is now firmly established that the Human T cell Leukemia Virus Type III which is specifically cytopathic for OKT4 helper cells is the cause of AIDS. There are many immunologic similarities between AIDS and SLE includ-

Table 1. Similarities Between AIDS and Autoimmunity

Polyclonal B cell activation
Immune complexes
Increased serum β-2-microglobulin
Acid-labile interferon
Decreased autologous mixed lymphocyte response
Decreased interleukin-2
Decreased natural killer cells

---

ing polyclonal B cell activation, serum immune complexes, increased serum β-2-microglobulin, acid-labile interferon, decreased AMLR, IL-2 and natural killer cell activity (Table 1). The active research and therapeutic trials being conducted in AIDS patients may soon bring information important also for autoimmune patients.

LESSONS FROM MURINE MODELS OF SLE

For over two decades certain inbred strains of mice genetically susceptible to generalized autoimmune disease resembling SLE have been invaluable models for study (6). The lessons learned from these animals (Table 2) indicate the complexity of the problem. There is no H2 or allotype association but only evidence for genetic heterogeneity among the several available strains. There is also an excessive Ia expression in the lpr mice. Sex hormones play an accelerating role in the female-predominant disease of B/W mice, and the Y chromosome has an accelerating influence in the male predominant disorder of BXSB mice. Lymphocytes from autoimmune mice have the ability to transfer the disease to histocompatible recipients. Some combination of a stem cell abnormality plus the inductive influence of the thymus probably confers this property on mature lymphocytes. Multiple lymphoid and lymphokine abnormalities are found as indicated in Table 2.

Table 2. Lessons from Murine Models of SLE

---

1. Genetic Heterogeneity (NZB, B/W, MRL/1pr, BXSB, gld)
   a. no H2 or allotype association
   b. excessive Ia expression

2. Accelerating Factors
   a. sex hormones – B/W
   b. Y chromosome – BXSB

3. Transmission of Disease by Lymphocytes
   a. bone marrow stem cells
   b. thymic induction

4. Multiple Lymphoid and Lymphokine Abnormalities
   a. polyclonal B cell activation
   b. IL-2 and T effector function decreased
   c. T suppressor cell deficiency
   d. T helper cell excess-1pr
   e. defective NK cell activity

Table 3. New Therapeutic Approaches to Autoimmune Disease

---

1. Specific Deletion or Suppression of Autoreactive Lymphocytes
   a. Monoclonal anti-Ia antibodies
   b. Monoclonal anti-idiotypic antibodies
   c. Attenuation with T cell lines

2. Less Specific Deletion or Suppression
   a. Antibodies to helper cells (anti-L3T4)
   b. Total lymphoid irradiation*

3. General Biologic Approaches
   a. Sex hormone modulation - androgen suppression*
   b. Dietary manipulation - calorie restriction, fish oil

4. Immunopharmacologic Approaches
   a. cyclosporin*
   b. immunomodulating drugs*

---

*Has been tried in patients

NEW THERAPEUTIC APPROACHES

The current biological revolution is not only bringing conceptual advances but also possibilities for new therapeutic interventions (2). To date, these therapeutic strategies have been tried predominantly in animal models of autoimmunity (except as indicated in Table 3). Monoclonal anti-Ia antibodies may act by interfering with cellular interactions involving class II molecules and have proven successful in several animal models. Monoclonal anti-idiotypic antibody specific for anti-DNA is less successful because of the emergence of private idiotypes which may be a significant problem with this potential form of therapy. Attenuated T cell lines specific for experimental autoimmune encephalomyelitis or arthritis have been used to vaccinate and protect against disease.

Antibodies to the L3T4 molecule of helper T cells has proved beneficial in murine lupus and allergic encephalomyelitis. This is an interesting refinement from older work with non-specific anti-lymphocyte antibodies. Total lymphoid irradiation, a treatment used in Hodgkins's Disease, has been tried successfully in a small number of patients with RA and SLE. It appears to deplete helper function and induces a non-specific suppressor.

General biologic approaches such as androgen suppression or dietary manipulation have been very successful in animal models. The attenuated androgen danazol has been used therapeutically in idiopathic thrombocytopenic purpura with some success. Fish oil fatty acids appear to interfere with arachidonic acid pathways and to suppress inflammation.

Immunopharmacologic approaches including interferon and IL-2 have been disappointing in AIDs patients. A variety of immunomodulating drugs are under development. Cyclosporin, a drug established as useful in transplantation, is being tried in autoimmune disease but its toxicity could be a problem.

REFERENCES

1. A. S. Ahmed, W. J. Penhale, and N. Talal, Sex hormones, immune responses and autoimmunity: mechanisms of sex hormone action, Am. J. Path. in press (1986).
2. S. Gupta and N. Talal, eds., "Immunology of Rheumatic Diseases," Plenum Publishing Corporation, New York (1985).
3. Y. Shoenfeld and R. S. Schwartz, Immunologic and genetic factors in autoimmune diseases, N. Eng. J. Med. 311:1019 (1984).
4. H. R. Smith and A. D. Steinberg, Autoimmunity: a perspective, Ann. Rev. Immunol. 1:175 (1983).
5. N. Talal, ed., "Autoimmunity: Genetic, Immunologic, Virologic, and Clinical Aspects," Academic Press, New York (1978).
6. A. N. Theofilopoulos and F. J. Dixon, Murine models of systemic lupus erythematosus, in: "Advances in Immunology," Volume 37, Academic Press, New York (1985).

SECTION V
IMMUNOLOGIC INTERVENTION WITH MONOCLONAL ANTIBODIES

Transfectomas Provide Antibodies with Novel Structures and Functions
Sherie L. Morrison, Letitia A. Wims, Polly D. Gregor,
Barry J. Kobrin, and Vernon T. Oi

The Use of Ricin A Chain-Containing Immunotoxins to Kill
Neoplastic B Cells
Jonathan W. Uhr, R. Jerrold Fulton, and Ellen S. Vitetta

Monoclonal Antibodies and Immunoconjugates as Anti-Cancer Agents
Robert K. Oldham

TRANSFECTOMAS PROVIDE ANTIBODIES WITH NOVEL STRUCTURES AND FUNCTIONS

Sherie L. Morrison, Letitia A. Wims, Polly D. Gregor,
Barry J. Kobrin, and Vernon T. Oi

Department of Microbiology and the Cancer Center/Institute
of Cancer Research, Columbia University College of
Physicians and Surgeons, New York, New York and
Becton Dickinson Monoclonal Center, Mountain View, California

The importance of antibodies in providing specific protection against disease has long been recognized. Antibodies can neutralize the effects of bacterial toxins, such as those causing tetanus and diptheria, can facilitate the killing of pathogenic bacteria, and can protect against viral infection of cells. The ability to specifically immunize and provide protection against infectious disease has had a major impact on public health. Indeed a coordinated program of immunization has led to the complete elimination of smallpox. It is perhaps fitting that smallpox should be the first disease to be eradicated in such a manner, because it was Jenner's work with this disease which can be considered to have been the beginning of modern immunology.

Antibodies have also been important for their many in vitro applications. The science of immunochemistry can be considered to have its beginnings with the development of the quantitative precipitin curve (19). Immunochemistry is now broadly applied in virtually all scientific disciplines. Immunochemical approaches have been used to investigate structural relationships between antigens by assessing their cross reactivity with different antibody preparations. Perhaps even more importantly antibodies are used to quantitate the amount of antigens present in various solutions. Initially quantitation was based on precipitin reactions; more recently radioimmunoassays and enzyme-linked immunoassays have been developed permitting the rapid quantitation of antigens present in small quantities.

Antibodies are also used in the in vivo diagnosis and assessment of disease states. By coupling tumor-specific antibodies with radionuclides, it has been possible to use scintography to identify and localize tumor metastases (23). A natural extension of these techniques is to use antibodies for the in vivo treatment of diseases. Such treatment can utilize antibodies as carriers of cytotoxic drugs to specific locations, such as a tumor where they can exert their effects (4,16,22,45). Alternatively antibodies can be used to directly kill tumors or other tissues by either complement-mediated mechanisms or by antibody-dependent cytotoxic cells (24). Antibodies can also potentially be used to intervene in such disease states as autoimmunity; preliminary experiments in animal model systems suggest great promise for such intervention (5,46).

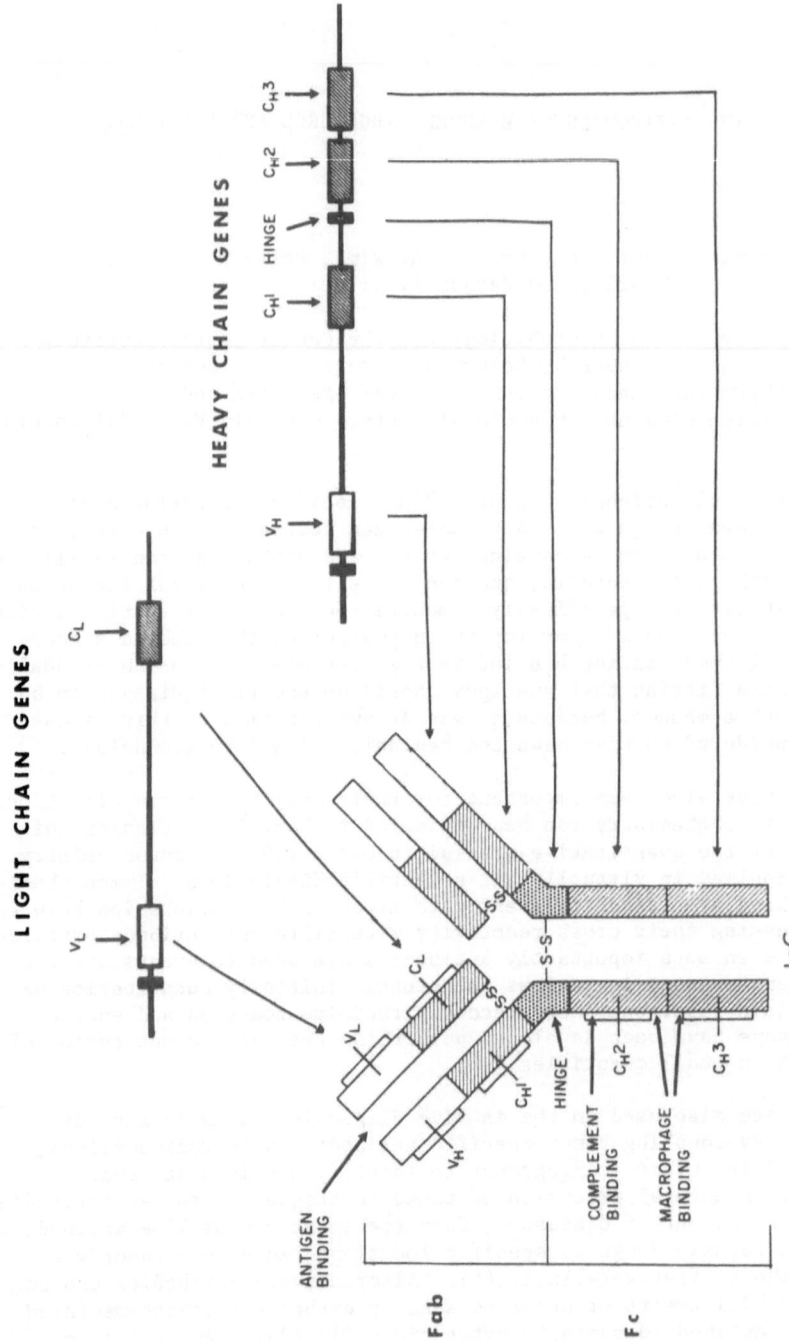

Figure 1.   Structure of the antibody molecule and the genes which encode the heavy and light chains.   The correspondence between the exons and the domains which they encode is indicated by arrows.   The hydrophobic leader sequence of both heavy and light chains is removed following translation and so is absent from the mature antibody molecule.   From (26).

Antibodies are the products of cells of the B lymphocyte lineage. B lymphocytes show an ordered pattern of immunoglobulin (Ig) gene rearrangement and expression as they develop. Rearrangement occurs first at the heavy chain locus; once a functional heavy chain protein is produced rearrangement of light chain genes takes place with kappa and then lambda rearranging if no functional kappa chains are produced. In addition, there is an increase in the amount of immunoglobulin produced as cells mature from B lymphocytes to plasma cells. The Ig produced by lymphocytes is largely membrane Ig while that produced by plasma cells is predominantly of the secreted form [reviewed in (47)].

Immunoglobulins are glycoproteins and in certain cases their biologic properties have been shown to require the presence of carbohydrate (32). Immunoglobulin molecules are made up of heavy chains and light chains both of which are required for immunoglobulin function. The antibody molecule folds into discrete functional domains, two for light chains, four or five for heavy chains. This domain structure of the protein is reflected in the structure of the genes encoding it (Figure 1). In most cases each functional domain has its own exon.

Each antibody molecule is divided into a variable region which reacts and binds antigen, and a constant region which contains the effector functions characteristic of antibody molecules. In the human there are nine different constant regions or isotypes (μ, δ, $\gamma1$, $\gamma2$, $\gamma3$, $\gamma4$, ε, $\alpha1$, and $\alpha2$); each constant region has its characteristic amino acid sequence and associated biologic properties.

In initial immunologic studies, antisera provided the source of antibody molecules. Animals, frequently rabbits, were injected with purified or partially purified preparations of antigen. The serum from such animals was either used directly or antibodies were purified using any of a large number of methods. Such sources however had inherent limitations since the antibodies they contained were heterogeneous both with respect to the binding specifics of the antibodies and their associated isotypes.

The discovery that multiple myeloma was a malignancy of plasma cells enabled a major breakthrough in immunology. Since myeloma is a monoclonal proliferation of plasma cells, the immunoglobulin produced is homogeneous. The availability of such homogeneous antibodies permitted the first structural studies of antibody molecules. However, this system suffered from the limitation that in most cases the myeloma proteins could not be shown to bind a known antigen.

These limitations were largely overcome when Köhler and Milstein (21) demonstrated that it was possible to generate a continuous cell line synthesizing antibodies of a defined specificity by fusing a myeloma cell line which grows continuously in tissue culture with a normal spleen cell. Such hybrids exhibit the immortality of their myeloma parent and synthesize the immunoglobulin produced by their normal spleen cell parent. However, hybridomas continued to have certain limitations in that it is not possible to conveniently produce hybridomas from all species. In addition you are limited to the specificity and isotype that the spleen cells were producing at the time of fusion.

Isolation and characterization of mutants has alleviated some of these shortcomings. Using a number of different selection techniques is has been possible to isolate isotype switch variants (25,37). These include variants in which the variable region has been moved to an entirely different constant region and variants in which the switch has occurred within the constant region to produce hybrid constant region (3,44). Mutants have also been isolated which show an altered affinity for antigen (8,9). Both increased affinity and decreased affinity for antigen has been found.

METHODS FOR PRODUCING STABLE TRANSFECTANTS

Gene transfection provides an alternative way to produce antibody molecules of the desired isotype and specificity (34,39). Since immunoglobulin genes can be altered before they are placed in the cell for expression, it is possible to create and express novel antibody molecules. In addition gene transfection can be used to identify regulatory sequences within Ig genes. Such sequences would include not only those sequences required for high level Ig expression but also would include those responsible for alternative forms of Ig such as membrane and secreted.

Several methods exist for introducing genes back into cells. Historically, $CaPO_4$ precipitates of DNA were first used to introduce DNA back into cells (7,17,48). This method works very well for some cells; however, lymphoid cells cannot readily be transfected using $CaPO_4$ precipitated DNA (33). Using protoplast fusion it has been possible to isolate stable transfections of lymphoid cells at frequencies approaching 1×10^{-3} (15,34). In this method, DNA of interest maintained as a plasmid in bacteria is amplified using chloramphenicol. The bacteria are then converted to spheroplasts using lysozyme, and the resulting spheroplasts fused to lymphoid cells using the same methods used to produce somatic cell hybrids (34,40). An alternative method to introduce DNA into lymphoid cells is electroporation in which cells in the presence of DNA in solution are subjected to a high voltage pulse (36).

Since even the most efficient methods only result in a very small percentage of the cells becoming stably transfected it is necessary to have a method to select such transfectants. In the initial studies, L cells deficient in thymidine kinase were transfected with herpes thymidine kinase and stable transfectants expressing the enzyme isolated using HAT selection (48). This method requires that the recipient cell line be drug-marked, e.g., deficient in thymidine kinase, often a laborious process. To circumvent this obstacle vectors were developed which contained genes providing dominant selectable markers (29,30,42). With dominant markers, the recipient cell line does not need to be drug-marked; hence they can potentially be used with any recipient cell line.

Two dominant selectable markers are frequently used. The first of these depends on the expression of the bacterial xanthine-guanine phosphoribosyl transferase (gpt); this enzyme unlike the endogenous hypoxanthine-guanine phosphoribosyl transferase can use xanthine as a substrate for purine nucleotide synthesis. When the conversion of IMP to XMP is blocked by mycophenolic acid, cells provided with xanthine can survive only if they express the bacterial gene (14).

The second dominant selectable marker relies on the expression of the phosphotransferase gene from Tn5 (designated neo). The antibiotic G418, which resembles gentamycin, neomycin and kanamycin in its structure interferes with protein synthesis in eukaryotic cells. The enzyme encoded by the bacterial gene neo inactivates drugs of this class and so will provide resistance to the action of G418 (10,11).

These two markers can be selected independently of each other. That is cells resistant to one drug can be sequentially selected for resistance to the other drug; alternatively cells resistant to both drugs can be selected in one step. This property of the two drugs can be very useful and permits the sequential or simultaneous transfection of the two different genes using the two independent selectable markers.

SEQUENCES WITHIN IMMUNOGLOBULIN GENES INFLUENCING THEIR EXPRESSION

Gene transfection provides a method to identify regulatory elements within immunoglobulin genes thus increasing our understanding of how specific gene sequences are controlled. In addition, if gene transfection is to be used as a way to produce large quantities of novel protein molecules, it is imperative that systems be optimized to produce the largest quantities possible.

An enhancer-like element has been identified within the major intervening sequence of heavy chain using gene transfection (1,15). This element of DNA has been shown to function in a position and orientation independent manner and enhances expression of the β-globin promoter in a transient assay. It has been shown to be required for both the transient and stable expression of transfected heavy chain genes (15). But in an apparent paradox, it has been demonstrated that when this sequence is deleted from the active endogenous heavy chain gene its continued expression is unaffected (49). However, when the genes with the enhancer deletions are cloned, they are not functional in transfection, verifying the importance of this enhancer sequence for the expression of transfected genes.

The level of expression of transfected H chain genes approaches that seen in the myeloma from which the gene was cloned. Thus when the γ2b MPC-11 H chain gene was transfected into the myeloma lambda chain producer J558L, stable transfectants with H chain mRNA levels 50 percent of that seen in the myeloma MPC-11 were obtained (20). It would thus appear that the H chain gene segments which are being used for transfection can reconstitute an active H chain transcription unit, when integrated into the chromosomal DNA of the recipient cell line. Variability in the level of H chains expression is seen among the different stable transfectants, but the contribution of the site of chromosomal integration to the level of expression would appear to be minor.

The heavy chain genes used for transfection extend beyond the secreted terminus of the gene and in many cases through the membrane exons. Recent studies of a spontaneous mouse myeloma mutant have suggested the importance of the sequences 3' of the heavy chain gene in influencing its expression (18). The mutant was identified because it synthesizes and secretes only about one tenth as much alpha heavy chain as the myeloma from which it was isolated. The expressed alpha chain gene was shown to be deleted of alpha sequences 11 bases beyond the 3' secreted terminus of the gene. Analysis of the nuclear and cytoplasmic RNA in the mutant demonstrated no differences in processing patterns, or in the sites and efficiency of cleavage and polyadenylation. Instead this mutant heavy chain gene was shown to be decreased in its transcription rate and demonstrates that sequences 3' of a heavy chain gene can influence its expression. The decreased transcription following the substitution of novel sequences 3' of the α chain gene could result from either the deletion of sequences that stimulate transcription or from insertion of sequences that depress transcription; the experiments performed did not distinguish between these two possibilities. It has not been demonstrated whether or not these changes 3' of the gene will exert an influence on the level of expression of an alpha heavy chain gene following transfection.

Heavy chain proteins can exist as either membrane or secreted immunoglobulins. In B lymphocytes heavy chains are primarily of the membrane form; as differentiation to plasma cells takes place, there is an increase in the level of heavy chain synthesis and a switch from being primarily of the

171

membrane form to being primarily of the secreted form [reviewed in (47)]. The processing of transfected heavy chain genes mirrors the processing seen in the recipient cell type. That is, when the recipient cell type is a lymphoma, processing is largely to the membrane form. When the recipient cell is of the plasma cell lineage, the heavy chain gene transcripts are processed primarily to the secreted form (20).

Alterations in the sequences 3' of Ig genes can lead to alterations in the processing of the transcripts to either the membrane or the secreted form. When a deletion of 830 bases beginning 22 base pairs beyond the AATAA poly A addition signal was made in the intervening sequence between CH_3 and the first membrane exon in the γ2b heavy chain gene, the processing pattern of this gene following transfection was found to be changed so that when this gene was transfected into a myeloma recipient it was processed primarily to the membrane form. A second deletion beginning 53 bases 3' of the first deletion was found to give rise to transcripts which were processed in the same pattern as transcripts from the unaltered gene (20). These experiments suggest that within 53 bases absent in the first deletion but present in the second, are signals important for heavy chain processing. The AATAA signal sequence for poly A addition is left intact in both deletions. However, the site at which cleavage and poly A addition takes place is absent from the first deletion. Absence of this sequence may change the processing pattern. Alternatively there may be a sequence which specifically directs processing to the secreted form. Examination of the 3' sequences shows that there is a sequence of 13 bases (GTCCTGGTTCTTT) which is highly conserved at the 3' secreted terminus of μ and γ chain genes of mouse and man but is missing from the membrane terminus. This conserved sequence is a candidate for a regulatory sequence which is specifically recognized to direct processing of heavy chain mRNA to the secreted form. Further experiments are required to verify a regulatory role for this sequence.

It has been difficult to determine what is required for efficient L chain expression following transfection. Using transient expression assays, an enhancer element has been identified in the major intervening sequence of the L chain gene (38). This enhancer element corresponds to a highly conserved sequence (35) present in mice, rabbits and man (13).

However, when the sequences required for L chain production in stable transfectants were determined, a slightly different result was found. The deletion of most of the major intervening sequence led to greatly decreased L chain production in stable transfectants. However, if only the region of the intervening sequence identified as an enhancer element was deleted, it was still possible to isolate stable transfectants synthesizing significant quantities of protein. In fact, several different sequences within the kappa light chain gene appeared sufficient to permit L chain expression in the stable transfectants (Morrison et al., in preparation). It is possible that gene sequences present near the site of integration substitute for those missing from the transfected gene and permit its expression.

However, it is clear that there is some aspect of the control of L chain expression following transfection which we do not understand. In most cases large amounts of sequences both 5' and 3' of the L chain have been included in the transfected gene. Thus it would be anticipated that any normal regulatory sequences would be included in these genes. However, unlike H chains, where expression of transfected genes approaches myeloma levels, expression of transfected L chains is usually much less than that seen in a myeloma. In most stable transfectants isolated with the entire S107A kappa light chains, the level of expression is only about five percent of that seen in the myeloma. In stable transfectants isolated using the MPC-11 L chain, the level of expression is even less. Recent results suggest that light chains differing only in their variable regions and 5' flanking are expressed to different levels following transfection. These results might suggest variability in promoter structure, or the contribution of either intragenic (V region) or 5' sequences to the level of expression.

It has been reported using a transient assay that the heavy chain enhancer is more powerful than the L chain enhancer. However, when chimeric genes were made in which V_H was joined to $C\kappa$ with either the H chain, L chain or both enhancers, no consistent differences in level of expression in the stable transfectants were seen. The frequency with which cell lines were isolated expressing the chimeric protein was increased with both enhancers present; however, the level of protein seen was approximately the same when either enhancer or both was present. Thus the enhancer strength differences readily observed in transient assays are not easily seen in stable transfectants. Once again flanking sequences may influence the level of expression of integrated genes. In addition, the level of expression in transient assays is usually determined by S1 analysis of the 5' end of the transcript. Expression in the stable transfectants has been assayed by the level of protein produced. These two different assays may in fact be looking at two different phenomena.

PRODUCTION OF NOVEL PROTEINS BY TRANSFECTOMAS

Once is was demonstrated that is was possible to produce both heavy and light chains by gene transfection (15,33,34) it became feasible to consider producing chimeric and other structurally altered immunoglobulins. The general approach to this problem is suggested by the structure of the Ig genes themselves. That is the various domains of the protein are contained on separate exons; the intervening sequences separating these exons become sites for joining the exons in novel combinations. In general this joining procedure is facilitated if there are novel restriction sites within the interven-

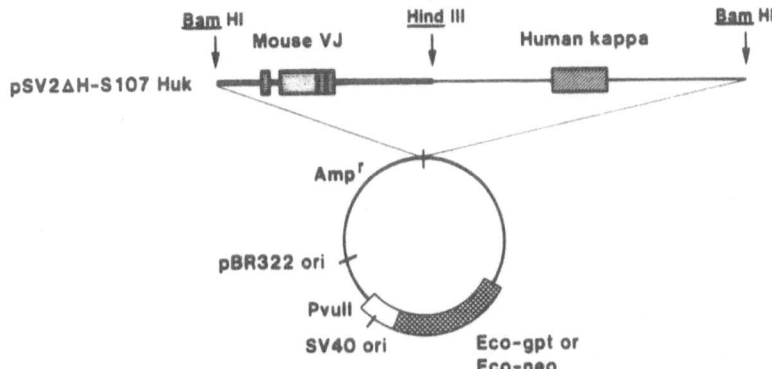

Figure 2.   Vector used for the isolation of stable transfectants synthesizing novel immunoglobulin molecules. The basic vector is pSV2 (29,30,42). Included within the vector is the pBR322 origin of replication (ori) and β-lactamase gene (Amr[R]) so these DNA segments can be replicated as plasmids in bacteria. The hatched region represents a gene contained within a eukaryotic transcription unit which provides a selectable marker in eukaryotic cells. The commonly used selectable genes are Eco-gpt and Eco-neo (see discussion). Inserted into non-essential regions in the vector is an immunoglobulin gene. In this example the gene is a chimeric gene in which the variable region from a mouse light chain gene has been joined to human Cκ using sequences within the major intervening sequence [Figure from (27)].

ing sequences. The novel sites may either be naturally occurring or may be generated by inserting synthetic linkers. A prototype vector is shown in Figure 2.

The first example of such a chimeric protein was the joining of the V_H from a mouse anti-azophenylarsonate hybridoma to C_K (41). When this construct was transfected into an L chain-producing variant of the hybridoma, the chimeric chain encoded by this gene assembled with the endogenous L chain. This L chain heterodimer bound antigen and was secreted. Such light chain heterodimers would be potentially used when an antigen binding molecule devoid of known biologic functions is needed. They would potentially be of use in neutralizing drug toxicity. A similar construction was made in which V region from the heavy chain of the anti-phosphocholine myeloma was joined to C_K. However in this case no antigen binding could be demonstrated for the heterodimer (Morrison and Oi, unpublished).

Chimeric L chains have also been produced in which the variable region from a human heavy chain was joined to mouse C_K (43). This construct was transfected into an L chain-producing mouse myeloma. The chimeric gene was efficiently transcribed and directed the synthesis of a protein of the expected molecular weight demonstrating that the human heavy chain promoter can function in mouse cells. However, the chimeric light chain did not assemble with the endogenous mouse lambda chain and the chimeric light chain was not secreted.

Gene transfection can also be used to effect isotype switching within a species. A cloned heavy chain variable region can be joined to any constant region and this protein can be produced by transfection. This method was

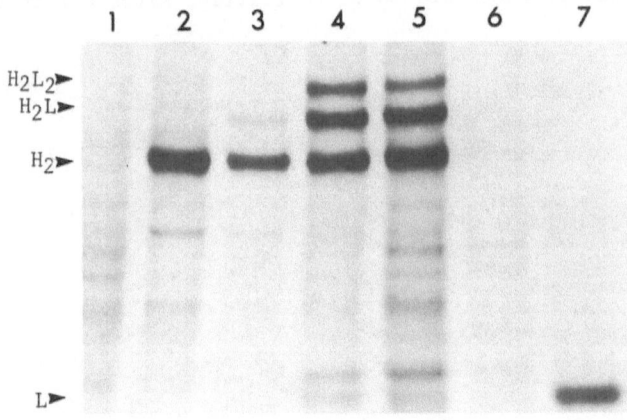

Figure 3. SDS-polyacrylamide gel analysis of immunoglobulin produced in transfectomas. A vector containing a chimeric immunoglobulin gene in which the variable region of a mouse heavy chain gene was joined to a human gamma chain constant region was transfected into a non-producing and a light chain producing mouse myeloma cell line. Transfectants were labeled for 60 minutes in the presence of ^{14}C-valine, threonine and leucine, cytoplasmic lysates prepared, and the immunoglobulins immunoprecipitated with anti-human Ig (lanes 1-6) and anti-mouse lambda (lane 7). Lane 1, non-producing myeloma; lanes 2 and 3, non-producing myeloma transfected with chimeric gene; lanes 4 and 5, lambda light chain producing myeloma transfected with chimeric gene; lanes 6 and 7, lambda light chain producing myeloma. [Reproduced from (28).]

used to produce a dansyl-specific IgA molecule; previous efforts to create such a molecule by standard isotype switching methods had been unsuccessful (J. Dangyl, personal communication). This approach may be especially useful when the available hybridomas are of an isotype, such as alpha, from which it is difficult to isolate switch variants.

Perhaps one of the most interesting classes of chimeric molecules are those in which V regions from mouse hybridomas are joined to human constant region genes. Such chimeric genes are efficiently synthesized in mouse cells (Figure 3). It has been demonstrated that molecules in which both the light and heavy chain constant regions are of human origin express the antigen specificity characteristic of the mouse myeloma from which they were cloned; however, this specificity is now associated with human constant regions and hence effector functions (6,27). Such molecules would be expected to be much less immunogenic in humans than is their totally mouse counterpart. They should therefore be more appropriate than totally mouse immunoglobulins for diagnostic and therapeutic applications in humans. These chimeric molecules can potentially be of any specificity since it is relatively easy to generate a mouse hybridoma of any specificity. Chimeric human-mouse antibodies may go a long way in overcoming many of the difficulties which have been encountered in producing human hybridomas.

The ability to produce altered molecules by gene transfection enables one to begin a fine structure-function analysis of the Ig molecule. The general applicability of such an approach has been eloquently demonstrated in the mouse system, where the availability of mouse myeloma mutants permitted a definition of the specificity of binding of Fc receptors in different cell types (2,12). In the human this approach has been limited by the availability of mutant protein and cell lines.

A general strategy for producing novel molecules by transfection is once again motivated by the structure of the genes. As noted above, structural domains are located in separate exons. By the use of linkers, each domain can be made into a cassette; cassettes can be inserted into, or removed from heavy chains, or aligned in novel sequences. Since the splicing signals between exons are conserved, mixing, matching or changing of exon order is straightforward. The great conservation of sequences between isotypes should also make it feasible to make recombinants within exons.

Once genes can be manipulated in vitro before they are expressed, they can also be altered. Therefore, in vitro mutagenesis will permit the making of small alterations within the Ig molecules whose effects can then be assessed. Potential applications of this general approach include an assessment of the function of carbohydrate in the Ig molecule. Up to now limited quantities of Ig lacking carbohydrate can be produced by cell lines grown in the presence of inhibitors of glycosylation. By using in vitro mutagenesis to remove the carbohydrate binding site, it should be feasible to produce large quantities of Ig deficient in carbohydrate. Functional analysis of the novel immunoglobulins should also define the precise specificity of the different cellular receptors for Ig, the precise sequence important for complement fixation, regions of the molecule determining serum half-life and placental passage. This knowledge will facilitate the production of Ig molecules with desired combinations of properties and effector functions.

ACKNOWLEDGMENTS

Work in the laboratories was supported by grants from the National Institutes of Health (CA 16858, CA 22736, CA 13696, and AI 19042) and the American Cancer Society (IMS-360) and a Research Career Development Award to Sherie L. Morrison.

REFERENCES

1. J. Banerji, L. Olsen, and W. Schaffner, A lymphocyte-specific cellular enhancer is located downstream of the joining region in immunoglobulin heavy chain genes, Cell 33:729 (1983).
2. B. K. Birshtein, R. Campbell, and B. Diamond, Effects of immunoglobulin structure on Fc receptor binding: a mouse myeloma variant immunoglobulin with a γ2b-γ2a hybrid heavy chain having complete γ2a Fc region fails to bind to γ2a Fc receptors on mouse macrophages, J. Immunol. 129:610 (1982).
3. B. K. Birshtein, R. Campbell, and M. L. Greenberg, A γ2b-γ2a hybrid immunoglobulin heavy chain produced by a variant of the MPC-11 mouse myeloma cell line, Biochemistry 19:1730 (1980).
4. H. E. Blythman, P. Casellas, O. Gros, P. Gros, F. K. Jansen, F. Paolucci, B. Pau, and H. Vidal, Immunotoxins. Hybrid molecules of monoclonal antibodies and a toxin subunit specifically kill tumor cells, Nature (London) 290:145 (1981).
5. C. Boitard, S. Michie, P. Serrurier, G. W. Butcher, A. P. Larkins, and H. O. McDevitt, In vivo preparation of thyroid and pancreatic auto-immunity in the BB rat by antibody to class II major histocompatibility complex gene products, Proc. Natl. Acad. Sci. U.S.A. 82:6627 (1985).
6. G. L. Boulianne, N. Hozumi, and M. J. Shuman, Production of functional chimeric mouse/human antibody, Nature (London) 312:643 (1984).
7. G. Chu and P. A. Sharp, SV40 DNA transfection of cells in suspension: analysis of the efficiency of transcription and translation of T-antigen, Gene 13:197 (1981).
8. W. D. Cook, S. Rudikoff, A. M. Giusti, and M. D. Scharff, Somatic mutation in a cultured mouse myeloma cell affects antigen binding, Proc. Natl. Acad. Sci. U.S.A. 79:1240 (1982).
9. W. D. Cook and M. D. Scharff, Antigen binding mutants of mouse myeloma cells, Proc. Natl. Acad. Sci. U.S.A. 74:5687 (1977).
10. J. Davies and A. Jiminez, A new selective agent for eukaryotic cloning vectors, Am. J. Trop. Med. Hyg. 29(5):1089 (1980).
11. J. Davies and D. I. Smith, Plasmid determined resistance to anti-microbial agents, Ann. Rev. Microbiol. 32:469 (1978).
12. B. Diamond, B. K. Birshtein, and M. D. Scharff, Site of binding of mouse IgG_{2b} to the Fc receptor on mouse macrophages, J. Exp. Med. 150:721 (1979).
13. L. Emorine, M. Kuehl, L. Weir, P. Leder, and E. E. Max, A conserved sequence in the immunoglobulin J_K-C_K intron: possible enhancer element, Nature (London) 309:447 (1983).
14. T. J. Franklin and J. M. Cook, The inhibition of nucleic acid synthesis by mycophenolic acid, Biochem. J. 113:515 (1969).
15. S. D. Gillies, S. L. Morrison, V. T. Oi, and S. Tonegawa, A tissue specific transcription enhancer element is located in the major intron of a rearranged immunoglobulin heavy chain gene, Cell 33:717 (1983).
16. D. G. Gilliland, Z. Steplewski, R. J. Collier, K. F. Mitchell, T. H. Chang, and H. Koprowski, Antibody-directed cytotoxic agents use of monoclonal antibody to direct the action of toxin A chains to colo-rectal carcinoma cells, Proc. Natl. Acad. Sci. U.S.A. 77:4539 (1980).
17. F. L. Graham and A. J. van der Eb, A new technique for the assay of infectivity of human adenovirus 5 DNA, Virology 52:456 (1973).
18. P. D. Gregor and S. L. Morrison, A myeloma mutant with a novel 3' flanking region: loss of normal sequence and insertion of repetitive elements leads to decreased transcription but normal processing of the alpha heavy chain gene products, Mol. Cell. Biol. in press (1986).
19. M. Heidelberger and F. E. Kendall, A quantitative theory of the precipitin reaction. III. The reaction between crystalline egg albumin and its homologous antibody, J. Exp. Med. 62:697 (1935).

20. B. J. Kobrin, C. K. Milcarek, and S. L. Morrison, Sequences near the 3' secretion-specific polyadenylation site influence the levels of secretion-specific and membrane-specific IgG_{2b} mRNA in myeloma cells, Mol. Cell. Biol. in press (1986).

21. G. Köhler and C. Milstein, Continuous cultures of fused cells secreting antibody of predefined specificity, Nature (London) 256:495 (1975).

22. K. A. Krolick, C. Villemez, P. Isahson, J. W. Uhr, and E. S. Vitetta, Selective killing of normal or neoplastic B cells by antibodies coupled to the A chain of ricin, Proc. Natl. Acad. Sci. U.S.A. 77:5419 (1980).

23. S. Larson, Radiolabeled monoclonal anti-tumor antibodies in diagnosis and therapy, J. Nucl. Med. 26:538 (1985).

24. R. Levy and R. A. Miller, Biological and clinical implications of lymphocyte hybridomas: tumor therapy with monoclonal antibodies, Ann. Rev. Med. 34:107 (1983).

25. B. Liesegant, A. Radbruch, and K. Rajewsky, Isolation of myeloma variants with predefined variant surface immunoglobulin by cell sorting, Proc. Natl. Acad. Sci. U.S.A. 75:3901 (1978).

26. S. L. Morrison, Transfectomas provide novel chimeric antibodies, Science 229:1202 (1985).

27. S. L. Morrison, M. J. Johnson, L. A. Herzenberg, and V. T. Oi, Chimeric human antibody molecules: mouse antigen-binding domains with human constant region domains, Proc. Natl. Acad. Sci. U.S.A. 81:6851 (1984).

28. S. L. Morrison, L. A. Wims, and V. T. Oi, Transfectomas: a new approach for the production of monoclonal antibodies, in: "Monoclonal Antibodies '84: Biological and Clinical Applications," A. Pinchera, G. Doria, F. Dammacco and A. Bargellesi, eds., Editrice Kurtis, Milano, Italy (1985).

29. R. C. Mulligan and P. Berg, Expression of a bacterial gene in mammalian cells, Science 209:1422 (1980).

30. R. C. Mulligan and P. Berg, Selection for animal cells that express Escherichia coli gene coding for xanthine-guanine phosphoribosyl-transferase, Proc. Natl. Acad. Sci. U.S.A. 78:2072 (1981).

31. M. S. Neuberger, G. T. Williams, and R. O. Fox, Recombinant antibodies possessing novel function, Nature (London) 312:604 (1984).

32. M. Nose and H. Wigzell, Biological significance of carbohydrate chains on monoclonal antibodies, Proc. Natl. Acad. Sci. U.S.A. 80:6632 (1983).

33. A. Ochi, R. G. Hawley, T. Hawley, M. J. Shulman, A. Traunecker, G. Kohler, and N. Hozumi, Functional immunoglobulin M production after transfection of cloned immunoglobulin heavy and light chain genes in lymphoid cells, Proc. Natl. Acad. Sci. U.S.A. 80:6351 (1983).

34. V. T. Oi, S. L. Morrison, L. A. Herzenberg, and P. Berg, Immunoglobulin gene expression in transformed lymphoid cells, Proc. Natl. Acad. Sci. U.S.A. 80:825 (1983).

35. D. Picard and W. Schaffner, A lymphocyte-specific enhancer in the mouse kappa gene, Nature (London) 307:80 (1984).

36. H. Potter, L. Weir, and P. Leder, Enhancer-dependent expression of human kappa immunoglobulin genes introduced into mouse pre-β lymphocytes by electroporation, Proc. Natl. Acad. Sci. U.S.A. 81:7161 (1984).

37. J.-L. Preud'homme, B. K. Birshtein, and M. D. Scharff, Variants of a mouse myeloma cell line that synthesize immunoglobulin heavy chains having an altered serotype, Proc. Natl. Acad. Sci. U.S.A. 72:1427 (1975).

38. C. Queen and D. Baltimore, Immunoglobulin gene transcription is activated by downstream sequence elements, Cell 33:741 (1983).

39. D. Rice and D. Baltimore, Immunoglobulin gene transcription is activated by downstream sequence elements, Proc. Natl. Acad. Sci. U.S.A. 79:7862 (1982).

40. R. M. Sandri-Goldin, A. L. Goldin, M. Levine, and J. C. Glorioso, High-

frequency transfer of cloned herpes simplex virus type 1 sequences to mammalian cells by protoplast fusion, Mol. Cell Biol. 1:743 (1981).

41. J. Sharon, M. L. Gefter, T. Manser, S. L. Morrison, V. T. Oi, and M. Ptashne, Expression of a V_HC_K chimeric protein in mouse myeloma cells, Nature (London) 309:364 (1984).

42. P. J. Southern and P. Berg, Transformation of mammalian cells to anti-biotic resistance with a bacterial gene under control of the SV40 early region promoter, J. Molec. Appl. Genet. 1:327 (1982).

43. L. K. Tan, V. T. Oi, and S. L. Morrison, A human-mouse chimeric immuno-globulin gene with a human variable region is expressed in mouse myeloma cells, J. Immunol. 135:3564 (1985).

44. S. A. Tilley, L. A. Eckhardt, K. B. Marcu, and B. K. Birshtein, Hybrid γ2b-γ2a genes expressed in myeloma variants: evidence for homologous recombination, Proc. Natl. Acad. Sci. U.S.A. 80:6967 (1983).

45. E. S. Vitetta, K. A. Krolick, M. Miyama-Inaba, W. Cushley, and J. W. Uhr, Immunotoxins: a new approach to cancer therapy, Science 219:644 (1983).

46. M. K. Waldor, S. Sriram, R. Hardy, L. A. Herzenberg, L. Lanier, M. Lim, and L. Steinman, Reversal of experimental allergic encephalomyelitis with monoclonal antibody to a T cell subset marker, Science 227:415 (1985).

47. R. Wall and M. Kuehl, Biosynthesis and regulation of immunoglobulins, Ann. Rev. Immunol. 1:393 (1983).

48. M. Wigler, S. Silverstein, L.-S. Lee, A. Pellicer, Y. C. Cheng, and R. Axel, Transfer of purified herpes virus thymidine kinase gene to cultured mouse cells, Cell 11:223 (1977).

49. D. M. Zaller and L. A. Eckhardt, Deletion of a B cell specific enhancer affects transfected, but not endogenous immunoglobulin heavy chain gene expression, Proc. Natl. Acad. Sci. U.S.A. 82:5088 (1985).

THE USE OF RICIN A CHAIN-CONTAINING IMMUNOTOXINS

TO KILL NEOPLASTIC B CELLS

Jonathan W. Uhr, R. Jerrold Fulton and Ellen S. Vitetta

Department of Microbiology
Southwestern Medical School
University of Texas Health Science Center
Dallas, Texas

INTRODUCTION

A cell-binding antibody conjugated to a plant or bacterial toxin has been termed an "immunotoxin." One such toxin, ricin, like most toxic proteins produced by bacteria and plants, has a toxic polypeptide (A chain) attached to a cell-binding polypeptide (B chain) (13). The B chain is a lectin that binds to galactose-containing glycoproteins or glycolipids on the cell surface. By mechanisms that are not yet well understood, the A chain of the cell-bound ricin gains access to the cell cytoplasm presumably by receptor-mediated endocytosis and penetration of the membrane of the endocytic vesicle. There is evidence that the B chain can also facilitate the translocation of the A chain through the membrane of the endocytic vesicle (4,5,12,20). In the cytoplasm, the A chain of ricin inhibits protein synthesis by enzymatically inactivating the EF-2 binding portion of the 60S ribosomal subunit. It is thought that one molecule of A chain in the cytoplasm of a susceptible cell can kill it (14).

The A and B chains of ricin can be separated, purified and covalently linked to antibodies derivatized with the thiol-containing cross-linker, SPDP. In the case of A chain-containing immunotoxins, the antibody portion substitutes for the lectin portion (B chain) thus allowing the specific targeting of the toxic A chain to the relevant target cells.

THE MURINE BCL$_1$ MODEL

This disease bears a close resemblance to the prolymphocytic form of chronic lymphocytic leukemia in the human, i.e., splenomegaly and severe leukemia (10,18). Injection of one BCL$_1$ cell into a normal BALB/c mouse results in leukemia in approximately one-half of the recipients 12 weeks later (24). Tumor-bearing mice usually survive for three to four months after receiving 10^5 to 10^6 tumor cells. The BCL$_1$ tumor cells bear large amounts of cell surface IgMλ and traces of IgDλ, both of which have the same idiotype.

The efficacy of immunotoxins in specifically killing subsets of cells in vitro has led to their application to deletion of particular cell types from suspensions of bone marrow cells. The ultimate objective is to facilitate bone marrow transplantation in the human as an approach to treatment of cancer and diseases of the hematopoietic system. Autologous bone marrow transplantation is used as an adjunct to treatment for certain types of cancer that are highly susceptible to x-irradiation and/or chemotherapy. The approach is to obtain bone marrow from a patient in remission (preferably in the first remission) and to freeze it. If the patient subsequently relapses, the patient is then subjected to "supralethal" therapy with x-irradiation and/or chemotherapy in order to eradicate the tumor. The patient is then rescued from death by infusion of his own bone marrow.

It would, of course, be highly desirable to purge such bone marrow of cancer cells by a cancer cell reactive immunotoxin. The only requirement of such an immunotoxin is that it should not damage the stem cells which are needed to reconstitute the patient's hematopoietic system.

In initial experiments, immunotoxins containing anti-idiotypic antibody directed against the tumor-derived Ig were incubated with populations of BCL$_1$ tumor cells and control cells. The specific immunotoxin decreased protein synthesis in the populations containing tumor cells by 70-80%; the percentage of tumor cells in these populations was also 70-80%. Control immunotoxins containing irrelevant antibodies had no effect on BCL$_1$ cells nor did specific immunotoxins have an effect on normal splenocytes, on T cell tumors, or on another B cell tumor bearing a different idiotype. Anti-idiotype antibody by itself did not affect protein synthesis in BCL$_1$ cells. These results indicate that immunotoxin-mediated killing of neoplastic B cells in a mixed population is specific (6).

Similar studies were performed using a tumor-infiltrated bone marrow (7) (containing 15% BCL$_1$ cells) because of the clinical implications of removing tumor cells from marrow. In addition, it was possible to evaluate the non-specific killing of stem cells by adoptively transferring the treated cells into lethally irradiated recipients. In these studies, anti-Ig immunotoxin was used since the only requirement for the specificity of the immunotoxin was that it kill all the tumor cells but not the stem cells. Thus, it was possible to use a polyvalent antibody against Ig rather than an anti-idiotypic antibody. The results of these experiments (Figure 1) indicate that 1) the hematopoietic system of all the animals was reconstituted because all lethally irradiated mice survived; and 2) 15 out of 20 mice treated with tumor-reactive immunotoxin did not develop tumors over a period of 25 weeks of observation. Of the five animals that relapsed, all had idiotype positive cells that were susceptible to the in vitro lethal effect of anti-Ig containing immunotoxins. Hence, no evidence was obtained for the emergence of an immunotoxin-resistant variant. Rather, the results of immunotoxin treatment in these studies were consistent with the survival of one cell per 1×10^6 cells injected. Results similar to ours have been obtained using antibody-ricin conjugates in the presence of lactose to delete tumor cells from rat bone marrow (21). We extended this approach to the removal of neoplastic B cells from human bone marrow and demonstrated that the tumor cells are killed but that the CFU$_{GM}$ BFU$_E$ are not (11).

Another approach to facilitating the bone marrow transplantation problem using immunotoxins is the elimination of T cells from HLA-matched bone marrow. The elimination of T cells is necessary to prevent the graft versus host disease (GVHD) that frequently accompanies such allogeneic transplantation (19). Prior studies have shown that antibody and complement is a highly effective maneuver to remove T cells and prevent GVHD. Studies by Kersey and his co-workers (2,23) over the past several years have shown the feasibility of using antibodies to T cells conjugated to intact ricin in the presence of 0.1 M galactose. This is a highly effective approach. Similar studies have been performed by Vitetta in collaboration with Martin and others in the Seattle Bone Marrow Transplantation Group using antibody A chain conjugates in which the antibody is specific to the CD3 antigen (Martin et al., unpublished). This conjugate is highly effective at killing T cells in human bone marrow (15). However, there are other problems with the use of such allogeneic marrow such as the emergence of late graft rejection and B cell lymphoma that have not yet been solved.

IN VIVO THERAPY OF BCL$_1$

The requirements for effective use of immunotoxins in vivo are considerably more formidable and stringent than their ex vivo use as described above for bone marrow transplantation. Potential problems include non-specific toxicity, specific toxicity due to cross-reactivity of the antibody in the immunotoxin with antigens present on life-supporting normal tissue, interaction of immunotoxin with tumor-associated antigens released into the circulation thereby forming antigen-antibody complexes, penetration of the immunotoxin into neoplastic tissue or into body compartments where there is a blood tissue barrier, and immune responses to the immunotoxin.

For the initial experiments, mice bearing massive tumor burdens (20% of body weight or approximately 10^{10} tumor cells) were employed (8). The strategy was to reduce the tumor burden by at least 95% using non-specific cytoreduction and to eliminate the remaining tumor cells with immunotoxins directed against either the idiotype or the δ chain of sIgD on the BCL$_1$ cells. The rationale for using anti-δ is that sIgD is present on a large proportion of B cell tumors and, therefore, would present a more practical reagent for clinical therapy. Furthermore, after cytoreductive therapy, there are virtually no sIgD-positive normal B cells or serum IgD to bind the immunotoxin. Normal B cells can also be regenerated from sIgD$^-$ cells. In these experiments, non-specific cytoreduction was accomplished with a combination of

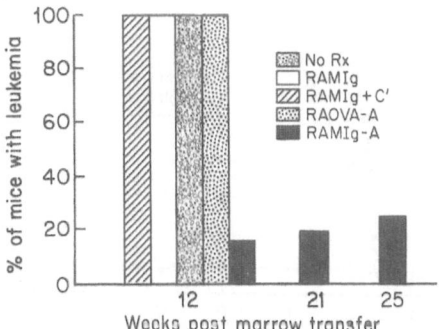

Figure 1. Adoptive transfer into lethally irradiated recipients of BCL$_1$-containing bone marrow cells treated with rabbit antibody to mouse Ig conjugated with A chain. Bone marrow cells containing 10 to 15 percent tumor cells were injected into groups of 20 mice at 10^6 marrow cells per mouse. Every two weeks after adoptive transfer the mice were examined for leukemia. At 25 weeks, all surviving mice were killed and 10^6 spleen cells were adoptively transferred into normal recipients. The spleen cells from one of the mice caused a tumor in these recipients ten weeks later. Thus, this mouse is scored as leukemic at 25 weeks.

splenectomy and fractionated total lymphoid irradiation (TLI). Animals receiving no further treatment other than TLI and splenectomy were dead within eight weeks (Figure 2). The injection of these cytoreduced mice with control immunotoxins or antibody alone did not prolong their survival. In contrast, animals receiving anti-immunotoxins appeared disease-free as judged by the absence of detectable idiotype-positive cells 10 to 18 weeks later in three of four experiments. In one experiment, treated mice relapsed at eight to ten weeks after immunotoxin therapy. It should also be noted that 14 weeks after such immunotoxin treatment, mice in remission had normal or above normal levels of sIgD-bearing B lymphocytes. Hence, stem cells, pre-B cells or sIgD⁻ lymphocytes had fully restored the virgin B cell compartment.

These results suggest that 1) either remaining tumor cells had been eradicated in the animals that appeared tumor-free or that some viable tumor cells remained but were "held in check" by host resistance mechanisms. 2) Immunotoxin to a normal tissue component, in this case sIgD, can be used to render animals disease-free and the host can survive the effects of such cross-reactivity and can reconstitute the B cell compartment. To determine whether the animals were disease-free, tissues were then transferred from disease-free animals 25 weeks after treatments. All animals adoptively transferred tumor into normal mice indicating that the animals were not tumor-free and suggesting that host resistance had developed.

The partial success of these experiments was probably due to the fact that non-specific cytoreduction was successful in reducing the number of remaining tumor cells to a level which could be effectively killed by a non-lethal dose of the immunotoxin. In addition, the immunotoxins in this instance did not kill all the remaining tumor cells yet prolonged remissions occurred. Presumably, the remaining viable tumor cells did not produce progressive disease because of a tumor-specific immune response.

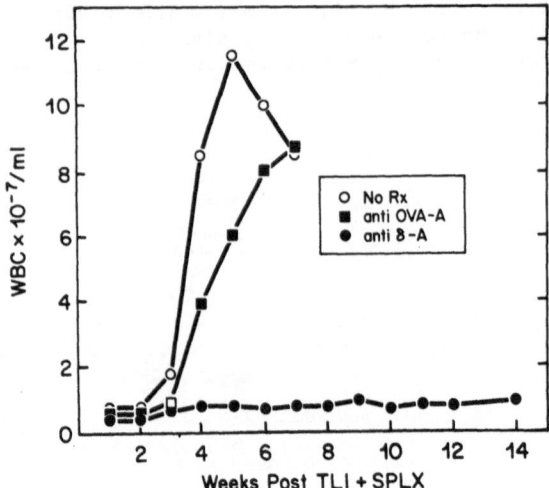

Figure 2. Effect of TLI, splenectomy, and administration of immunotoxin on leukemic relapse of BCL$_1$-bearing mice. After nine doses of TLI and splenectomy, mice were injected with two doses of 20 µg of anti-δ or control immunotoxin or were not injected. There were nine mice per group. Leukemic relapse was monitored by determining the number of white cells in the blood of the treated mice. The control mice were all dead at 7 weeks after TLI. The rabbit anti-mouse δ-A chain treated group was monitored for a period of 12 weeks post-TLI, at which point the experiment was terminated. 0 = no treatment; ■ = anti-OVA-A; ● = anti-δ-A.

USE OF B CHAIN-CONTAINING IMMUNOTOXINS TO POTENTIATE A CHAIN-CONTAINING IMMUNOTOXINS

It is known that in many cases ricin conjugates are significantly more toxic than antibody-A chain conjugates (4,5,12,20). In addition, free B chains can synergize in vitro with A chain-containing immunotoxins in specifically killing target cells (12). It is postulated, therefore, that the greater toxicity of ricin-containing immunotoxins as compared to A chain-containing immunotoxins is due to the capacity of the B chain to facilitate the entry of A chain into the cytoplasm (12). It would be desirable to develop a strategy in which the putative transport role of the B chain could be preserved while eliminating and minimizing its function as a lectin. One approach would be to utilize two types of immunotoxins. Tumor reactive antibodies could be conjugated to either ricin A chain or ricin B chain. Affinity purification of the immunotoxins on their respective antigens would be used to remove free A and B chains. Using the two immunotoxins, the two subunits of the ricin toxin could, thereby, be delivered independently to the same target cell.

To test this approach, a human neoplastic B cell line (Daudi) was treated with a low concentration of RAHIg-A that did not inhibit their protein synthesis. A goat anti-rabbit Ig-B chain conjugate also did not affect Daudi cells. However, when the cells were treated with RAHIg-A, washed, and then treated with different concentrations of GARIg-B, there was significant potentiation of cytotoxicity (26). When GARIg alone was used or when GARIg was mixed with 1% free B chains (the maximum estimated contamination of the secondary IT), no potentiation of the killing by RAHIg-A was observed. These experiments demonstrate that the potentiation of killing is dependent upon the covalent attachment of the B chain to the secondary antibody.

An irrelevant secondary IT (GA-OVA-B) was ineffective at potentiating killing by the RAHIg-A. In addition, an irrelevant primary IT (RA-OVA-A) or antibody (RAHIg) followed by the GARIg-B did not inhibit protein synthesis (data not shown).

We can only speculate on the subcellular events that underlie the synergy. It is likely that a portion of the two immunotoxins that bind to the same target cell are endocytosed together and are present in the same endosome. Therein, interchain disulfide bonds may be split and free A and B chains may be released into the endocytic vesicle. The B chain would then facilitate translocation of the A chain into the cytoplasm with resultant cell death. These results represent a new strategy for utilizing the toxic property of the A chain and the translocating ability of the B chain in a way that retains the specificity conferred by the antibody of A chain immunotoxin.

ADDITIONAL STRATEGIES TO OPTIMIZE THE USE OF A CHAIN IMMUNOTOXINS

There are four problems with the use of A chain immunotoxins that have been studied and in which progress has been made. 1) Lack of specific target cell toxicity of some A chain immunotoxins. So-called lysosomotropic agents that raise the pH of endocytic vesicles have been shown to potentiate A chain immunotoxins (1,16) and, in our laboratory, to markedly potentiate the potentiation of B chain-containing immunotoxins (3). These agents include ammonium chloride, chloroquine and monensin. The above studies have been carried out in vitro. It remains to be determined whether such agents can be used successfully in vivo and, in particular, if they potentiate target cell toxicity, do they potentiate non-specific toxicity as well. 2) Rapid uptake of A chain and B chain-containing immunotoxins by the liver due to their mannose-containing carbohydrates. It is known that Kupffer cells have receptors for

mannose (17) and these undoubtedly account in large measure for the rapid
uptake of immunotoxins by the liver and their consequent divergence from
target cells. Thorpe and colleagues (22) have developed a chemical procedure
to remove the majority of mannose residues from ricin. Such partially deglycosylated molecules are not taken up rapidly by the liver and, hence, have a
longer half-life in the circulation. It has been shown that such partially
deglycosylated A and B chains function quite effectively as immunotoxins
(27). A chain immunotoxins appear unaffected by the deglycosylation whereas
B chain immunotoxins are reduced three- to five-fold in effectiveness. It
may be helpful to use such deglycosylated immunotoxins in vivo, but further
studies will be needed again to determine the effect of deglycosylation on
therapeutic index. 3) The lectin binding site on the B chain may affect the
specificity of B chain immunotoxins in vivo. It has been shown biochemically
that inactivation of the lectin binding activity of the B chain can be
achieved by chloramine T-mediated iodination with virtually full retention
of the capacity of B chain as an immunotoxin to potentiate A chain immunotoxin
killing (28). It should be possible, therefore, to generate B chains by
recombinant DNA techniques in which the lectin binding site has been inactivated by site-directed mutagenesis and the potentiating activity retained.
4) Stability of the disulfide bond in vivo. There is conflicting evidence
regarding the stability of the SPDP linkage of A chain to antibody in vivo.
Our own studies (Inaba et al., unpublished) suggest that there is some instability in vivo. The problem of reduction of this bond in vivo is that
not only is some of the immunotoxin inactivated, but the free antibody generated from such immunotoxins then compete with the immunotoxin for antigenic
sites on the target cell. Hence, even a modest instability can result in a
significant reduction of specific target cell toxicity. We have recently
made immunotoxins using the F(ab) fragment of monoclonal or polyvalent antibody directed against particular immunoglobulin isotypes such as IgD. A
chains can be directly bound to the cysteine on the heavy chain that forms
the inter H chain disulfide bond on the intact molecule. Thus, using Ellman's
reagent, one can directly bind the sulfhydryl group on the A chain to the
cysteine in question resulting in a disulfide bond without an amino acid
spacer. This bond appears to be more stable in vivo. In addition, it has
recently been shown that F(ab) antibody directed against the immunoglobulin
of B lymphocytes has a different intracellular fate than intact antibody of
the same specificity (9). The F(ab) fragment after binding to surface Ig
and endocytosis of the complex does not go directly to lysosomes. In contrast, intact antibody and its bound surface Ig do go to lysosomes. Hence,
this different intracellular pathway could allow F(ab)-A chain immunotoxins
to translocate the A chain into the cytosol before destruction by lysosomal
enzymes.

IN VIVO THERAPY OF THE BCL_1 TUMOR WITH UNIVALENT VS. DIVALENT ANTI-δ
A CHAIN IT

We have compared the effectiveness of the IgG-A and F(ab)-A ITs in mice
bearing the BCL_1 tumor. The original model of the in vivo BCL_1 tumor has
been modified in order to obtain results more rapidly. We have shown that
one to three weeks after the injection of 10^6 to 10^7 BCL_1 cells into normal
BALB/c mice, approximately 40% or 4 to 8 x 10^7 cells in the spleens of these
mice, bear the BCL_1 idiotype. Since the spleen is the primary site of early
tumor growth, an enumeration of the number of idiotype-positive spleen cells
represents a fairly accurate measurement of the tumor burden in these animals.
These mice were injected with different doses of the IgG or F(ab)-A chain.
The antibody was a monoclonal rat anti-mouse chain of the IgG_{2b} isotype.
Twenty-four to 48 hours after injection of the IT, the spleens were removed
and analyzed for the presence of idiotype-positive cells. As shown in Figure
3, as determined by the number of idiotype-positive cells remaining in the
spleen, both univalent and divalent ITs eliminated the majority of the tumor

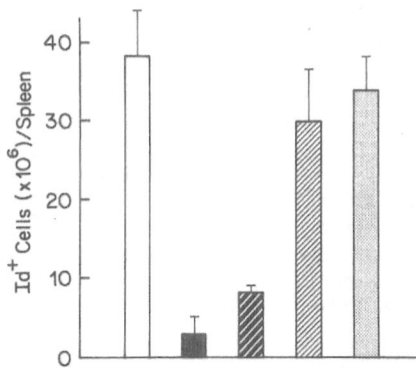

Figure 3. In vivo treatment of BCL_1 leukemia with a rat monoclonal antibody to mouse δ chain, JA12-A or F(ab)'-JA12-A. Mice were injected i.p. with 5×10^6 BCL_1 tumor cells. Three weeks after injection of tumor cells, groups of four mice were treated with a single i.v. injection of PBS (□) or 0.5 mg of JA12-A (▨), F(ab)'-JA12-A (■), JA12 (▨) or F(ab)'-JA12 (▨). Twenty-four hours after treatment spleens were removed and tumor cells were quantified by FACS analysis after staining with rabbit anti-idiotype and FITC-goat anti-rabbit antibody.

cells in a period of 24 hours following injection of a single dose of 0.5 mg IT. The F(ab) IT-A appeared more effective than the divalent IT-A and this difference has been observed in additional experiments. Tumor cell number did not decrease further after another 24 hours. Antibody alone or a control IT (R+Ig-A chain) did not induce killing (data not shown). This dose of IT gave maximal killing with both ITs. Although the observed killing represents only 80 to 90% of the initial tumor cells, the total number of tumor cells killed was 3 to 3.5×10^7. It should also be noted that the status of the remaining BCL_1 cells is not known. These cells could be programmed for death. Adoptive transfer assays will be necessary to quantify the number of viable tumor cells present in the remaining population of idiotype-positive cells. There was no evidence of liver or kidney damage in these animals. Further work will be aimed at optimizing the killing of BCL_1 cells by the F(ab) A anti-IT by varying the method of administration (bolus injection vs. slow infusion) and the number of treatments. We will then determine whether the piggyback B-IT can enhance the killing of A-IT-treated cells in vivo.

ACKNOWLEDGMENTS

We thank our colleagues Drs. Krolick, Villemez, Isakson and Cushley who collaborated with us on these studies; our technicians Mr. Y. Chinn, Ms. S. Gorman, Ms. R. Nisi, Ms. L. Trahan and Mr. T. Tucker and Ms. F. Hall for secretarial assistance. These studies were supported by National Institutes of Health grant CA-28149.

REFERENCES

1. P. Casellas, B.J.P. Bourrie, P. Gros, and F. Jansen, Kinetics of cyto-toxicity induced by immunotoxins: enhancement by lysosomotropic amines and carboxylic ionophores, J. Biol. Chem. 259:9359 (1984).
2. A. H. Filipovich, R. J. Youle, D. M. Neville, Jr., R. Vallera, R. Quinones, and J. H. Kersey, Ex vivo treatment of donor bone marrow

with anti-T cell immunotoxins for prevention of graft–versus–host disease, Lancet 8375:469 (1984).

3. R. J. Fulton, J. W. Uhr, and E. S. Vitetta, The effect of antibody valency and lysosomotropic amines on the synergy between ricin A chain and ricin B chain-containing immunotoxins, J. Immun. 136:3103 (1986).

4. L. L. Houston, Transport of ricin A chain after prior treatment of mouse leukemia cells with ricin B chain, J. Biol. Chem. 257:1532 (1982).

5. F. K. Jansen, H. E. Blythman, D. Carriere, P. Casellas, O. Gros, P. Gros, J. C. Laurent, F. Paolucci, B. Pau, P. Poncelet, G. Richer, H. Vidal, and G. A. Voison, Immunotoxins: hybrid molecules combining high specificity and potent cytotoxicity, Immunol. Rev. 62:185 (1982).

6. K. A. Krolick, C. Villemez, P. Isakson, J. W. Uhr, and E. S. Vitetta, Selective killing of normal or neoplastic B cells by antibodies coupled to the A chain of ricin, Proc. Natl. Acad. Sci. U.S.A. 77:5419 (1980).

7. K. A. Krolick, J. W. Uhr, S. Slavin, and E. S. Vitetta, In vivo therapy of a murine B cell tumor (BCL$_1$) using antibody-ricin A chain immuno-toxins, J. Exp. Med. 155:1797 (1982).

8. K. A. Krolick, J. W. Uhr, and E. S. Vitetta, Selective killing of leu-kemia cells by antibody-toxin conjugates; implications for autologous bone marrow transplantation in the treatment of cancer, Nature 295:604 (1982).

9. P. Metezeau, I. Elguindi, and M. Goldberg, Endocytosis of the membrane immunoglobulins of mouse spleen B cells: a quantitative study of its rate, amount and sensitivity to physiological, physical, and cross linking agents, EMBO J. 3:2235 (1984).

10. M. J. Muirhead, M. H. Holbert, J. W. Uhr, and E. S. Vitetta, BCL$_1$, a murine model of prolymphocytic leukemia, Amer. J. Pathol. 105:306 (1981).

11. M. J. Muirhead, P. J. Martin, B. Torok-Storb, J. W. Uhr, and E. S. Vitetta, Use of an antibody-ricin A chain conjugate to delete neo-plastic B cells from human bone marrow, Blood 62:337 (1983).

12. D. M. Neville, Jr. and R. J. Youle, Monoclonal antibody ricin or ricin A chain hybrids: kinetic analysis of cell killing for tumor therapy, Immunol. Rev. 62:75 (1982).

13. S. Olsnes and P. Pihl, Different biological properties of the two con-stituent peptide chains of ricin. A toxic protein inhibiting protein synthesis, Biochemistry 12:3121 (1973).

14. S. Olsnes and A. Pihl, Chimeric toxins, in: "Pharmacology of Bacterial Toxins," J. Drews and F. Dornes, eds., Pergamon Press, New York (1981).

15. O. Press, E. Vitetta, A. Farr, J. Hansen, and P. Martin, Efficacy of ricin A chain immunotoxins directed against human T cells, Cellular Immunol. in press (1986).

16. S. Ramakrishnan and L. L. Houston, Inhibition of human acute lympho-blastic leukemia cells by immunotoxins: potentiation by chloroquin, Science 223:58 (1984).

17. P. D. Stahl, J. S. Rodman, M. J. Miller, and P. H. Schlesinger, Evidence for receptor-mediated binding of glycoproteins, glycoconjugates, and lysosomal glycosidases by alveolar macrophages, Proc. Natl. Acad. Sci. U.S.A. 75:1399 (1978).

18. S. Slavin and S. Strober, Spontaneous murine B cell leukemia, Nature 272:624 (1977).

19. E. D. Thomas, The role of marrow transplantation in the eradication of malignant disease, Cancer 49:1963 (1982).

20. P. E. Thorpe, D. W. Mason, A.N.F. Brown, S. J. Simmonds, W.C.J. Ross, A. J. Cumber, and J. A. Forrester, Selective killing of malignant cells in a leukemic rat bone marrow using an antibody ricin conjugate, Nature 297:594 (1982).

21. P. E. Thorpe and W.C.J. Ross, The preparation and cytotoxic properties of antibody toxin conjugates, Immunol. Rev. 62:119 (1982).

22. P. E. Thorpe, S. I. Detre, B.M.J. Foxwell, A.N.F. Brown and E. Mayes, Modification of the carbohydrate in ricin and metaperiodate–cyanoborohydride mixtures: effects on toxicity and in vivo distribution, in press (1986).

23. D. A. Vallera, R. J. Youle, D. M. Neville, Jr., and J. H. Kersey, Bone marrow transplantation across major histocompatibility barriers. V. Protection of mice from lethal graft-vs.-host disease by pretreatment of donor cells with monoclonal anti-Thy 1.2 coupled to the toxin ricin, J. Exp. Med. 155:949 (1982).

24. E. S. Vitetta, K. A. Krolick, and J. W. Uhr, Neoplastic B cells as targets for antibody-ricin A chain, Immunol. Rev. 62:159 (1982).

25. E. S. Vitetta, W. Cushley, and J. W. Uhr, Synergy of ricin A chain-containing immunotoxins and ricin B chain-containing immunotoxins in in vitro killing of neoplastic human B cells, Proc. Natl. Acad. Sci. U.S.A. 80:6332 (1983).

26. E. S. Vitetta, R. J. Fulton, and J. W. Uhr, The cytotoxicity of cell-reactive immunotoxin containing ricin A chain is potentiated with an anti-immunotoxin containing ricin B chain, J. Exp. Med. 160:341 (1984).

27. E. S. Vitetta and P. E. Thorpe, Immunotoxins containing ricin A or B chains with modified carbohydrate residues act synergistically in killing neoplastic B cells in vitro, Cancer Drug Delivery 2:191 (1985).

28. E. S. Vitetta, Synergy between immunotoxins prepared with native ricin A chains and chemically modified ricin B chains, J. Immunol. 136:1880 (1986).

MONOCLONAL ANTIBODIES AND IMMUNOCONJUGATES

AS ANTI-CANCER AGENTS

Robert K. Oldham

Biological Therapy Institute
Franklin, Tennessee

INTRODUCTION

The use of antibodies in the treatment of human solid tumors is supported
by sufficient preclinical and clinical data to suggest that this approach
will be of real value in the development of selective biotherapy (1). Most
of the early antibody trials focused on the use of unconjugated antibody to
determine toxicity, tolerance, the localization in solid tumor deposits.
These studies defined the distribution of antibody in normal and neoplastic
tissues (2-8).

Murine monoclonal antibodies have been reasonably well tolerated in
patients. Doses from one milligram to several grams have been administered,
serum antibody levels have been determined, antiglobulin effects have been
assessed and the biodistribution analyzed. Although the clinical responses
to unconjugated antibody have not been striking, there is unequivocal evidence
that antibody does localize on individual cells and finds tumor deposits
after intravenous injection (9). Biodistribution studies utilizing antibody
conjugated to tracer quantities of isotope have demonstrated that antibody
will also go to the liver, spleen and other organs of the reticuloendothelial
system (10). Selective retention of the murine monoclonal antibody or the
antibody isotope conjugate have been demonstrated in the tumor bed.

These findings give a great deal of support to the concept that antibody
may be useful in the selective targeting of isotopes, drugs, toxins and biologics to solid tumors. Several reviews now exist on the use of monoclonal
antibody in the treatment of human solid tumors along with reviews of the
historical data on heteroantisera in cancer treatment (1,11-13).

DEVELOPMENT OF MONOCLONAL ANTIBODIES FOR THERAPY

There are already in existence many different monoclonal antibodies
which may be assessed in clinical trials in patients with solid tumors (14).
For tumors such as melanoma, lung, breast and colon cancer, there are more
than twenty antibodies each which have been described and characterized.
IgM, IgG and IgA preparations are available as are various subclasses of
IgG's. No doubt there will be a large variety of new monoclonal antibodies
described in the future, both murine and human. Thus, it is already apparent

that the limitation for the use of monoclonal antibody preparations in the clinic will not be due to a shortage of antibody preparations (1).

The "perfect" antibody (unconjugated or as a targeting agent) has not been identified for any human solid tumor. There is now more evidence that a single antibody or fixed extra antibody cocktail, just right for each class of cancer, may be possible. The problem becomes how does one prepare antibodies and conjugates for the clinic? There are no striking limitations on preparatory methods for manufacturing high purity, homogenous preparations of monoclonal antibodies. Techniques are available to produce preparations of greater than 90% purity which can be characterized as to antibody isotope, level of purity, degree of contamination by other substances, stability, and other pertinent physical/chemical characteristics.

Given a wide menu of antibody preparations and the ability to prepare them for the clinic, the next consideration is how does one select preparations for clinical trials and which preparations should be used in the first patient studies? Human solid tumors come in many shapes, sizes and types. It seems unlikely that hard and fast rules can be made on the selection of antibody preparations for all solid tumors. Obviously, the distribution of the tumor, its vascularity, its sensitivity to drugs and radiation and the quantitative expression of antigens on the tumor cell surface are all significant factors in antibody selection. The availability of other immunologically active cells within the tumor bed may be an important consideration for the use of conjugated antibody. There are data to support the use of certain classes of antibody relative to the activation and use on in situ immune mechanisms with the infusion of antibody. In terms of antibody as a targeting agent for isotopes, drugs, toxins and biologics, the issue may be more than one of biodistributions within the tumor bed and access of the toxic agent to the tumor cell within each tumor nodule. This may bring forth a whole different set of principles for immunoconjugates as opposed to using unconjugated antibody in the activation of in situ tumor immunity. Thus, it is apparent what while certain principles in the use of monoclonal antibody for human solid tumors may be important, each tumor type and, in fact, each individual patient may have to be individually evaluated for the optimal use of a monoclonal antibody preparation (15).

The antibody, whether conjugated or not, presumably must reach the tumor bed to be effective. One general principle has been that smaller antibody or antibody fragments may be more likely to diffuse from the vascular compartment out into the tumor bed. Early data from our studies have indicated that the more antibody one infuses into the vascular compartment, the more antibody one delivers to the tumor cell bed (9). While access to the tumor bed is clearly quite important, retention within the tumor bed may be more important. Preparations of antibody fragments may diffuse more quickly into the tumor nodule, but larger molecules may be retained for a longer period of time within the same nodules. Therefore, at the level of these very elementary principles, there is much to be learned about the use of antibody preparations in clinical trials. It does not seem reasonable, at this point in time, to presume that sufficient evidence is available to proceed with these clinical trials based on hard and fast rules as to which antibody preparation should be tested and which should not (15).

There are certain important principles in the design and execution of clinical trials using monoclonal antibodies for the treatment of patients with solid tumors (1,16,17). To learn from these early trials, it is necessary to have an active and competent laboratory to demonstrate that the antibody reached the tumor nodule and the techniques of immunohistology using biopsy specimens subsequent to infusion of antibody has been quite valuable (9,18,19). This has allowed investigators to characterize the distribution of antibody within the tumor nodule and to contrast it with that in surrounding normal tissues. The use of tracer labeled antibody preparations using diagnostic isotopes has also been very valuable in characterizing the biodistribution of antibody in these early studies. It is well recognized that as one conjugates antibody to anything, the biodistribution of the antibody may change and this requires some cross checking between studies using conjugated and unconjugated antibodies. Thus, these two techniques, immunohistology and immunoradiolocalization are complementary and have sometimes been synergistic in the performance of these early phase studies. A laboratory to measure circulating antibody after injection is critical to an understanding of the pharmacokinetics in these antibody trials (9). In addition, one should be able to measure circulating antigen, if such exists, and the importance of being able to measure antigen antibody complexes and antibody complexes is equally obvious (9). Finally, it is now known that low levels of "natural" antimurine antibodies may exist in human serum prior to the infusion of murine monoclonal antibodies (9). The ability to quantitate antiglobulin responses is also very important in the development of these clinical trials since antiglobulin responses may be important in the biodistribution of the infused antibody.

Careful clinical observations need to be made in the context of monoclonal antibody studies in patients with solid tumors. A daily dialogue between the laboratory scientist and the clinician is essential to maximize the information flow and to protect the patient during these early phase trials. Antibodies are biologic substances and require laboratory and clinical expertise. These preparations should not be considered as just another class of drugs to be given by individuals or groups expert in the use of chemotherapy. Biotherapy is very different from chemotherapy. The immune system and tumor cells may have receptors and/or mechanisms for dealing with biologic substances in a very different manner than a chemical compound. Therefore, the use and development of monoclonal antibody therapy requires expertise in immunology and biotherapy.

It seems prudent to continue studies with monoclonal antibody to try to derive the maximum amount of information without strong preconceived notions on the design of such studies or on potential therapeutic results. In these early phases, the selection of antibodies may be largely empirical and the clinic and laboratory are critical. Even issues such as the prediction of in vivo activity is very difficult at the moment. In our studies of antibody conjugates, those conjugates with the greatest activity in vitro did not always have the strongest activity in vivo (20). While the cytotoxic capability in the test tube is an important piece of information for a conjugated antibody, other factors such as biodistribution, antibody retention in the tumor bed, the metabolic translation through the membrane and a host of other factors may be equally or more important for in vivo activity.

CLINICAL TRIALS

Within the Biological Response Modifiers Program (BRMP), National Cancer Institute (NCI) (Table 1) we focused on three different diseases. The fourth disorder under study is poorly differentiated lymphoma with anti-idiotype antibodies. One patient with this disorder has been treated with antibody preparations at the time of this report. This report will focus on our solid tumor experience. Our results on leukemia/lymphoma have been previously reported (8).

Melanoma patients were treated with 9.2.27 IgG_{2A} murine monoclonal antibody developed by Dr. A. C. Morgan, Jr. This antibody recognized a 250 proteoglycan antigen on the surface of melanoma cells. It shows a high degree of specificity for melanoma and was considered an excellent candidate for early clinical trials. As is illustrated by Table 2, we performed a series

Table 1. Monoclonal Antibody Protocols at the BRMP - NCI

Antibody	Disease	No. of Patients	Dose (mg)	Schedule	Length of Infusion (hr)	Dose Escalation[a]
T101	CLL	7	1, 10, 50	biweekly	2	fixed
T101	CLL	6	50, 100	biweekly	50	fixed
T101	CTCL	8	1, 10, 50	biweekly	2, 50	fixed
T101	CTCL	3	100, 200, 500	biweekly	2[b]	escalating
9.2.27	melanoma	13	1, 10, 50, 100, 200, 500	biweekly	2	escalating
9.2.27	melanoma	7	100 mg x 5, 500 mg[c]	daily	2	fixed
anti-idiotype	CLL	1	10, 20, 50, 100, 200, 500	biweekly	4	escalating
111In-T101	CTCL	10	1 mg T101 + 5 mCi 111In[d]	once daily	2-10	
111In-9.2.27	melanoma	8	1 mg 9.2.27 + 5 mCi 111In[d]	once only	2	

[a]Fixed, dose fixed for each patient with escalation between patients. Escalating; each patient receives multiple dose levels.

[b]Patients received 2 mg T101/hr for 4 hr to modulate the T65 antigen from circulating cells and then received a 6-hr infusion of high dose T101 (100 mg, first week; 200 mg, second week, 500 mg, third week).

[c]Patients received five daily doses of 100 mg of antibody, four weeks off therapy followed by a single infusion of antibody.

[d]Some patients received 10-50 mg of unlabeled T101 or 9.2.27 in addition to immunoconjugate.

Table 2. In Vitro[a] and In Vivo[b] Reactivity of 9.2.27 Antibody with Melanoma Cells in Cutaneous Skin Lesions

| | | | 9.2.27 Reactivity | | | |
| | | | Flow Cytometry (%) % Positive Cells | | Immunoperoxidase[c] Score | |
Patient	Dose 9.2.27	Days Post-Treatment	In Vitro	In Vivo	In Vitro	In Vivo
A.F.	Pretreatment		80	ND	++	−
	1 mg	1	92	0	++	−
D.F.	Pretreatment		83	ND	++	−
	1 mg	1	0	0	+	−
	50 mg	1	72	0	++	+
	200 mg	1	ND	ND	++	+
M.F.	Pretreatment		97	ND	++	−
	10 mg	1	98	2	+	−
	100 mg	1	72	50	+	+
	200 mg	4	98	91	+	+
B.C.	Pretreatment		90	ND	++	−
	200 mg	1	73	71	+	+
C.S.	Pretreatment		76	ND	++	−
	1 mg	1	91	0	++	−
	200 mg	1	41	35	++	+
A.T.	Pretreatment		0	ND	+	−
	50 mg	1	ND	ND	++	++
	200 mg	1	14	50	++	++
M.G.	Pretreatment		76	1	++	−
	50 mg	4	97	1	++	−
J.S.	Pretreatment		ND	ND	++	−
	50 mg	1	ND	ND	++	+
	100 mg	1	ND	ND	++	++

[a]In vitro reactivity refers to reactivity when excess 9.2.27 was added during the staining procedure.
[b]In vivo reactivity refers to endogenously bound 9.2.27 after IV antibody therapy.
[c]Staining of melanoma cells with 9.2.27 was graded on a + to ++ scale which represents a combination of both percent positive cells and intensity of staining.

of studies looking at the delivery of antibody to the tumor bed with two separate techniques. After infusion of antibody intravenously, skin nodules were removed and stained for mouse antibody using the immunoperoxidase technique. Additionally, a portion of the tumor was disassociated into single cell suspensions and the tumor cells assessed by flow cytometry for the presence of antibody and antigen on the tumor cell surface. From these studies, it became clear that 200-500 milligrams of antibody was necessary to saturate the tumor cell surface antigens. Obviously, saturation has two phases. One can saturate all of the cells within the tumor nodule with at least some antibody on each cell and at a second level one can saturate all the antigen on all the cells in a particular nodule. Flow cytometry is very helpful at looking at saturation of individual viable cells in a disassociated cell preparation whereas immunoperoxidase is an excellent technique to give a better sense of saturation across a histological section from a tumor nodule (9).

Following the studies of antibody alone and the localization by tissue analysis, radioimmunolocalization using 9.2.27 conjugated to Indium-111 or Iodine-125 was done to analyze biodistribution. Labeled antibody went to the reticuloendothelial system but over time it showed selective retention in tumor cell sites (21).

Phase I studies have also been performed with antibody to the P97 kilodalton antigen on the surface of melanomas and other tumors (28). Less extensive studies were also done with antibody 48.7 directed at the same antigen recognized by 9.2.27 (18). These studies were confirmatory of the results discussed above. Immunohistologic confirmation of antibody in the biopsy site with selective binding to the melanoma cells, was seen. Pharmacokinetic parameters were measured which defined the peak antibody concentration and the half-life of the antibody in these studies. Peak level and half-life were affected to antiglobulin levels and trace labeled antibody preparations were very useful in making these measurements.

Larsen and co-workers have labeled antibodies of P97 with therapeutic doses of I-125 in attempts to show therapeutic activity for isotope conjugates in patients with melanoma. Localization of the labeled antibody has been seen and evidence of minor tumor regression was noted (22).

Trials with monoclonal antibody in patients with melanoma are now ongoing at several centers. These clinical trials are moving very rapidly from antibody alone to therapeutic attempts with antibody coupled to a variety of toxic agents. Early reports of therapeutic activity using ricin A chain anti-melanoma antibody have been encouraging (L. Spitler, personal communication).

Gastrointestinal carcinoma has been the other major cancer type treated with monoclonal antibody. Studies by Sears and co-workers in over twenty patients with gastrointestinal malignancies using antibody 17-Ia IgG_{2A} gave definitive evidence of localization of the antibody in the tumor (19). Doses from 15-1000 milligrams per patient have been given without severe side effects. Circulating immunoglobulin has been seen for as long as fifty days and they reported antiglobulin responses were dependent on the amount of antibody given (not confirmed in recent studies). They reported evidence of clinical antitumor responses in at least three of twenty patients. They postulated these effects may be related to antibody-macrophage interactions within the tumor bed and they suggested that a combination of high doses of antibody to reduce the antiglobulin responses and the use of an IgG_{2A} subclass might be a reasonable approach to study further patients with antibody.

Dillman and co-workers have given infusions of anti-CEA monoclonal antibody and reported localization without antitumor response (23). Further studies are now underway with unconjugated antibody 17-1A in Philadelphia and with a variety of antibodies to gastrointestinal carcinoma by other investigators using conjugated reagents.

A brief report on the use of IgG_3 monoclonal antibody which had in vitro cytotoxicity on human gastrointestinal carcinoma was reported by Lemin and co-workers in abstract form (24). Eight patients were treated by infusion with this antibody preparation. Complement consumption and fever were noted and murine antiglobulins appeared to produce mild serum sickness. Immunohistologic evidence of antibody localization was seen but no clinical responses were observed.

Melino and co-workers from London reported on the use of human antibody produced by allogeneic immunization in 12 volunteers. These antibodies were then used to target Daunorubicin and Chloroambucil in 12 neuroblastoma patients over the age of two. These preparations were well tolerated and no antiglobulin, allergic or toxic effects were noted. Marked antitumor responses were reported in nine of twelve patients and all responding patients were said to be disease-free after more than three years. This unique and striking report is the first study where allogeneic immunization of normal volunteers was used to create a heteroantiserum with resultant therapeutic effects. Clearly, follow-up on these studies will be very important to confirm these results (25).

Finally, Houghton and co-workers using an antibody to cell surface GD induced responses in some of their 12 patients with melanoma (26). Many studies are in progress with the use of unconjugated antibody and with conjugated antibody in vitro and in Nu/Nu mouse xenograft models (37). Many of these preparations show excellent toxicity in vitro and in vivo for human tumor cells. It is anticipated that within the next year there will be a large number of studies initiated with antibody conjugates in man.

PROSPECTS FOR THE FUTURE

The application of unconjugated antibody and of antibody immunoconjugated as therapeutic anticancer agents in man has just begun. However, even with the early information available, there are some principles for the optimization of monoclonal antibody therapy which may be important in the design of future studies (Table 3). The antibodies have been murine in origin, which are foreign proteins in man. Depending on the factors such as circulating cells bearing antigen or antigen in the serum, there may be seen a spectrum of clinical toxicities in association with monoclonal antibody therapy (Table 4).

From the early trials of antibody, it is apparent that there are some strategies that can be entertained to approach certain problems and enhance the potential therapeutic activity of these preparations (Table 5).

A sumary of recent serotherapy trials using monoclonal antibody for solid tumors is shown in Table 6. No attempt has been made to summarize

Table 3. Optimization of Monoclonal Antibody Therapy

---

1. Antibody Specificity
   a. immunoperoxidase
   b. radiolocalization
2. Antigen Characterization
   a. biochemical nature
   b. topography
   c. epitope
   d. heterogeneity
3. Antibody-Antigen Interaction
   a. turnover of antibody bound to tumor cells
   b. degree of antibody internalization
   c. antigen levels in serum
4. Antibody Delivery
   a. dose
   b. regimen
   c. route
   d. pharmacokinetics
   e. comparison of various cytotoxic agents conjugated
      to the same antibody

Table 4. Clinical Toxicity in MoAb Trials

Fever	Dyspnea
Chills	Hypotension/tachycardia
Flushing	Anaphylactic/analhylactoid reactions
Emesis	Serum sickness
Urticaria	Increased creatinine
Rash	Headache
Nausea/Vomiting	Bronchospasm*

*Pulmonary toxicity (dyspnea, bronchospasm, etc.) has been
 mainly observed with circulating antigen-bearing cells
 during MoAb infusion.

the older data with heteroantisera as this has been reviewed (12). More
recent reports with rabbit, goat and even human allogeneic serums have not
been summarized here. While these approaches may be of value and are of
interest, they lack the essential features of reproducibility, high titer,
unlimited quantity and molecular purity needed to proceed with the large
scale clinical trials. Emerging evidence on the use of antibodies derived

Table 5. Problems with MoAb Therapy

Problem	Possible Solutions
Antigenic modulation	Not all antibodies cause modulation; use 2 MoAb recognizing same antigen (different epitopes*) or different antigens; choose different antigen.
Release of free antigen	Plasmapheresis; plasmapheresis over immuno-absorbent column; schedule MoAb treatments appropriately.
Antibody to mouse cells	Human antibodies, low dose cyclophosphamide plasmapheresis with immunospecific absorption, effect of antibody dose and schedule on antimurine response, induction of tolerance.
Non-sustained reduction of leukemic cells	Repeated, intermittent MoAb infusions
Neoplastic cells outside blood less sensitive with few clinical responses	Infuse more than one MoAb directed toward different epitopes on the same antigen. Infuse more than one MoAb directed toward different antigens on the same cell. Infuse more than one MoAb using different subclasses (IgG1, IgG2, IgM, etc.). Conjugate MoAb to drugs, toxins or isotopes.

*Epitopes are different parts of the antigen molecule. Each epitope can
 stimulate and react with antibody directed toward that part of the antigen
 molecule. Thus, different antibodies can be generated to the same "antigen."

Table 6. MoAb Serotherapy Trials in Patients with Solid Tumors

Institution	Disease	MoAb[b]	References
Univ. of Pennsylvania (Wistar)	GI[a] cancer	17-1A	(19)
Univ. of California at Los Angeles	GI cancer	CCOLI	(24)
Univ. of California at San Diego	Colon Cancer	065	(33)
Univ. of California at San Diego	Melanoma	Ab to p97 Ab to p240	(4)
Fred Hutchinson Cancer Center	Melanoma	Ab to p97	(22)
Swedish Hospital Medical Center-Seattle	Melanoma	48.7 and Ab to p97	(18)
National Cancer Inst.	Melanoma	9.2.27	(1,9)

[a]GI = gastrointestinal; [b]Ab or antigen designation

by in vitro or in vivo immunization of humans for the purpose of producing human monoclonal antibody are of interest, but no clinical trials have been carried out with human monoclonal antibodies. These preparations possess certain advantages but may also have certain inherent disadvantages (1). Certain conclusions from monoclonal antibody serotherapy trials are summarized in Table 7.

Based on current data, the future does not look very bright for the use of unconjugated antibody. Minor clinical effects with conjugated antibody have been seen in leukemia and certain lymphomas. In solid tumors, only the report of Sears and co-workers on possible clinical effects of unconjugated

Table 7. Summary - MoAb Serotherapy Trials

1. IV murine-derived MoAb can be given safely by prolonged infusion (>1 hr) without immediate side effects.
2. Bronchospasm and hypotension have followed rapid infusion (5 mg per hr) and higher doses of monoclonal antibody to T cells at higher doses (>20 mg).
3. Dosages from 1 mg to 3 gms have been given safely with careful monitoring.
4. A sustained decline in leukemic cells requires multiple MoAb treatments over several weeks.
5. Skin lesions and lymph nodes can regress following MoAb treatment.
6. There has been no reduction in the bone marrow leukemia cells.
7. Antigenic modulation sometimes occurs following MoAb treatment.
8. Free antigen may be detected in the serum following MoAb treatment.
9. Clear evidence of selective localization of infused antibody in solid tumors is available.
10. Antibodies to mouse cells may develop following MoAb therapy.
11. There is considerable variation with respect to toxicity, bio-availability, and activity related to immunoglobulin class, antigen, and distribution to tumor.

antibody in gastrointestinal carcinoma (16) and the Houghton report in
melanoma are encouraging (26). The major conclusion to be drawn from all of
these studies is that antibody alone confirms the targeting capability of
these biological substances. At a second level of consideration, the in
vitro activity and the in vivo preclinical activity of immunoconjugates are
indeed encouraging (27). Very early studies with the use of immunoconjugates
of antibody and isotopes in human solid tumors have shown encouraging localization and even some evidence of therapeutic effects (22). There are those
who are searching for the "perfect" immunoconjugate. That is, a conjugate
with complete specificity for the tumor and without problems of side effects
with reference to localization of the antibody in organs not containing tumor.
However, all of the early data would indicate that mouse antibody conjugates
are going to go to the reticuloendothelial system and that tumor-associated
antigens are not absolutely specific. Therefore, it is important to judge
immunoconjugates as one would judge any other systemic therapy. Is the toxicity worth the therapeutic effect? At the bottom line, one is looking for
therapeutic approaches with selectivity and activity superior to the currently
available approaches. Given the lack of selectivity for the available modal-
ities of treatment and in particular given the very poor selectivity of
systemic chemotherapy, any improvement in the selective delivery of toxic
substances to tumor cells through monoclonal antibody technology will be a
step in the right direction (28,29). In spite of these encouraging data for
the use of antibody as a targeting agent, the heterogeneity of cancer is an
important consideration (17). If one uses a single antibody or a fixed combination of a few antibodies that cover only a portion of the tumor cells
and, if that preparation does not eliminate the true replicating cell population (stem cell) from the tumor population, eventual outgrowth of viable
cells and perhaps resistant cells will be inevitable. Therefore, it seems
logical to proceed with attempts to type human tumors and to deliver toxic
substances to them utilizing "cocktails" of antibodies sufficient to cover
all the tumor cells known to exist in each patient. This type of approach
may require a considerable amount of testing for each patient and a "typing"
of one or more tumors from each patient. Such approaches may be much more
custom tailored than is easily approachable through the product development
paradigm which has been used with some success in the development of new
cancer drugs (30). If indeed the spectrum of human tumor heterogeneity is
great, the possibility of the ideal antibody conjugated to the ideal toxic
agent may not be achievable. Investigators in this area should not despair
because the heterogeneity of the immune system is also great and theoretically
can be used to provide adequate coverage for the heterogeneity of cancer
cell population. However, the difficulties in preparing antibodies and immunoconjugates for clinical use are obvious and these approaches will be
complex and time-consuming. Testing of various antibodies and immunoconjugates is now underway. Investigators and patients alike can anticipate an
improvement in the selective delivery of toxic agents to the cancer cell in
the near future (30-35).

REFERENCES

1. R. K. Oldham, Monoclonal antibodies in cancer therapy, J. Clin. Oncol.
    1:582 (1983).
2. S. M. Larson, J. P. Brown, P. W. Wright, J. A. Carrasquillo, I. Hell-
    strom, and K. E. Hellstrom Imaging of melanoma with I-labeled mono-
    clonal antibodies, J. Nucl. Med. 24:123 (1983).
3. J. Ritz and S. F. Schlossman, Utilization of monoclonal antibodies in
    treatment of leukemia and lymphoma, Blood 59:1 (1982).
4. R. E. Sobol, R. O. Dillman, and J. D. Smith, Phase I evaluation of
    murine monoclonal anti-melanoma antibody in man: preliminary obser-
    vations, in: "Hybridomas in Cancer Diagnosis and Treatment," M. S.
    Mitchell, and H. F. Oettgen, eds., Raven Press, New York (1981).

5. H. F. Sears, J. Mattis, D. Heryln, P. Hayry, B. Atkinson, C. Ernst, Z. Steplewski, and H. Koprowski, Phase I clinical trial of monoclonal antibody in treatment of gastrointestinal tumors, Lancet i:762 (1982).

6. R. A. Miller and R. Levy, Response of cutaneous T cell lymphoma to therapy with hybridoma monoclonal antibody, Lancet ii:226 (1981).

7. R. A. Miller, D. G. Maloney, R. Warnke, and R. Levy, Treatment of B cell lymphoma with monoclonal anti-idiotype antibody, N. Eng. J. Med. 306:517 (1982).

8. K. A. Foon, R. Schroff, P. A. Bunn, D. Mayer, P. G. Abrams, M. F. Fer, J. Ochs, G. Bottino, S. A. Sherwin, D. J. Carlo, R. B. Herberman, and R. K. Oldham, Effects of monoclonal antibody therapy in patients with chronic lymphocytic leukemia, Blood 64:1085 (1984).

9. R. K. Oldham, K. A. Foon, A. C. Morgan, C. S. Woodhouse, R. W. Schroff, P. G. Abrams, M. Fer, C. S. Schoenbeck, M. Farrell, and E. Kimball, Monoclonal antibody therapy of malignant melanoma: in vivo localization in cutaneous metastasis after intravenous administration, J. Clin. Oncol. 2:1235 (1984).

10. D. M. Goldberg and F. H. Deland, History and status of tumor imaging with radiolabeled antibodies, J. Biol. Resp. Modif. 1:277 (1983).

11. K. A. Foon, M. I. Bernhard, and R. K. Oldham, Monoclonal antibody therapy: assessment by animal tumor models, J. Biol. Resp. Modif. 1:277 (1983).

12. S. A. Rosenberg and W. D. Terry, Passive immunotherapy of cancer in animals and man, Adv. Cancer Res. 25:323 (1977).

13. R. O. Dillman, Monoclonal antibodies in the treatment of cancer, Crit. Rev. Hemat. Oncol. 1:357 (1984).

14. B. D. Boss, R. Longman, I. Trowbridge, and R. Dulbecco, eds., "Monoclonal Antibodies and Cancer," Academic Press, New York (1983).

15. R. K. Oldham, Therapeutic monoclonal antibodies: effects of tumor cell heterogeneity, Cancer Treatment Symposium (Germany) (1986).

16. R. K. Oldham, Biologicals and biological response modifiers: new strategies for clinical trials, in: "Interferons, IV" N. B. Finter and R. K. Oldham, eds., Elsevier Science Publishers (1985).

17. R. K. Oldham, Antibody-drug and antibody-toxin conjugates, in: "Immunity to Cancer," A. E. Reif and M. S. Mitchell, eds., Academic Press, New York (1985).

18. G. E. Goodman, P. Beaumier, I. Hellstrom, B. Fernyhough, and K. E. Hellstrom, Phase I trial of murine monoclonal antibodies in patients with advanced melanoma, J. Clin. Oncol. 3:340 (1985).

19. H. F. Sears, D. Herlym, Z. Steplewski, and H. Koprowski, Effects of monoclonal antibody immunotherapy in patients with gastrointestinal adenocarcinoma, J. Biol. Resp. Modif. 3:138 (1984).

20. A. C. Morgan, J. W. Pearson, and R. K. Oldham, In vivo models for preclinical evaluation of immunotoxins, in: "Immunotoxins: The Current Status of Antibody Conjugates for Radioimaging and Therapy of Cancer," C. W. Vogel, ed., Oxford University Press (1986).

21. J. A. Carrasquillo, P. G. Abrams, R. Schroff, J. Reynolds, A. C. Morgan, A. Keenan, K. A. Foon, P. Perentesis, M. Horowitz, Y. Szimendera, R. K. Oldham, and S. Larson, Imaging of metastatic melanoma with 111 in 9.2.27 anti-melanoma monoclonal antibody (1986).

22. S. M. Larson, J. A. Carrasquillo, and K. A. Krohn, Radiotherapy with "anti-P97" iodinated monoclonal antibodies in melanoma, in: "Proceedings of the Third World Congress of Nuclear Medicine and Biology," C. Raynaud, ed., Pergamon Press, New York (1982).

23. R. O. Dillman, J. C. Beauregard, D. L. Shawler, et al., Results of early trials using murine monoclonal antibodies as anticancer therapy, in: "Protides of the Biological Fluids," H. Peeters, ed., Pergamon Press, New York (1983).

24. S. Lemkin, K. Tokita, G. Sherman, et al., Phase I-II study of monoclonal antibodies (MCA) in gastrointestinal cancer, ASCO Abstracts (1984).

25. G. Melino, P. Elliott, K. B. Cooke, et al., Allogeneic antibodies (abs.) for drug targeting in human neuroblastoma (nb.) ASCO Abstracts (1984).

26. A. N. Houghton, D. Mintzer, C. Gordon-Cardo, S. Welt, B. Fliegel, S. Vadhan, E. Carswell, M. R. Melamed, H. F. Oettgen, and L. J. Old, Mouse monoclonal IgG3 antibody detecting GD3 ganglioside: a phase I trial in patients with malignant melanoma, Proc. Natl. Acad. Sci. 82:1242 (1985).

27. A. C. Morgan, Jr., G. Pavonasassivam, K. M. Hwang, C. S. Woodhouse, R. W. Schroff, K. A. Foon, and R. K. Oldham. Preclinical and clinical evaluation of a monoclonal antibody to human melanoma-associated antigen, in: "Protides of the Biological Fluids," H. Peeter, ed., Pergamon Press, London 32:773 (1985).

28. R. K. Oldham, Biologicals and biological response modifiers: fourth modality of cancer treatment, Cancer Treat Rep. 68:221 (1984).

29. M. G. Hanna, Jr., M.E. Key, and R. K. Oldham, Biology of cancer therapy: some new insight into adjuvant treatment of metastatic solid tumors, J. Biol. Resp. Modif. 4:295 (1983).

30. R. K. Oldham, Biologicals: new horizons in pharmaceutical development, J. Biol. Resp. Modif. 2:199 (1983).

31. M. E. Key, M. I. Bernhard, L. C. Hoyer, K. A. Foon, R. K. Oldham, and M. G. Hanna, Guinea pig 10 hepatocarcinoma model for monoclonal antibody in normal and malignant tissues, J. Immunol. 139(3):1451 (1983).

32. M. I. Bernhard, K. A. Foon, T. N. Oeltmann, M. E. Key, K. M. Hwang, G. C. Clarke, W. L. Christensen, L. C. Hoyer, M. G. Hanna, and R. K. Oldham, Guinea pig line 10 hepatocarcinoma model: characterization of monoclonal antibody and antibody conjugated to diptheria toxin A chain, Cancer Res. 43:4420 (1983).

33. M. I. Bernhard, K. M. Hwang, K. A. Foon, A. M. Keenan, R. M. Kessler, J. M. Frincke, D. J. Tallam, M. G. Hanna, L. Peters, and R. K. Oldham, Localization of 111-In and 125-I labeled monoclonal antibodies in guinea pigs bearing line 10 hepatocarcinoma tumors, Cancer Res. 43:4429 (1983).

34. K. M. Hwang, K. A. Foon, P. H. Cheung, J. W. Pearson, and R. K. Oldham, Selective antitumor effect of a potent immunoconjugate composed of the A chain of abrin and monoclonal antibody to a hepatocarcinoma associated antigen, Cancer Res. 44:4578 (1984).

35. R. K. Oldham, Does sufficient selectivity of monoclonal antibodies to cancer cells exist for therapeutic application? in: "Clinical Use of Monoclonal Antibodies in Cancer Therapy and Imaging: Current Status, Controversies and Future Directions," R. Dillman, I. Royston, D. Carlo, eds., Martinus Nijhoff Publishing (1986).

SECTION VI
OVERVIEW AND COMMENTS

Overview and Comments
Gregory W. Siskind

OVERVIEW AND COMMENTS

Gregory W. Siskind

Division of Allergy and Immunology, Department of Medicine
Cornell University Medical College
New York, New York

Since in the space available I cannot truly summarize a meeting of this
sort which covers such a broad area of immunology, I would like instead to
share with you some of the thoughts and reactions I had while listening to
the presentations.

Our understanding of immunoglobulin structure is progressing rapidly
(K. J. Dorrington, E. A. Kabat, S. L. Morrison). It is now clear that each
immunoglobulin domain has a basic configuration consisting of two layers of
anti-parallel pleated sheets with hypervariable regions at the turns in the
chain, so that they are brought together to form the antigen combining region.
While allosteric changes do not seem important, in most cases, in the expression of the effector functions of antibodies, the possibility that shifts in
fine structure in the combining site region contribute to binding potential
of an antibody molecule has not, to my knowledge, been ruled out. Clearly
the old rather mechanical "lock and key" concept of the binding site must be
replaced by a more dynamic view which sees the site as a three dimensional
distribution of chemical groups on the surface of the molecule. This display
of chemical groups, with their varied potential to form different types of
chemical bonds (hydrophobic interactions, electrostatic interactions, hydrogen
bonds, etc.) undoubtedly accounts for the specificity of the molecule.
Thought of in this manner, that is as a display of potential sites for interaction with other molecules, the recent findings of unexpected cross-reactivities (multispecificity) or what we referred to some time ago as degeneracy,
becomes a logical indeed expected result. The old observation of the exqui-
site specificity of antibody may well result, not from the binding properties
of individual antibody molecules, but rather from the overal binding properties of the population of molecules present in the usual heterogeneous immune
serum. With the impact of "monoclonal technology" we should not forget these
specificity problems. Unexpected cross-reactions (multispecificity or degeneracy) may well be the rule with monoclonals. Greater apparent specificity
may at times be obtained by using a mixture of several monoclonals. With
each monoclonal a different set of cross-reactions exists. In a mixture,
the common specificity dominates (as in a typical immune serum), and the
cross-reactivities present with individual molecules are, in effect, diluted
out: thus, the mixture appears highly specific. I would suggest that degeneracy is the usual situation, although it is very difficult to probe.

I would like to point out that some years ago my laboratory demonstrated that a large amount (at times over 5 mg/ml) of very low affinity antibody is produced by animals immunized with dinitrophenylated proteins. This antibody precipitates poorly with antigen and can be detected only by a direct binding assay (such as equilibrium dialysis). Its association constant for the dinitrophenyl hapten is, in some cases, only slightly higher than the "nonspecific" binding of the hapten by normal IgG (approximately 10^3). Despite its low affinity, this binding activity, which is absent from pre-immune serum, appears in response to the antigen and can therefore be defined as antibody. It seems inevitable that such extremely low affinity antibody can bind numerous other ligands with higher affinity and is thus undoubtedly degenerate (multispecific). I would point out that this low affinity antibody can be present in very high concentrations (5-10 mg/ml) emphasizing the marked degree of degeneracy (multispecificity) which probably exists and may well contribute to the protective function of our "normal" serum antibody. Obviously certain particular types of degeneracy (e.g., an antibody which also binds the Fc portion or an idiotope on another antibody molecule) might have special biological effects, but degeneracy as a concept should not be limited to these.

Thus the antibody response is typically both redundant and degenerate. Redundant in that a number of clones reacting with a particular epitope are usually stimulated. Degenerate in that individual antibody molecule undoubtedly bind multiple distinct epitopes.

For the first century of immunologic investigation, the mechanism for the generation of diversity was a centeral theoretical issue. During the past few years we have come to understand the general principles underlying the molecular processes involved in the generation of diversity (L. E. Hood). Combinatorial mechanisms involving bringing together V and J gene segments for light chains and V, D and J gene segments for heavy chains result in a marked degree of diversity. This diversity is expanded by introduction of variation at joining sites and by somatic hypermutation. Further diversity is probably generated by bringing together different heavy and light chains. The detailed molecular mechanisms whereby a given VDJ unit can be combined with any of the various constant region gene segments is still uncertain; however, the general principles are clear and it seems likely that progress in this area will be rapid (R. Wall). Some developmental data (M. Cooper) suggest that these isotype shifts may be programmed events which occur, at least in the chicken, relatively early in development. Despite the sophistication of the molecular biology in this area, the biology of isotype selection is still poorly understood. Clearly the different isotypes have evolved to handle different biological needs. Most would agree, for example, that IgE antibodies are useful in handling parasitic infestation. But how infestation with a parasite turns on IgE production is not understood. To put it another way, how does the body identify something as a parasite to which it should produce IgE antibodies. The same questions could be raised, but not answered, for each of the other isotypes. In many cases we do not even understand the biological benefits of a particular isotype.

A variety of data have suggested that somatic hypermutation (L. E. Hood) may be important in contributing to affinity maturation (increase in antibody affinity for the antigenic determinant with time after immunization). While random mutation certainly may lead to higher affinity for a given epitope, it seems to me equally or even more likely that any given mutation could lead to lower affinity for the test ligand. Furthermore, what may be low affinity for one ligand may be high affinity for another. Thus, how we see and interpret the role of somatic mutation as related to affinity maturation may well depend upon details of the procedures we use to probe the system and the particular antigen studied (for example, with antigens such as phosphorylcholine which tend to elicit very dominant idiotypes, the situation may differ from antigens to which idiotypic dominance is not so prominent a feature of the response). Further, the question of whether hypermutation continues after the cell has matured, that is whether hypermutation occurs during the proliferative response to antigen, is still not definitively answered.

The general pattern of B cell differentiation (M. Cooper, N. Klinman) seems clear. Comparisons of birds with mammals indicate differences which highlight the limits of our knowledge: the extent of somatic mutation, when the somatic mutations occur, the degree to which the generation of diversity is programmed and ordered and the degree to which it is stochastic, the cellular and molecular processes involved in isotype switching and differentiation to produce antibodies of different isotypes are all still poorly understood. Clearly, B cell differentiation must be divided into pre-antigen receptor, antigen-independent events and post-antigen-receptor development, potentially environmentally influenced events. The extent to which the antigen-independent events are stochastic versus programmed is still uncertain. It seems likely that after development of a receptor for antigen, the B cell population repertoire distribution can be shifted by either tolerance induction, antigen stimulation or idiotype network interactions.

The regulation of B cell differentiation is being actively investigated (R. Wall). The possible importance of dominant negative transacting factors in blocking positive signals was discussed. The interesting possibility was raised that the turning off of dominant blocking factors, that block differentiation-inducing factors from acting, may play a key role in regulating gene activation during differentiation.

Progress in understanding both the cellular and the biochemical processes involved in B cell activation was described (E. S. Vitetta, W. E. Paul). As in certain other cell activation systems, the activation of B cells (by cross linking surface immunoglobulin) seems to involve increases in inositol phospholipid metabolism, in free intracellular Ca^{++}, in inositol phosphates, in phospholipase C and in protein phosphorylation (W. E. Paul). The mechanism for transfer of the signal across the membrane is still not understood. Data are developing which suggest an auto-regulation of B cells at the signal transmission level.

Purified, antigen-specific B cells can be activated directly by a T-independent antigen or by a T-dependent antigen in the presence of carrier specific T cells (E. S. Vitetta). Formation of conjugates of T and B cells can be directly visualized. Their formation requires that there is Ia identity between the B and T cells, that the B cells are specific for the hapten and that the T cells are specific for the carrier. Processing of antigen by B cells appears necessary in some systems. Memory B cells are being better defined. They are probably characterized by having higher affinity antigen receptors and an increased concentration of Ia on their surface. Both factors would tend to make them more efficient in binding antigen and interacting with T cells.

A number of papers were presented on idiotype networks, their properties, and possible role in manipulating the immune system constructively or destructively (A. Nisonoff, C. A. Bona, H. Kohler, G. W. Siskind, B. F. Erlanger, L. D. Kohn, R. S. Geha). It seems highly probable that a network of idiotypes and anti-idiotypes does exist at the B cell, T cell and serum antibody levels. It is reasonable to assume that the network normally exists in a type of steady state. Introduction of antigen expands specific clones, perturbing the steady state. There follows a shift in distribution of idiotypes and anti-idiotypes until a new steady state is achieved. This shift in distribution of idiotypes is in effect the immune response. The stability of the system, resulting from its self-regulatory potential, provides for long-term memory in the absence of continuing antigen exposure. Biologically, I believe it provides a way for the animal to constantly respond to its microenvironment and, over a long period of time, to develop and maintain a useful distribution of antibodies to prevent infection. In this regard, I would like to remind you that an agammaglobulinemic patient can be maintained free of infection with passively administered gammaglobulin. Thus, an immune response (antibody production) is really not necessary to protect from infectious disease. I would suggest that we remain free of infections, not by responding to potential pathogens when exposed to them, but by having responded to them or to cross-reacting antigens some time in the past. If no appropriate response has been made in the past, disease occurs and the immune system must respond so as to bring about recovery. Thus infectious disease can be viewed as a failure of the immune system which when operating ideally, keeps us free from infections. I would suggest that it is in the maintenance of a useful distribution of antibodies and T cells, to prevent disease, that the idiotype network fulfills its primary biologic function. It is fashionable to point out that elderly persons have reduced antibody and T cell responses and therefore increased infections. While true, I would suggest that perhaps one should be more impressed by how free of infection elderly people generally remain despite their reduced immune response. Possibly this is because the idiotype network has maintained the production of a population of antibodies and T cells that are appropriate for protection against the usual environmental pathogens to which the individual is exposed.

The potential for use of anti-idiotypes to shift the distribution of idiotypes and anti-idiotypes in the network has opened a new approach to vaccine development (A. Nisonoff, H. Kohler). Its practical potential is still uncertain. However, in situations where the nominal antigen is either toxic, potentially contaminated with virulent virus, or unstable, the anti-idiotype approach may be valuable.

Applying the idiotype-anti-idiotype concepts it is clear how one can obtain antibodies specific for receptors as a result of an immune response to a ligand for the receptor (B. F. Erlanger, L. D. Kohn). Thus the anti-idiotype antibody to antibody specific for the ligand may be an internal image of the ligand and bind the receptor. This concept provides new insight into a route by which one can develop autoimmune disease. On the other hand this also provides a route through which control of autoantibody responses and perhaps also undesirable IgE responses may be achieved.

With respect to development of autoimmunity (N. Talal) several points were discussed which should be mentioned. The possibility of inducing auto-antibody as a result of exposure to an environmental agent (infectious or chemical) which cross-reacts with a host antigen was discussed. Furthermore, anti-idiotype antibody to an anti-virus antibody might react with a cell surface receptor for the virus and offer another route to autoimmunity. However, I would like to emphasize that the presence of auto-antibodies is not sufficient to cause disease. Auto-antibodies are seen in relatives of patients with autoimmune disease and in the aged without causing disease. Thus it is clear that additional factors, possibly not immunologic in nature, are important in the etiology of autoimmune disease.

Observing the application of the concepts of basic immunology to therapeutic intervention in disease is always exciting (N. Talal, J. W. Uhr, R. K. Oldham). It is one of the ultimate gratifications to workers in science. A number of approaches, including anti-idiotype vaccines, idiotype network manipulations, use of sex hormones, and use of toxin-conjugated antibodies (immunotoxins) were discussed and hold out great promise for future meetings.

CONTRIBUTORS

BARAK, Zahava, Department of Microbiology, Mount Sinai School of Medicine, One Gustave Levy Place, New York, New York 10029

BEAVEN, Michael A., Ph.D., Dep. Chief, Laboratory of Chemical Pharmacology, National Heart, Lung, and Blood Institute, National Institutes of Health, Bethesda, Maryland 20205

BEN-PORAT, Tamar, Department of Microbiology, School of Medicine, Vanderbilt University, Nashville, Tennessee 37232

BONA, Constantin A., M.D., Ph.D., Professor of Microbiology, Mount Sinai School of Medicine, One Gustave Levy Place, New York, New York 10029

BONILLA, F. A., Department of Microbiology, Mount Sinai School of Medicine, One Gustave Levy Place, New York, New York 10029

BRISKIN, Michael, Molecular Biology Institute and Department of Microbiology and Immunology, UCLA School of Medicine, University of California, Los Angeles, California 90024

CARTER, Carla, Molecular Biology Institute and Department of Microbiology and Immunology, UCLA School of Medicine, University of California, Los Angeles, California 90024

CAYANIS, E., Department of Biochemistry, Columbia University College of Physicians and Surgeons, New York, New York 10032

CLEVELAND, W. Louis, Ph.D., Assistant Professor, Department of Microbiology, Columbia University College of Physicians and Surgeons, New York, New York 10032

COOPER, Max D., M.D., Professor of Pediatrics and Microbiology, University of Alabama in Birmingham, School of Medicine, Birmingham, Alabama 35294

DORRINGTON, Keith J., Ph.D., D.Sc., Director and Vice President, Research and Technology, Connaught Research Institute, Willowdale, Ontario, Canada M2R 3T4

EDELMAN, I. S., M.D., Professor and Chairman, Department of Biochemistry, Columbia University College of Physicians and Surgeons, New York, New York 10032

ERLANGER, Bernard F., Ph.D., Professor of Microbiology, Columbia University College of Physicians and Surgeons, New York, New York 10032

FASEL, Nicolas, Molecular Biology Institute and Department of Microbiology and Immunology, UCLA School of Medicine, University of California, Los Angeles, California 90024

FROSCHER, Barbara G., Department of Immunology, Scripps Clinic and Research Foundation, La Jolla, California 92037

FULTON, R. Jerrold, Ph.D., Department of Microbiology, Southwestern Medical School, University of Texas Health Science Center, Dallas, Texas 75235

GEHA, Raif S., M.D., Chief of the Division of Allergy, Department of Pediatrics, Harvard Medical School, The Children's Hospital, Boston, Massachusetts 02115

GOIDL, Edmond A., Ph.D., Associate Professor of Microbiology, University of Maryland School of Medicine, Baltimore, Maryland 21201

GOVAN, Herman, Molecular Biology Institute and Department of Microbiology and Immunology, UCLA School of Medicine, University of California, Los Angeles, California 90024

GREGOR, Polly D., Department of Microbiology and Cancer Center/Institute of Cancer Research, Columbia University College of Physicians and Surgeons, New York, New York 10032

GURISH, Michael F., Department of Biology, Rosentiel Research Center, Brandeis University, Waltham, Massachusetts 02254

HERMANSON, Gary, Molecular Biology Institute and Department of Microbiology and Immunology, UCLA School of Medicine, University of California, Los Angeles, California 90024

HILL, B. L., Department of Microbiology, Columbia University College of Physicians and Surgeons, New York, New York 10032

HOOD, Leroy E., M.D., Ph.D., Bowles Professor and Chairman, Department of Biology, California Institute of Technology, Pasadena California 91125

HORNBECK, Peter, National Institute of Allergy and Infectious Diseases, National Institutes of Health, Bethesda, Maryland 20892

KABAT, Elvin A., Ph.D., Professor, Departments of Microbiology, Human Genetics, and Neurology, Columbia University College of Physicians and Surgeons, New York, New York 10032 and National Institute of Allergy and Infectious Diseases, National Institutes of Health, Bethesda, Maryland 20892

KIEBER-EMMONS, Thomas, Department of Molecular Immunology, Roswell Park Memorial Institute, Buffalo, New York 14263

KIM, Young Tai, Ph.D., Associate Professor of Medicine, Cornell University Medical College, New York, New York 10021

KLEIN, Michel H., M.D., Associate Professor, Department of Immunology, University of Toronto, Toronto, Canada M5T 2S8

KLINMAN, Norman R., M.D., Ph.D., Department of Immunology, Scripps Clinic and Research Institute, La Jolla, California 92037

KOBRIN, Barry J., Department of Microbiology and the Cancer Center/Institute of Cancer Research, Columbia University College of Physicians and Surgeons, New York, New York 10032

KOHLER, Heinz, M.D., Ph.D., Head, Department of Molecular Immunology, Roswell
Park Memorial Institute, Buffalo, New York 14263

KOHN, Leonard D., M.D., Chief, Section on Biochemistry of Cell Regulation,
National Institute of Arthritis, Diabetes, and Digestive and Kidney
Diseases, National Institutes of Health, Bethesda, Maryland 20892

KU, H. H., Department of Microbiology, Columbia University College of
Physicians and Surgeons, New York, New York 10032

LAW, Ronald, Molecular Biology Institute and Department of Microbiology
and Immunology, UCLA School of Medicine, University of California,
Los Angeles, California 90024

MIZUGUCHI, Junichiro, Laboratory of Immunology, National Institute of Allergy
and Infectious Diseases, National Institutes of Health, Bethesda,
Maryland 20892

MORRISON, Sherie L., Ph.D., Professor of Microbiology, Columbia University
College of Physicians and Surgeons, New York, New York 10032

NISONOFF, Alfred, Ph.D., Professor of Biology, Rosenstiel Research Center,
Brandeis University, Waltham, Massachusetts 02254

OI, Vernon T., Becton Dickinson Monoclonal Center, Mountain View, California
94040

OLDHAM, Robert K., M.D., Director, Biological Therapy Institute, Franklin,
Tennessee 37064

PAUL, William E., M.D., Chief, Laboratory of Immunology, National Institute
of Allergy and Infectious Diseases, National Institutes of Health,
Bethesda, Maryland 20892

PENN, A. S., Department of Neurology, Columbia University College of
Physicians and Surgeons, New York, New York 10032

RAJAGOPALAN, R., Department of Microbiology, Columbia University College of
Physicians and Surgeons, New York, New York 10032

SARANGARAJAN, R., Department of Microbiology, Columbia University College of
Physicians and Surgeons, New York, New York 10032

SISKIND, Gregory W., M.D., Professor of Medicine, Division Head, Division of
Allergy and Immunology, The New York Hospital-Cornell Medical Center,
New York, New York 10021

TALAL, Norman, M.D., Professor of Medicine and Microbiology, Head of the
Division of Clinical Immunology, The University of Texas Health Science
Center at San Antonio, San Antonio, Texas 78284

THORBECKE, G. Jeanette, M.D., Professor of Pathology, New York University
School of Medicine, New York, New York 10016

TSANG, Wayne, National Institute of Allergy and Infectious Diseases,
National Institutes of Health, Bethesda, Maryland 20892

UHR, Jonathan W., M.D., Professor and Chairman, Department of Microbiology,
University of Texas Southwestern Medical School, Dallas, Texas 75235

VICTOR-KOBRIN, Carol, Department of Microbiology, Mount Sinai School of
Medicine, One Gustave Levy Place, New York, New York 10029

VITETTA, Ellen S., Ph.D., Professor of Microbiology, University of Texas Southwestern Medical School, Dallas, Texas 75235

WALL, Randolph W., Ph.D., Professor of Microbiology and Immunology, UCLA School of Medicine, University of California, Los Angeles, California 90024

WAN, K. K., Department of Biochemistry, University of Toronto, Toronto, Canada M5S 1A8

WASSERMAN, N. H., Department of Microbiology, Columbia University College of Physicians and Surgeons, New York, New York 10032

WEKSLER, Marc E., M.D., Wright Professor of Medicine, Department of Medicine, Cornell University Medical College, New York, New York 10021

WIMS, Letitia A., Department of Microbiology and the Cancer Center/Institute of Cancer Research, Columbia University College of Physicians and Surgeons, New York, New York 10032

Myasthenia gravis, 156
  experimental, 157
  sex variations in incidence of,
    159
Myeloma, mouse, 21

National Cancer Institute, 191
Network theory, 11, 12, *see also*
    Idiotype network
Neuroblastoma, 194
Neutrophils, low affinity receptors,
    8
Nitrophenyl, 21

Original Antigenic Sin, 23
Ovalbumin gene, transcription
    termination in, 56

pp62, 73
pp65-70
2-Phenyloxazolone, 21
Phorbol myristate acetate
  B cell and, 74
  membrane-associated phospho-
      proteins and, 73
Phosphatidyl inositol bisphosphate,
      hydrolysis, B cell activa-
      tion and, 71-72
Phospholipase C, receptor cross-
      linkage and, 72
Phosphoproteins
  isoelectric points, 73
  membrane-associated
    anti=immunoglobulin M and, 73
    phorbol myristate acetate and, 73
Phosphorylcholine, idiotypes
      elicited from, 204
Pocket concept, 11
Pokeweed mitogen, synthesis of
      auto anti-idiotype, 144
Poliovirus type II, antigen, 83
Pompa proteins, V regions of
      rheumatoid factors, 137
Protein(s)
  lay, 137
  Pompa, 137
Protein kinase C, 72
Pseudogenes, 19
Pseudorabies virus, antibodies,
      induction, 84-87

QUPC52, 22

Rabies virus glycoprotein, antigen,
    82
Radioimmunoassay, idiotype, 95
Reovirus type 3, antigen, 82
Retinol-binding protein, antibodies,
    84
Rheumatoid arthritis
  DR4 positivity, 157
  sex variation in incidence of, 160
  total lymphoid irradiation in, 162

Ricin, 179-185, *see also* Immunotoxins
  conjugates with antibody, 180
  conjugates, versus antibody-A chain
      conjugates, 183
  deglycosylation, 184

Schistsoma mansoni, antigen, 83
Seattle Bone Marrow Transplantation
      Group, 181
Sendai virus, antigen, 82
Staphylococcus aureus, protein A, 6
Streptococcus pneumoniae, antigen, 83
Systemic lupus erythematosus, 137,
    155
  AIDS and 160-161
  C4 null genes, 157
  murine models, 161
  total lymphoid irradiation in, 162

T cell
  antigen receptor, 157
  graft-versus-host disease and, 180
  helper, 155
  interleukin-2 receptors, 157
  regulatory idiotopes on, 15
  suppressor, 155
Testosterone, immune response nad,
    159
Tetanus, antibodies, 135-150
  auto anti-idiotype, 145
Tetanus toxoid, immune response, 135
Thyroglobulin
  immunization, 125
  monoclonal autoantibody, 30
Thyroiditis, chronic, sex variation
      in incidence of, 160
Tobacco, mosaic virus, 144
Total lymphoid irradiation, 162
Transcription, 56, *see also* Gene
      expression
Trinitrophenyl, 62
Trypanosomes, antigen, 82
Tumor cells, antibody-ricin con-
      jugates and, 180
Tumors, antibodies in treatment of,
    189

Vaccines
  anti-idiotypic antibodies as, 84
  idiotype, 15

W3129, 22
Waldenstrom macroglobulin, monoclonal
      antibodies, 21
Western blot assay, 127